"Jorge continues to inspire and make losing weight fun and part of your life forever."

—Mariel Hemingway, author of *Healthy Living from the Inside Out*

"Jorge Cruise has done it again! Long at the forefront of teaching people how to live healthy lives, his new book shows you how to exercise effectively, safely, and efficiently. A great guide to a healthier you!"

—John Robbins, author of *Healthy at 100* and the internationally acclaimed bestseller *Diet for a New America*

"I agree with Jorge wholeheartedly. Along with a sound eating plan, strength training is the key to overall health improvement. And, as the saying goes, 'Slow and steady wins the race!'"

—Frederick Hahn, celebrity trainer, author, and owner of Serious Strength NYC

"Jorge Cruise defines how to maximize results in a short amount of time—which is invaluable in this fast-paced world. With traditional strength training, there are reps. With Jorge's program, there are *REPS*! With this technique, you can shape your body faster than you ever thought possible."

—Kathy Smith, fitness expert and author of *Feed Muscle, Shrink Fat*

"You'll love the results: boosting your metabolism, increasing your stamina, and easily fitting into your jeans again."

—Lucy Beale, author of *The Complete Idiot's Guide to Glycemic Index Weight Loss*

"In this chaotic world where dozens of new diet and exercise books seem to pop up every year, it's all too easy to get confused and to give up hope. This book clearly details the 'basics' that should form the foundation to any healthy lifestyle. Read the first few pages and you'll soon discover that you can have the body you've always dreamed of in half the usual time."

—Christopher Guerriero, founder of MaximizeYourMetabolism.com and host of *The Energy Factor* health television show

BODY AT
HOME

OTHER BOOKS BY JORGE CRUISE

The 12-Second Sequence™

The 12-Second Sequence™ Journal

The 3-Hour Diet™

The 3-Hour Diet™ Cookbook

The 3-Hour Diet™ for Teens

The 3-Hour Diet™ On-the-Go

8 Minutes in the Morning®

8 Minutes in the Morning®: Extra-Easy Weight Loss

8 Minutes in the Morning®: Flat Belly

8 Minutes in the Morning®: Thinner Thighs and Hips

BODY AT
HOME

A Simple Plan to Drop 10 pounds

JORGE CRUISE

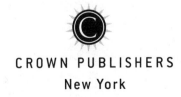

CROWN PUBLISHERS
New York

Published in the United States by Crown Publishers, an imprint of the Crown Publishing Group,
a division of Random House, Inc., New York.

www.crownpublishing.com

CROWN and the Crown colophon are registered trademarks of Random House, Inc.

Library of Congress Cataloging-in-Publication Data

Cruise, Jorge.

Body at home / Jorge Cruise.

p. cm.

Includes bibliographical references and index.

ISBN 978-0-307-38333-4

1. Physical fitness. 2. Reducing exercises. 3. Reducing diets. I. Title.

RA781.C785 2009

613.7'1—dc22

2008050634

Printed in the U.S.A.

10 9 8 7 6 5 4 3 2 1

First Edition

Notice:

The information given here is designed to help you make informed decisions about your body and health. The suggestions for specific foods, nutritional supplements, and exercises in this program are not intended to replace appropriate or necessary medical care. Before starting any exercise program, always see your physician. If you have specific medical symptoms, consult your physician immediately. If any recommendations given in this program contradict your physician's advice, be sure to consult your doctor before proceeding. Mention of specific products, companies, organizations, or authorities in this book does not imply endorsement by the author or the publisher, nor does mention of specific companies, organizations, or authorities in the book imply that they endorse the book. The author and the publisher disclaim any liability or loss, personal or otherwise, resulting from the procedures in this program. Internet addresses and telephone numbers given in this book were accurate at the time the book went to press.

Product pictures, trademarks, and trademark names are used throughout this book to describe and inform the reader about various proprietary products that are owned by others. The presentation of such pictures and information is intended to benefit the owner of the products and trademarks and is not intended to infringe upon trademark, copyright, or other rights, or to imply any claim to the mark other than that made by the owner. No endorsement of the information contained in this book has been given by the owners of such products and trademarks, and no such endorsement is implied by the inclusion of product pictures or trademarks in this book.

Trademarks:

Body at Home
12-Second Sequence
12Second.com
3-Hour Diet
3HourDiet.com
8 Minutes in the Morning
Controlled Tension
Instant Health
Jorge Cruise
JorgeCruise.com
Time-Based Nutrition
Jorge's Packs
Priority Solution

THIS BOOK IS DEDICATED TO YOU

Investing in your health *always* pays off. And in these difficult
economic times, it is an absolute necessity. Your ability to be
fit and healthy will give you the greatest advantage
at home and at work.

CONTENTS

ACKNOWLEDGMENTS

Without the support of my wife, Heather, I would not be the man I am today. Thank you, sweetheart, for bringing beauty, style, balance, and joy into my life, and for magnifying the magic of it all for me. Thank you for always believing in me. I love you with all my heart.

To my wonderful sons, Parker and Owen: You both are the light in my eyes. You keep me on my toes and full of wonder as I watch you grow.

To my dad, Mel, who over twenty years ago was diagnosed with prostate cancer and overcame it through a commitment to a healthy lifestyle. You are my original motivation to make health my mission. Thank you, Dad.

To Jade Beutler, James E. Williams, OMD, Dr. James Novak, and Dr. Mehmet Oz for showing me how to personally continue to be the best man I can be physically, no matter what my age: You are part of my family and true sources of inspiration for me. Thank you.

To Jared Davis and Gretchen Lees for being the creative force behind all my books. You guys are the best, and I am very grateful for all your effort and hard work on this book. Thank you, team. A special thank you as well to Oliver Stephenson and Chance Miles for helping me work with all the extraordinary people in this book each week as we ran our test groups; and to Chance, for being one of our Body at Home™ Stars. Thank you to Auriana Albert for your culinary creations in this book.

A special thank you to Lacie Weddle, our cover model and a Body at Home™ Star mom. And to Miguel Garcia, our fitness model for the men's exercises.

My great appreciation also to Steve Hanselman, my literary adviser and invaluable support system. And, of course, to my amazing editor Heather Jackson and assistant editor Heather Proulx for their continued support and commitment to making this book truly extraordinary. I feel so very lucky for your belief in me. Also a very big special thank you to Jenny Frost, Tina Constable, Kristin Kiser, Christine Aronson, Carrie Thornton, Philip Patrick, Jill Flaxman, Amy Metsch, Linda Kaplan, Andrew Leibowitz, Donna Passannante, Shawn Nicholls, and Penny Simon.

Thank you to Jack Curry and TJ Walter at *USA WEEKEND Magazine* for your extraordinary efforts in helping me get my message out to America every week; I am so grateful for your support and friendship.

My special thanks to Dr. David Katz, Jane Friedman, Steve P. Murphy, Ardath Rodale, Bob Wietrak, Edward Ash-Milby, Richard Galanti, Terry Goodman, and Natalie Farage for their outstanding support and friendship throughout the years.

And thanks to Cathie Black, Cathy Chermol, Hilary Estey McLoughlin, Tyra Banks, John Redmann, Sheila Bouttier, Katie Couric, Lisa Gregorisch-Dempsey, Meredith Vieira, Amy Rosenblum, Marc Victor, Diane Sawyer, Chris Cuomo, Patty Neger, Monica Escobedo, Wendy Whitworth, Linda Evans, Karen Katz, Emeril Lagasse, Barbara Walters, Bill Geddie, Donald Berman, Dusty Cohen, Cherie Bank, Ivorie Anthony, Jennifer Austin, Kelli Gillespie, and Richard Doutre Jones for allowing me to share my message with the public.

And finally to our newest partners and friends who have provided essential support for this project. Thank you to Jack Hogan, Brian Hogan, Ron Caporale, and Laurie Berger at LifeScript®. To Reid Tracey, Stacey Smith, and Louise Hay at Hay House. To Charles Caswell, Richard Davis, and Paul Goldberg at GoFit™. To Brent Brookes, Jim Zahniser, and Daniel Schwerin at Precor®. To Bruce Barlean and Jade Beutler at Barlean's Organic Oils. To Richard Galanti, Sharron Rugh, Ginnie Roeglin, Anita Thompson, Tim Talevich, Pennie Clark Ianniciello, David W. Fuller, and Pat Volchok at Costco.

BODY AT HOME™ FOR WOMEN

PART 1

FOREWORD FOR HER

By Mariel Hemingway, author of Mariel Hemingway's **Healthy Living from the Inside Out** *and creator of Mariel's Kitchen*

I am dedicated to helping people—especially women—find the system that works for *them* individually. Because I think achieving health and fitness for us as women is so specific and unique, it is important to create the right environment to let your fitness flourish. This means it has to work in your life, not pull you out of your life. And let me tell you, Jorge gets it! He has nailed what it takes for you to get the most from the time and energy that you spend on your exercise and nutrition. With *Body at Home™* you can transform your life in a doable and sustainable way. *Trust me: This is a crash course on getting gorgeous that works.*

We all want to look good in our clothes and wear those skinny jeans, but there is a way to do it that lasts a lifetime. When you train your inner self as well as your body, you create lasting fitness habits. When you build your inner strength, you are creating the motivation that will drive you to enduring health and happiness.

What I love about this program is that you can do it anywhere and you can see results immediately. I also love that you are your own trainer. I am always telling people that they can be their own trainers, nutritionists, and healers. This is the fitness program that makes you the boss, yet you are totally guided through a system that works. So take your book to the gym or your personal workout room (even your living room!) and get busy. Feel great and have the body you are meant to have and love and enjoy this life with. Let Jorge Cruise be your guide. He won't fail you.

1 Drop 10 Pounds in Two Weeks at Home!

"Trust me: This is a crash course on getting gorgeous *that works.*"

—MARIEL HEMINGWAY

The most critical thing you can do over the next two weeks is drop 10 pounds—or about one jean size. This might sound simplistic, but whether you are a grandma, mom, single business professional, or college student—or any combination of these—*no matter what your age,* your life and health will dramatically transform when you lose 10 pounds from your belly, butt, thighs, and hips. How do I know this? I have worked with thousands of clients at my JorgeCruise.com website and hundreds of women in person in San Diego to develop this women's at-home program, and their success stories, which are featured throughout this book, confirm it. My clients not only end up looking slimmer, but also feel their confidence soar by the end of their very first workout (and many times within the first 90 seconds). And when it comes to overall good health, my clients have used the plan to reduce stress and even start to reverse the effects of life-threatening diseases such as cancer, stroke, high blood pressure, and diabetes. Bottom line: The next two weeks will be one of the most important times for you; you'll see some extraordinary transformations!

So my challenge to you right now is to make a decision that you and your health will come first for the next two weeks. Let's get started.

I wrote this section for one reason—to help women at any age firm and flatten their trouble zones at home. I received countless e-mails from women, and they asked me to help them shrink and sculpt those biggest trouble zones *at home:* their belly, butt, hips, and thighs. They wanted to get into their stylish jeans—without ever stepping foot in the gym! I knew what I had to do.

This new plan can be done 100 percent at home and requires no costly equipment. Everything you will need, from the exercises to the eating plan, to an important method of connecting with your motivation is here. You will truly love it no matter how many pounds you need to burn or what age you are. Are you ready to get started right now? Well, if you are short on time and want to start immediately, then jump to Chapter 2 to read my Priority Solution™, a women's-only strategy to ensure your success on this plan. But if you can, I strongly recommend you read on for an essential overview of the program.

My Story

As a kid and young man I struggled with my weight. I had no confidence and felt hopeless. I was raised in a Mexican American family, and I was always taught that food was love—and my mom loved me a lot! As I got older I realized that food had become my best friend and I needed to find a way to change my lifestyle and develop a healthy relationship with food and fitness.

Today I run JorgeCruise.com, write my weekly column for *USA WEEKEND Magazine,* and have a super-busy personal life. My wife, Heather, and I are always on the go with our two small boys, Parker and Owen. I am almost 40 years old and I can tell you this: I have never been in better shape. Because of Body at Home™ I can see my abs and I feel proud to take my shirt off at the beach! Bottom line: This plan will prove to you the only thing that matters is the quality of the workout, not the number of reps. It will be a huge learning lesson that will keep you fit and in shape for the rest of your life!

HOW BODY AT HOME™ FOR WOMEN WORKS

With this program, you will use the resistance-training method from my *New York Times* best seller *The 12-Second Sequence™.* It's truly the most effective method I have ever created to burn fat *at rest*. This method is designed to rev your *resting* metabolism. Imagine burning fat at the computer, in the car, and even when you are watching TV. What's the secret? The secret lies in the *after-burn*. Almost every woman I have ever trained has not been aware of the after-burn and its power to shrink and sculpt her body. The after-burn is what happens when you restore lean muscle tissue—this muscle puts your body into a fat-burning state 24/7. You see, lean muscle tissue is the most metabolically active tissue on the body and burns calories all day (see sidebar, page 7). This is the secret that I use to keep my abs looking good and my workouts super effective.

What is the key to restoring lean muscle tissue on your body? The most effective way to restore it is through resistance training. That's it. The challenge is that most resistance-training programs are so time-consuming that you never commit to the program and, worst of all, you end up never really seeing dramatic results. Another thing that can make other programs tough is that they often require you to go to a gym as well. Don't get me wrong: I love going to the gym, but sometimes it's not as practical if you've got kids or no time to travel there. Well, this book will solve that for you! You can do everything at home with just a few basic items.

With my Body at Home™ for Women program you will truly discover the most effective way to create lean muscle tissue—not big bulky muscles, but long lean shapely muscles, which consume calories and burn fat while you're doing absolutely nothing.

What makes it so effective is something I call Controlled Tension™. This method forces your muscles to fatigue in just four reps, by slowing each exercise to a 10-second count and a 2-second hold. This is critical because in order to restore lean muscle tissue, you must force it to the point of fatigue. With Controlled Tension™ you are using a unique and powerful combination of two resistance-training methods that are proven effective at restoring lean muscle tissue. By combining *slow cadence lifting* and *static contraction,* I created the ultimate body-sculpting, time-saving method available. Before the 12-Second Sequence™, these two techniques had never been combined. Now, I have built upon this core technique and created the ultimate in fitness customization for women with Body at Home™ for Women. If you want more on the science behind the original technique, make sure to pick up a copy of my *12-Second Sequence™* book.

The Cardio Myth

I love cardio because it's excellent for your health. But if you are like many women, I know you have relied on jogging or the elliptical machine or a step aerobics class to change your body—and I bet you've been disappointed. As wonderful as cardio is for your heart, it isn't the most efficient or effective way to sculpt your body. If the average woman did an entire hour of moderately paced walking, she would burn about 150 calories. If you consider that there are approximately 3,500 calories in just 1 pound, you can imagine all the walking you would have to do to burn the equivalent of 1 pound.

The other problem with doing only cardio is that once you stop exercising, your body essentially stops burning calories. This is not true with resistance training. When you strength-train, you take advantage of your body's natural ability to maintain an after-burn, the scientific term for which is *excess post-oxygen consumption (EPOC).* Remember, the after-burn is the extra calories your body burns after you complete a workout.

Many studies have shown that strength training creates a significantly longer after-burn than aerobic activity. One study published in the *International Journal of Sport Nutrition and Exercise Metabolism* analyzed the EPOC of women who had completed a strength-training session. The study came up with amazing results. The researchers determined that the women experienced a 13 percent increase in their EPOC after exercising. Not only that, but their after-burn stayed elevated for *16 hours after they finished exercising.* Another study conducted at Colorado State University compared the EPOC effects of aerobic exercise to strength training. That research revealed that strength training generated a much longer-lasting EPOC compared to the aerobic activity: Strength training was still burning calories 14½ hours post-workout.

FOR WOMEN ONLY

This program is designed exclusively for women, and it incorporates my brand-new life strategy: the Priority Solution™. This strategy is so important that I've given it its own chapter (Chapter 2), and I want to tell you it will be a critical tool for sculpting your body. Be sure not to miss that chapter. It's truly vital to your success.

For now, I simply want to challenge you to make a commitment to yourself to see this program all the way through to the end. Remember, *in only two weeks you will drop 10 pounds*—mostly from your waist. I also recommend measuring your waist to track your success—a lot of my successful clients recorded amazing losses in inches and felt that was the most effective way to gauge their progress. Also remember, there's nothing more dangerous than extra fat in your abdominal area, so big losses there can be even more important than those made on the scale. By shrinking your waist to a healthy 32.5 inches or less, you'll reduce your risk for developing life-threatening diseases.

Are you ready to change your body? I know you are. Let's start together and move on to Chapter 2.

(10) BODY AT HOME™ STAR   Amber Grant

Height: 5'7" | **Age:** 29 | **Lost:** 10 pounds (Plus restored 1 pound of lean muscle)

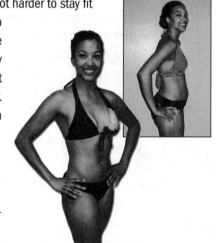

"I've always been pretty active and into fitness, but as I got older it got harder to stay fit and trim. When I heard about Body at Home™, I was really excited to get started and see if it could really turn out the results that were promised. The program was pretty easy to incorporate into my lifestyle and wasn't too time-consuming. I dropped 4 pounds the first week and had consistent drops in weight every week thereafter. Needless to say, I'm happier with a firmer, healthier body. This is a program that I can use as a foundation for my life."

Amber's Secrets to Success

· Start a workout group to help keep you motivated and on track.
· Pick out motivational pictures and use them for inspiration—visualize the body you want and you're sure to get there.
· Make the full commitment to the program for eight weeks, knowing it's going to change your entire life!

2 A Woman's Best Friend: The Priority Solution™

"I'm so happy with the results, and I now have the confidence to go out and achieve the rest of my dreams. I love music and aspire to be a professional singer. Being confident with my new toned body will help me with my career and will give me confidence in my upcoming audition. Thanks, Jorge! I finally feel sexy again!"

—MARIBEL GIL, BODY AT HOME™ STAR, LOST 24 POUNDS

Get ready to meet your new best friend. In order to ensure you will be on the fast track to dropping 10 pounds in two weeks at home, it's *essential* for you to maximize two critical elements: your physical focus and inner drive. In this chapter you will discover my secret that customizes my Body at Home™ method for women. I call it the Priority Solution™. The Priority Solution™ is without question one of the most important techniques I have created to help you get visible results quickly. And here's the great news: There are only two simple steps. The first will empower you physically—I call it the "Body Priority." And the second, the "Life Priority," will help you create a powerful inner focus.

STEP 1: YOUR BODY PRIORITY

The *Body Priority* is a highly customized method of resistance training that allows you to increase your resting metabolism while giving special focus and priority to your trouble zones—hips, thighs, butt, and abs. This specialized focus is why I can guarantee you will drop 10 pounds in two weeks at home. And your time commitment will be just three 20-minute at-home workouts per week. So your investment is only one hour a week. It's really that simple.

As you already know from Chapter 1, all your workouts on this program are resistance-training based, which means they will efficiently restore precious fat-burning lean muscle tissue. Here, unlike in my *12-Second Sequence™* book (a more "advanced" program that requires gym time—an ideal plan for when you are done with this book), you will not use a circuit-training method as your base. Don't get me wrong: Circuit training is great, but it doesn't allow you to focus on specific body parts.

If you followed the 12-Second Sequence™ program, you may notice that there are three workouts a week with the Body at Home™ plan instead of two. This critical third day is added to create the maximum results in your specific trouble zones. It's going to guarantee you sculpt your belly, butt, and thighs with strategic focus. It's just an extra 20 minutes a week, and I promise it will be worth it!

Bottom line: When you want to shrink and sculpt *specific areas,* you need something much more focused—a structure in which your overall effort is not divided into various muscle groups during a session. A structure of training in which you focus on one muscle group for three or four exercises before moving on to the next body part is ideal. You'll also get a little rest time in between sets to maximize your recovery. This kind of strategic focus and structure will give you extreme precision and your sexiest body ever.

This is how the training cycle will look: Day one will be your most important day because this is when you will focus on some of the most critical trouble zones. This is the day you will focus on legs (thighs/hips/butt), triceps, and abs. Doing this workout at the start of the week and in this exact order will be critical. Ideally it will be on a Monday. Why? Doing this workout on Mondays will ensure you have six days of rest before hitting these essential body parts again. And if you recall from Chapter 1, during the workout is when you break your muscles down, and only when you rest do you create beautiful, new, fat-burning tissue. During each workout we can work on only one primary "large" muscle group. That means each 20-minute workout will pair a "large" muscle group with a secondary "smaller" muscle group. Abs will end every workout. You can work your abs more frequently than other muscle groups because they have a unique resilient power to recover quickly. On day one, the small muscle group you focus on will be your triceps—without question the top trouble zone for women after the hips, thighs, and butt.

After this 20-minute workout you might be thinking, "I don't need to exercise more body parts, right, Jorge? I hit those lower body parts to help me drop 10 pounds and get into my jeans, and I worked my triceps as a bonus." I know that might sound good, but while half of the secret to getting into those jeans is to focus on your trouble zones, the *other* half of the secret lies in maximizing your resting metabolism. Remember, increasing your overall amount of lean muscle tissue is the key to burning fat *all over* your body. Since you have lean muscle everywhere, you've got to work all those different muscle groups: There are muscles in your back, chest, biceps, and shoulders that we will focus on. Neglecting these other parts will not allow you to achieve the best results. That's why on day two you will hit back and biceps, which I recommend you do on a Wednesday. And then on day three, which ideally will be a Friday, you will work your chest and shoulders.

By following this three-day structure, you will be revving your resting metabolism to its maximum and sculpting those trouble zones most effectively. And as a major bonus you will be creating beautiful, balanced symmetry in your body. You will truly look and feel your sexiest.

STEP 2: YOUR LIFE PRIORITY

The second part of the Priority Solution™ is what I call the "Women's Life Priority." The key is to empower yourself from the inside. The only way you will truly transform your body in 14 days is by being *consistent*. The customized 20-minute workouts won't be beneficial unless you do them consistently. That means sticking to the workouts on Mondays, Wednesdays, and Fridays for two weeks—at least. Committing to exercise for two weeks, even from home, can be extremely challenging if you are not prepared and your inner drive is not turned on. So get ready to discover my secret for creating a powerful and positive inner edge that will help you achieve success quickly and, perhaps even more important, help draw you toward long-term success.

How does it work? In ten-plus years of working with a mainly female clientele, I have discovered that one of the best methods to empower a woman is to create a customized "key" to unlock the door to her critical *inner drive*. While that key may be different for every woman, there are shared goals or obstacles that women face at different stages in their lives. It's difficult to generalize, but chances are if you are in your twenties, your priorities are likely to be very different from the priorities of someone who is in her forties or fifties. Customized direction reflecting these core differences will help you create and maintain a strong inner drive.

The first step is for you to come up with your own Life Priority *without* my support. Fill out the chart on the next page to the best of your ability. Don't spend more than 10 minutes doing this. Respond from your heart and keep it short and sweet. And I suggest you write your responses in pencil in case you want to change something later.

All right, now that you have filled out your current top Life Priority, let's make it stronger and

SUCCESS CONTRACT

Photocopy and place on refrigerator, pantry, and bedside.

My Name: _____

My Goal: To drop 10 pounds by _____
(Ideally, pick a Monday to start, and count out 14 days from that date.)

My Method: Three 20-minute workouts per week for two weeks—just one hour a week.

My Top Priority and Reason: Beyond looking your sexiest and being healthier . . . Think of what's driving you at the core: Ask yourself, "What's my ultimate motivation for getting fit?"

_____

_____

_____

_____

_____

_____

Signature

perhaps even better. The stronger the items on that list are for you, the stronger your inner drive will become.

Now, for the second step! Depending on your age, jump down to the decade section that best applies to you. There are common lifestyle challenges that all women face; these may come for you at a different decade than for others, or maybe you are experiencing several challenges at the same time. So I encourage you to read the motivation factors of every decade. But if you want to save time, skip to your decade and let's get started planting some new potent seeds to strengthen your inner drive.

Twenties: Increase Confidence

If you are in your twenties, then first I want to congratulate you for being so ahead of the game. You should be very proud of yourself for taking charge of your life's most important asset—your physical body. By taking action now to shrink and sculpt your body, you will have a critical advantage for the rest of your life. You might be thinking, "But that's the rest of my life. What's in it for me *right now?*" I know the immediate rewards will probably be the most powerful for you. So what's the greatest advantage you need to be aware of right now? Here it is: Dropping 10 pounds in the next two weeks will directly *increase your confidence.* And when you feel confident, you immediately have an advantage in life. Healthy self-esteem will help you excel in your personal and your professional life.

When you use the Body at Home™ plan, it will create for you a level of fitness and health that will translate into a strong sense of self-worth, which can dramatically impact your relationships on every level. Whether you are just starting to date, have a serious relationship, or are married, this plan will help boost your level of confidence. And this higher level of confidence will positively transform your personal life. This result has been documented in various university studies. A study done at the University of Minnesota considered the effect of body image on a woman's sexual behavior. Researchers discovered that women who were more satisfied with their physical bodies were more likely to initiate relationships on an intimate level; they enjoyed sex more and felt more comfortable when they were naked than women who were dissatisfied with their bodies. Of course this doesn't mean that it's all about sex—it can mean you're more comfortable approaching someone you think is attractive at a bar or even just wearing a cute swimsuit to the beach. It's all about creating a level of confidence that you carry with you all the time.

Let's talk about your professional life. If you are just starting out in the workforce, here is something critical for you to know. It might not be fair, but it's a fact that people who are physically fit and "attractive" will earn more money than those who are not. Since attractiveness is subjective, it can come down to your level of fitness, your personal hygiene, and even how you wear your clothes. Let's just say it's all about how you present yourself. If you appear to care about yourself and respect yourself, then others will follow suit. As Cathie Black, president of Hearst Magazines, points out, "You have a lot of power to shape the public perception of yourself."

There are university studies that confirm this, but you will never read about them in your employee handbook. In one study, researchers asked students at a university to judge the appearance of 94 members of the faculty. The researchers then compared those ratings with classroom teaching ratings given by students in 463 courses taught by those professors. The latter ratings were used to help determine the professors' salary increases. The more physically fit and attractive a professor was, the higher was his or her student rating—and salary. Why is this? Well, when you are more fit and take care of yourself, you are more confident. This could be due to the natural endorphins your body releases when you exercise regularly or to the extra energy you feel when you are fit—you are just a more vibrant person. Confidence grows when you know you look good and feel good. You carry your head high, you initiate and lead conversations, and you create magnetism that draws people to you. And that spark is invaluable in the workplace and in your personal life.

So here is what I invite you to do. If creating that crucial inner confidence is something that would motivate and drive you, simply add that to your Life Priority chart on page 12. Select areas in which you want to build confidence—hopefully, some from both the personal and the professional perspectives—and take the first step toward achieving that level of confidence with your first workout. You can do it!

 BODY AT HOME™ TWENTIES SUPERSTAR Maribel Gil

Height: 5'5" | **Age:** 27 | **Lost:** 24 pounds

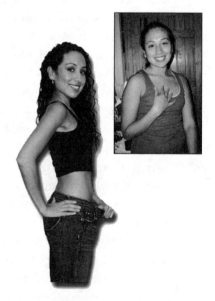

"Growing up, I was always able to eat what I wanted and never gained a pound. My friends used to call me 'Mari-Flaca,' which means 'skinny Mari' in Spanish. But once I got into my twenties, my metabolism slowed way down. All of a sudden I was packing on the pounds! No matter how much I exercised, I was never able to get the results that I wanted. Then I heard about Jorge's Body at Home™! I can finally fit back into my skinny clothes! I love the exercises in the book because they make me look great and feel strong. I learned that less really is more! I used to exercise for two hours a day, five times a week and see minimal results. With this program, however, I work out less and get the best results I've ever seen!"

Maribel's Secrets to Success

· Look in the mirror and see the difference in the way your clothes fit and how your muscles are more defined. Each week, you will look better and better!

· Make the morning cardio like your cup of coffee. It's the first thing you do when you get up so it will become a routine part of your day that you can't live without. It helps you start the day on a healthy note!

· Be flexible and make a schedule that you can stick to. For example, I can't get to a treadmill at the gym in the morning before work, so I do a power walk in my neighborhood as soon as I wake up. I also try to get the workouts done as early in the week as possible.

Thirties: Manage Stress

If you are in your thirties, then there is one word that I bet is constantly coming up for you: STRESS. Even just looking at that word probably makes all the busy thoughts that need attention travel to the front of your mind. I know stress is not a pretty part of life, but it's part of living so we must figure out the best way to manage it. Part of managing stress is learning to accept it and, on some level, appreciate it for the fire it adds to our lives—it's the pressure that shapes and drives us. Without stress, nothing would ever get done!

Every woman in her thirties that I know feels she must be a superwoman. Many of them have to balance growing career responsibilities while simultaneously maintaining strong intimate relationships and close friendships, taking care of kids, and purchasing their first big items such as a home. This whirlwind of responsibility and activity can have a debilitating effect if it becomes overwhelming—it can make you feel paralyzed! It can stop you from achieving results and accomplishing your goals. What's going to be your number-one weapon against debilitating stress? Exercise. Yep, the exercises in your Body at Home™ workouts are going to help you fight stress. Each workout is designed to sculpt your muscles and burn fat and, in the process, give you an emotional advantage that immediately will help alleviate stress.

Studies indicate that exercise increases the body's concentration of the neurotransmitter *norepinephrine* in the regions of the brain involved in stress response. Scientists believe this means that exercise can enhance the body's ability to respond to stress. People who strength-train also sometimes experience the euphoria that results from an exercise-induced release of opiate-like compounds called *endorphins.* An endorphin rush can make you feel exhilarated as well as calm and relaxed, and is a potent stress reliever.

In addition to producing chemical reactions, exercise is a great way to get some alone time—and even blow off steam. If you experience some tension, burn it off with your morning cardio or take it out on your resistance bands. You'll feel more relaxed and peaceful at home, you will sleep better, and you'll be happier throughout the day.

So here is what I will ask you to do if managing stress sounds like something that would help you move to a level of accomplishment at which you can stay consistent, feel fulfilled, and see results that continue to keep you motivated. Add "endorphins" to your list on the Life Priority chart on page 12. Write down that your Body at Home™ workouts will help promote the release of stress-reducing, energizing endorphins and will help you feel good and face daily challenges head-on. I guarantee you'll feel a difference even after your first workout. I've had clients share with me the peace of mind and sense of accomplishment they feel after just one amazing 20-minute workout!

18 BODY AT HOME THIRTIES SUPERSTAR Carrie Wang

Height: 5'5" | **Age:** 37 | **Lost:** 18 pounds

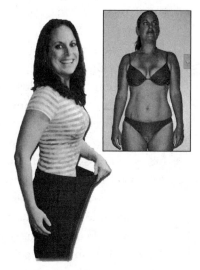

"Like many women, I have battled with my weight my whole life. As a mother of two and an elementary teacher, I'm very busy! I would see women who succeeded on other programs and think, 'Yeah, right!' But with the Body at Home™ program, you can do it! Since you work out only 20 minutes, three times a week, you can make it fit into any schedule! Now I am finally that person I never thought I could be. I look in the mirror and I absolutely love what I see! I look so much younger, I love my body, and I feel and look better now than I ever have in my whole life. Now I am the one in the cute outfits I used to envy on other women. And knowing this, I will never go back to that old, overweight person I used to see in the mirror ever again."

Carrie's Secrets to Success

· Be sure to plan ahead. Make sure you have your meals for the week planned and prepared at least the day before.

· Don't be a slave to the scale! You will notice results in how your clothes fit and how you feel and look in the mirror sooner than you will on the scale.

· Set achievable goals! Don't make goals that are unrealistic. Set goals that you can achieve in a few weeks instead of a huge goal that will take you much longer. Have that big goal for yourself, but set smaller ones to reach along the way so you will continue to be successful.

Forties: Prevent Decline

If you've just hit 40 or you are in your mid-to-late forties, you're probably noticing some changes in your body—and I bet they're not all ones you like. These physical changes occur because of hormonal ones and the natural effects of life—it's just a fact that no one can escape the effects of age. Although I'm not talking about the kind of visible changes that happen at puberty, you may be noticing changes in where you carry your weight and how your body metabolizes food. According to my good friend Dr. Mehmet Oz, since women's bodies are optimally designed to have children in their 20s, they can handle a lot and bounce back quickly. In your 30s, you may have had kids and put your body through pregnancy and childbirth; but even if you didn't, I bet you were constantly bombarded with stress. And now you might be feeling a bit worn down and you're looking for a rejuvenating force. But in addition to that, you have reached a decade where letting your health decline can lead to life-threatening diseases such as diabetes, breast cancer, and stroke. That's why the focus for you in this decade will be prevention. One study done at the University of British Columbia found "irrefutable evidence of the effectiveness of regular physical activity in the prevention of several chronic diseases (e.g. cardiovascular disease, diabetes, cancer, hypertension, obesity, depression, and osteoporosis)."

Beyond disease prevention, making a commitment to this program will help you manage other health-related issues that can arise in your forties. Of course you know that you are likely to start experiencing symptoms of menopause in your fifties. But did you know that the symptoms of perimenopause—the stage that occurs several years before menopause when the ovaries start producing less estrogen—are likely to start in your forties? Symptoms of perimenopause include hot flashes, breast tenderness, worsening of PMS, decreased sex drive, fatigue, mood swings, irregular periods, and difficulty sleeping. Around this time, women generally start to gain weight, especially around their bellies, which can lead to a host of problems, including the metabolic syndrome.

The *metabolic syndrome* is a group of related disorders that can increase the likelihood of heart disease and diabetes. Symptoms include excess weight, particularly around the midsection, high levels of bad cholesterol, insulin resistance, high blood sugar, and high blood pressure.

Starting Body at Home™ and dropping 10 pounds in your forties can help prevent you from developing the metabolic syndrome. In fact, one study of 118 women conducted in Canada found that those who performed physical activity were less likely than inactive women to develop symptoms of metabolic syndrome. Another study, conducted in Germany, found that regular exercise not only trimmed women's waistlines but also reduced cholesterol levels, maintained bone density, and reduced the incidence of migraines and mood swings.

I challenge you right now to prevent the decline of your body by committing to three Body at Home™ workouts each week. This time will be invaluable to your health and will help you prevent potentially serious health problems in the years to come. It's vital to your health and longevity! Go to page 12 and jot down your deepest motivation for making a commitment to your fitness today.

Height: 5'6" | **Age:** 46 | **Lost:** 10 pounds (Plus restored 2 pounds of lean muscle)

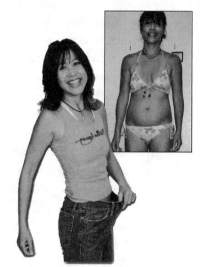

"This year my goal was to get rid of my tummy fat that I've been carrying around with me for over five years.

"I now eat healthier and am more aware of what I put into my body. I don't crave any of the fatty foods that I used to crave. I love eating every three hours! I also love working out—I actually started to crave the workouts. It's amazing and rewarding to work out my body. I feel great every day.

"I love being able to wear all of my clothes—now some of them are even too baggy! My favorite old jeans at the bottom of the closet that I couldn't wear before are now my favorite everyday jeans!"

Sharon's Secrets to Success

· Make a commitment to stay committed for the eight weeks.

· Don't cheat! You will not get to your goal by cheating.

· Write down what you ate each day for at least a week.

Fifties-Plus: Reverse Decline

If you are in your fifties and beyond, now is the time for you to proactively bounce back into a life of health and fitness—one that doesn't stop you from participating in any activity you wish or experiencing your life to the fullest. If you are already fit and you've picked up this book to stay in shape or maybe drop a few pounds, then congratulations on continuing to make your health a priority! Dropping a jean size will help you start to dramatically improve your vitality. If you are like a lot of women in their fifties and up, years of neglect might have caught up with you—but you have the power to take back control of your life right now. Studies have even shown that exercise can practically take years off your age. One study done at the University of Wisconsin revealed that previously sedentary women in their fifties who participated in an exercise program increased their fitness level by 23 percent. Even more important, they reduced the occurrence of functional decline often attributed to age. That's right—you can actually maintain and even improve your quality of life as you get older. And guess what? The book you hold in your hands is going to help you take control and create quality that lasts.

If you've been experiencing symptoms of menopause, you may feel they get in the way of your fitness goals. Some days you just can't bear the thought of exercising because you feel so lousy. But I have some great news for you. Your Body at Home™ workouts are going to help you manage those symptoms. A study done by the University of Granada, in Spain, revealed that menopausal women who exercised improved their menopausal symptoms substantially and "significantly improved their health-related quality of life." Many of the women in this study admitted to not having exercised in five years. This means that even if you haven't picked up a weight or put on your sneakers in a long time, you too can still experience the incredible effects of exercise.

One of the greatest risks to your health after menopause is osteoporosis. Osteoporosis reduces bone mineral density (BMD) and compromises the strength of the bone. Women with osteoporosis are at greater risk for bone fractures that can severely reduce their quality of life. Women are particularly vulnerable to osteoporosis after menopause because the ovaries stop producing estrogen, which in turn accelerates bone loss.

Exercise—strength training in particular—can halt and even reverse the loss of BMD. Researchers funded by the National Institute of Arthritis and Musculoskeletal and Skin Diseases (a part of the Department of Health and Human Services) conducted a trial of 320 postmenopausal women between the ages of 45 and 65 to determine whether exercise alone had an effect on BMD. They found that the women who exercised demonstrated significant improvement after one year of resistance training.

Besides improving BMD and reducing the risk of injury as women age, exercise can improve quality of life in other ways. Regular exercise can increase heart and lung capacity, lower blood pressure, increase strength, reduce body fat, and reduce susceptibility to depression and disease. You're never too old to reap the benefits of exercise!

My challenge to you right now is to realize that, by fully embracing the Body at Home™ for the next two weeks, *you can take control of your health* and even reverse damage done by previous neglect. Think of that training time as a magical time that will transform your body and help you recover some of your youthful vitality. So go to page 12 and add to your list key words from this section that have motivated you. You can do it!

Height: 5'5" | **Age:** 50 | **Lost:** 10 pounds (Plus restored 2 pounds of lean muscle)

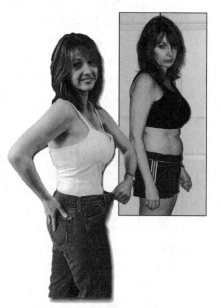

"I'm a single mom with two sons, 7 and 13. They are my angels, and I want to be around for them for a long time. I am turning 50 this year, and when I looked in the mirror, I realized I was turning into a 'dumpy' older woman—and I want to be proud of how I look at 50.

"I really only needed to lose 10 pounds, but those last 10 pounds had been around for quite a while! I had no idea that working out only 20 minutes three times a week could make such an amazing difference in such a short time. Within the first two weeks, I could tell a big difference in how my jeans fit! I have lost 3 inches in my waist, 2 inches in my hips, and I really feel sexy again! I actually have definition in my arms and legs again. I am very happy with how I look, and I owe it to the Body at Home™. I am wearing shorts that I never would have worn in the last two years. I have a lot of energy and I just feel fabulous!"

Sallie's Secrets to Success

· Pack snacks in sandwich bags with right portions so you're not tempted to eat the whole bag at once.

· When the cravings come and you are tempted to eat outside of the plan, brush your teeth and drink 8 ounces of water.

· Fast-food places have a lot of good choices now. Be sure to ask for low-fat dressing. One favorite is Arby's® Market Fresh® Santa Fe Salad with low-fat ranch dressing and extra chicken.

Remember, to get on the fast track to shrinking and sculpting your belly, butt, hips, and thighs, it's essential for you to maximize both your *physical focus* and your *inner drive*. The Priority Solution™ will be your best friend in identifying these elements and allowing the Body at Home™ program to work for you.

So my invitation to you is to take a deep breath and commit to this program right now by reading the next chapter. There you'll learn about all the important eating strategies that will accelerate your success.

Following these steps will ensure you drop 10 pounds in two weeks at home and continue through to the eight-week point, where you will reveal your best body ever. With Body at Home™ and the Priority Solution™ you will learn how to keep the weight off long-term, and you will discover the healthiest and sexiest you. You're going to love it!

3 Eating Right

It's time to eat! In this chapter I've included vital information that will help you achieve optimum health through the ages. There are just two key secrets to eating right to drop that jean size in two weeks at home: timing and ingredients.

SECRET 1: TIMING

A crucial component of this eating plan is *eating approximately every three hours*. Ideally you'll eat breakfast within one hour of waking up; then, three hours later, you'll eat a snack. Three hours later, you'll eat lunch, followed by a snack—yes—three hours after lunch. Finally, you'll eat dinner three hours after your afternoon snack; and before you go to bed, you'll have your last snack.

Many of my clients ask how many calories they will be eating. And the truth with this program is that the quality of your meals is more important than the calories you consume. So here's the big distinction for you right now: Don't worry about counting calories. Yes, you heard me right. Calories are not going to be as important as the quality of what you are eating. This eating plan is fiber-dense and nutrient-rich and will leave you feeling completely satisfied. If at first it doesn't feel quite right for your appetite, give it a few days and you will love how fulfilled, fresh, and energized you feel.

Why is eating every three hours so crucial? Essentially, it does three vital things: reduces cortisol hormone levels that contribute to belly fat; helps you maintain a high metabolic rate so you stay energized and continue to burn fat; and helps you control your appetite so you don't binge and sabotage all your hard work. Bottom line: Numerous research studies support that eating small meals throughout the day, instead of one or two large meals, reduces hunger and enhances weight loss. For more details on why eating every three hours is so beneficial, visit JorgeCruise.com or pick up a copy of my book *The 3-Hour Diet*.

SECRET 2: QUALITY NUTRIENTS

You know that you're going to eat every three hours, but which foods from the endless supermarket shelves and fast-food drive-throughs do you choose? Our society offers so many choices that we're often confused about what's healthy and will help us reach our goals. Well, I've simplified it for you in this section. Remember, there's no deprivation, and no food group has been omitted. This plan is about a quality, delicious, filling, and balanced diet that will help you burn fat and restore lean muscle tissue.

A quality diet is comprised of three macronutrients: protein, carbohydrate, and fat. All three are essential to good health. On this plan, aim to get about 40 percent of your calories from protein, 40 percent from carbohydrate, and 20 percent from fat. You don't have to divide every meal so specifically, but by the end of the day, you should be as close to a 40/40/20 ratio as possible. Let's take a look at each of these macronutrients to discover why it is so crucial to your success on this program.

Protein

Protein is going to be a very important nutrient for you to consume on this program. Proteins are made up of chains of amino acids. Our bodies manufacture some amino acids on their own, but others we need to get from the foods we eat. Amino acids that we have to get from our foods are called *essential amino acids*. Our bodies use amino acids to build and repair tissue. If you don't consume enough protein, your body actually cannibalizes lean muscle and uses it to fix and create other tissue. As you know, that's bad because it will slow your metabolism.

When choosing sources of protein, look for high-quality, low-fat options like skinless white-meat poultry; lean beef and pork; fatty, cold-water fish like salmon and tuna; eggs; and low-fat dairy like 2 percent milk, cottage cheese, and yogurt. Choosing lean protein sources, instead of fatty ones like rib-eye steak, will ensure that you get all the protein you need without consuming excess calories. Portion size is important too. If you weigh more than 150 pounds, you should eat 5 ounces of protein at every meal. If you weigh less than 150 pounds, eat 3 ounces at each meal. A 3-ounce portion is roughly the size of a deck of cards; 5 ounces, about a deck and a half.

And here is one other thing you need to know about protein. It's the ideal snack as well. As I mentioned earlier, you're going to have three daily snacks. I highly recommend that you drink whey protein shakes for these snacks. Why is whey so important? Whey is the most bioavailable source of protein you can consume. Your body can absorb its nutrients more easily than it can absorb protein from other sources. As a result, your muscles can use whey protein right away to repair and create new tissue, and you'll have the greatest nutritional advantage for creating a lean and sculpted figure.

In addition to helping you build lean muscle, whey protein has other health benefits. It can help reduce the risk of developing preventable illnesses, such as cardiovascular disease. It has been found to help prevent or reduce high blood pressure and elevated cholesterol, which are among the leading causes of heart disease and stroke. High levels of cysteine, found in whey protein, have been correlated with lower risk of developing breast and prostate cancers. Whey protein is also high in immunoglobulin, alpha-lactalbumin, and beta-lactalbumin, all of which boost your immune system. Just one more reason to make sure you drink your whey protein shakes! Look for a brand that provides about 20 grams of protein per serving and has between 100 and 150 calories. You can check out the brand I helped create, called Jorge's Packs™, at jorgespacks.com. It's delicious. For more ideas and protein snack options, be sure to check the Snacks section in the Ideal Foods List on page 342.

Carbohydrate

Carbs are an important source of energy when you are active and exercise, so you don't want to omit them from your diet. The secret is knowing which carbs to eat and when. Your body responds differently to various types of carbs. Some, like potato chips, white bread, white rice, pasta, and sugar (also known as simple carbohydrates), cause your blood sugar to spike quickly and dramatically. When your blood-sugar level is roller-coastering, it's difficult to control your appetite and avoid bingeing. So it's best to limit your consumption of *simple* carbs as much as possible.

Other carbs cause a slow and steady release of sugar into your bloodstream and therefore help you control your appetite. These are called *complex* carbohydrates, and they're found in most vegetables, fruits, and whole grains, such as whole-wheat flour and bread, whole-wheat pasta, brown rice, oatmeal, air-popped popcorn, barley, millet, and quinoa (pronounced "keen-wa"). In addition to helping you regulate your appetite, complex carbs provide vitamins, minerals, and, most important, fiber. Fiber not only helps you stay full longer but also aids digestive health and reduces your risk of developing colon cancer.

Although fruits, vegetables, and grains are all carbohydrates, I've divided them into starchy and nonstarchy categories for this eating plan. *Starchy* carbs include grains, bread, rice, potatoes, and corn. *Nonstarchy* carbs include fruit and most vegetables (except potatoes, sweet potatoes, beets, and rice), such as lettuce, cucumber, celery, spinach and other dark greens, broccoli, green beans, bell peppers, onions, and garlic. See the Ideal Foods List on page 342 for a more extensive list of starchy and nonstarchy carbs.

On this program, you'll eat starchy carbs with breakfast and lunch, but you'll stop eating them after lunch. For breakfast and lunch, you'll have one serving of starchy carbs (a half cup or one slice of bread). For dinner, you'll omit starchy carbs and double your serving of vegetables. Why do we omit carbs at night? They provide a lot of energy that you won't use as you wind down from your day, and your body will store that unused energy as fat. A typical serving of vegetables is 1 cup cooked or 2 cups raw. So for dinner you should have 2 to 4 cups of veggies. Since fruit is a little denser in calories than veggies, I like to eat them with breakfast instead of later in the day. Keep your servings of fruit to about 1 cup diced or one item, such as an apple. These serving sizes will ensure that you receive the ideal number of calories and nutrition and keep you from feeling hungry.

Fat

A lot of people think *fat* is a scary word, but fat is a crucial component of any healthy eating plan. Fats are made up of chains of fatty acids, some of which, like some proteins, can't be generated by the body (and are called *essential fatty acids*). Fat serves as a storage system for your body to tap into for energy when food is scarce. Fat keeps you insulated against cold, helps you digest and absorb vitamins and minerals, and helps cells and organs function properly.

Not all fats are created equal, however. Food contains several different kinds of fat: saturated fat, trans (or hydrogenated) fat, and unsaturated fat. Most foods with high levels of *saturated fat* come from animal sources. Examples include beef, lard, chicken skin, butter, whole milk, and cheese. Some plant oils also contain saturated fat—coconut oil, palm kernel oil, and palm oil. Saturated fat is considered bad because research shows that it raises cholesterol levels and can help clog your arteries. You can usually tell that a fat is saturated because it's solid at room temperature.

Trans (or *hydrogenated*) *fat,* also solid at room temperature, is considered even worse for your health than saturated fat. Health experts contend that hydrogenated fat, a relatively modern invention, is the most dangerous kind of fat you can eat. There is no safe recommended daily allowance of trans fat, and the Institute of Medicine suggests that people avoid it as much as possible. *Hydrogenation* is a process that adds hydrogen molecules to liquid fats such as vegetable oils to make them solid at room temperature. Hydrogenated fat, and the products made with it, stay fresh on supermarket shelves much longer than products made from natural fats, which is why food manufacturers use hydrogenated fat so much. Foods containing trans fat include margarine and shortening and most store-bought cookies, cakes, crackers, and other baked goods.

The healthiest kind of fat is unsaturated. *Unsaturated fat* helps keep your arteries clear, decreases cholesterol levels, and reduces the risk of developing cardiovascular disease and many types of cancers. It is found in olive, peanut, canola, sunflower, corn, and soybean oils and in avocados.

Omega-3 fats are a special type of unsaturated fat. They are true gems when it comes to your health and weight management. Omega-3s help suppress your appetite, help you feel more full on less food, and even maintain lean muscle tissue. They also have an amazing ability to unlock stored body fat so you can burn it for fuel. Omega-3s improve the health of cell membranes, which allows more oxygen to circulate throughout your body. This additional oxygen helps your muscles convert stored body fat for energy. Omega-3s are the only fats that have this special ability! Lastly, they are able to regulate the body's ratio of insulin to glucagons. Insulin tells your body to store fat, and glucagons tell your body to burn it. Because omega-3 fats increase the ratio of glucagons to insulin, you burn fat more easily.

You'll find omega-3 fats in flaxseed products, olives and olive oil, fatty cold-water fish like salmon and tuna, avocados, seeds, almonds and other nuts, and soybeans. My personal favorite source of omega-3s is flax oil or fish oil. I've tried a few different brands, but my favorite by far is Barlean's® Organic Omega Swirl Oil Supplement—with a fruit-smoothie look and taste. You can find more info about Barlean's® in the Approved Products list on page 347. Whatever your favorite fat, aim to have one serving or approximately 45 calories of it with every meal. That's about 1 teaspoon of any fat in liquid form, such as flax or olive oil, one slice of avocado, or a small handful of almonds.

Water

Though not exactly a food, water is an essential nutrient that you need enough of every day. Your body is made up of 55 to 75 percent water, and each of your cells requires daily replenishment to function properly. You lose water through your normal daily perspiration, from going to the bathroom, and even through the air you exhale. When you're only slightly dehydrated, you feel sluggish and tired and you may not be able to think very clearly. Regularly depriving yourself of water increases your risk of developing kidney stones and becoming constipated. Not drinking enough water can even make you overeat! The body sometimes misinterprets the signal for thirst as hunger, which makes you want to nibble when you really don't need food.

Many people recommend that you drink 8 cups of water every day, but I think it's a good idea to drink even more, especially when you're exercising regularly. Try to drink at least half of your body weight (in pounds) in water (in ounces) each day. That means that if you weigh 160 pounds, you should drink 80 ounces, or 10 cups, of water each day. It sounds like a lot, but drinking that much really isn't hard. If you have any health conditions, be sure to ask your doctor about the appropriate amount of water for you. The secret is to spread your drinking out throughout the day and make the water taste great. Or you can do something as simple as add a squeeze of lemon to your water—it's so refreshing!

Here's a quick overview of a sample day; see the Resources for Her section for recipes.

SAMPLE DAY

Breakfast 7:00 a.m.	Snack 10:00 a.m.	Lunch 1:00 p.m.	Snack 4:00 p.m.	Dinner 7:00 p.m.	Bedtime Snack 10:00 p.m.
Vegetable Frittata	1 whey protein shake or alternative protein snack (See the Ideal Foods List for options.)	Grilled Ham and Cheese with Tomato Soup	1 whey protein shake or alternative protein snack (See the Ideal Foods List for options.)	Beef Tenderloin Salad with Garlic Vinaigrette	1 whey protein shake

EATING RIGHT AT ANY AGE

Due to hormonal changes and maybe some experiments with unhealthy or unbalanced diets, you are more likely than your male counterparts to develop a nutrient deficiency at some point in your life. But don't worry, you can prevent—and even reverse—dietary deficiencies by eating the right nutrient-rich foods and taking the appropriate supplements when you need to. Here, I've outlined some important dietary considerations for you as you travel through your life. Think of these as critical road signs you should follow to help keep you on the right course. If you miss a sign, you could end up heading right toward the hospital—and I know you don't want that! One simple way to make sure you're getting a steady supply of vitamins and minerals is to take a daily multivitamin.

WHAT TO DO IF YOU'RE . . .

In Your Twenties

If you're in your twenties, you might think paying attention to things like vitamins and nutrients is something only your mom does, but the truth is, now is the perfect time to adopt some good habits. If you do, your body will thank you later!

Balancing your social life, work, and maybe even school is tough, so eating on the go is probably one of your main dietary defaults. Fast food and eating out normally don't go well with following an eating plan, but the Body at Home™ plan takes your hectic life into consideration. Check out the Fast and Frozen Foods List on page 344 for some options that will help keep you on track even when you're on the go. Make your best effort to eat fresh foods whenever you can, but remember you always have the foods on this list to fall back on in a pinch.

Stock up on calcium now. Your body pretty much stops building up your bones at around age 30, so it's crucial to build up reserves while you still can. Aim for about 1,200 milligrams a day from food sources like milk and cheese or from a quality supplement. Vitamin D helps your body absorb calcium, so eat eggs and fish and other foods rich in Vitamin D, and get a little bit of sun each day—but not during peak hours!

There's a mineral too that should be on your list: iron. Getting enough iron will help you feel energized and keep your mind and body sharp. Eat lean meats and dark green vegetables like kale and broccoli, or look for iron-enriched whole-wheat pastas.

Lastly, when you pick up a good multivitamin, look for one that you have to take only once daily. To be effective, some multivitamins have to be taken twice a day, which I know can be tough to remember sometimes.

In Your Thirties

Chances are if you're in your thirties, you've started to take nutrition a bit more seriously. You've probably gotten to know the produce section of the grocery store by now, but maybe you want to know a little more about maximizing your nutrition from foods. If you're thinking about getting pregnant during this decade of your life, there are some specific things you want to be sure to get into your diet. Omega-3 fatty acids have great health benefits all the time, but they also are known to be essential to the development of a baby's eyes and brain. Salmon and some other fish, eggs, and flax oil—my favorite—are rich in omega-3s.

If you've already had kids or you take birth control pills, your body could be deficient in key vitamins and minerals, such as some B vitamins, vitamin A, and magnesium. These deficiencies can lead to more severe PMS symptoms and a weakened immune system, among other things. Eat more carrots, potatoes, and peas for B6; get vitamin A from squash and sweet potatoes; and get magnesium from whole-wheat bread or brown rice and vegetables such as artichokes and spinach.

Folate is another important vitamin to get plenty of during years in which you may be considering getting pregnant. Folate is a B vitamin that you can find in asparagus, green peas, and fortified cereals. Having the right amount of folate in your body can help prevent birth defects. Be sure to take it *before* you start trying to conceive; ask your doctor for specific recommendations. Even if you're not planning on pregnancy, folate plays a crucial role in producing new cells and helping keep them strong, so it's good for everyone.

In Your Forties

As you get older, your metabolism does slow down a bit. I know we all hate to hear this, but you can make an adjustment just by being smarter with your food choices. Minimize fast-food trips and processed foods—they can wreak havoc on your system and rapidly add empty calories to your diet.

One of the best friends to have in your forties is fiber. First off, it's been shown to help balance your estrogen levels, which can alleviate some symptoms of perimenopause. It has also proven effective at lowering your risk of heart disease and lowering your cholesterol, and helping keep your blood glucose levels balanced. Bottom line: Fiber is good for you. Quality sources of fiber include kidney beans, split peas, and raspberries. Add the berries to your oatmeal for breakfast and you've got a great fiber-filled start to your day.

While you can no longer build your bones up, you can help fight a decline in their density by getting the proper amount of calcium. Stick to about 1,200 milligrams a day. Also, remember to keep your sodium intake down and your soda and alcohol consumption to a minimum. These three things don't do your bones any favors!

Boost your immune system by getting plenty of foods rich in vitamin E, such as spinach and almonds. Also, try wheat germ, which is an excellent source of this powerful antioxidant. Vitamin E helps your cells fight against free radicals and helps keep your skin and hair healthy.

In Your Fifties-Plus

You may be noticing a trend here, but guess what you should be getting plenty of in your fifties: calcium! Once you've reached menopause or are very close to it, your estrogen levels continue to drop, and this means you have less natural prevention against bone loss. Experts recommend upping your daily intake of calcium to 1,600 milligrams. It's crucial to help keep your bones as strong as possible—especially as you get older.

When you reach your fifties, your body doesn't absorb B12 as readily as it used to, so it's important to consider taking a supplement. B12 helps make DNA and keeps your nerve and blood cells in shape. It's also been shown to prevent plaque buildup that can lead to heart disease and stroke. Plus, when you're lacking in B12, you may feel sluggish—so stay energized by staying on top of this important vitamin.

Since you're going to be eating every three hours on this plan, you'll already be on a schedule that will keep your blood sugar levels balanced and your hunger satiated. It's especially critical for you to follow this if you're 50 or over. A structured eating schedule will help keep your body from storing unexpected calories as fat—the last thing you want to do!

To make sure you're ready to face all the challenges that menopause and life after menopause bring, look for a multivitamin packed with plenty of good stuff that will help you weather hormonal imbalances and the rising risk of disease. It's also imperative for you to eat disease-fighting sources of antioxidants, such as dark green vegetables, beans (pinto beans and kidney beans are surprising sources), and plenty of berries. Blueberries, cranberries, and blackberries deliver powerful doses of antioxidants to help prevent unwanted cell damage.

FREE DAY

The idea of committing to a specific eating plan for an entire eight weeks may make you a little nervous. How can you possibly go eight weeks without your favorite ice cream or pizza? Well, I have great news for you: You don't have to! On one day each week—your free day—you can eat whatever you want. Really—whatever you want!

Are you thinking, "How can I have a free day and still lose weight?" Well, studies have shown that if you eat double the amount of calories you normally eat in one day, you will actually speed up your metabolism by 9 percent for the following 24 hours. That doesn't mean you get to double the number of calories you're eating on the other days; it just gives you complete freedom with your food choices for one day. I believe deprivation will only lead to bingeing, so this gives you a small break to make sure you don't feel deprived of your favorite things.

There's only one catch to having a free day: It means no cheating on the other days of the week! But I think you're going to be surprised at how you feel after your free day. Because you are being so good to your body every other day of the week, you will be amazed at how lethargic and unhealthy you'll feel. In fact, I bet after a few free days, you actually will cut back to one free meal or even just a small dessert. Once you realize the power and energy you have when you're fueling your body with the right foods from the Body at Home™ eating plan, you won't want to feel any other way.

You may not need a free day, or you may worry that a free day will allow you to get off course too much. Don't worry—the free day is completely optional. If you want to remain committed to the eating plan every day of the eight weeks, that's great. The best thing is, it's up to you—the Body at Home™ plan is made to work for everyone, so customize it to fit your own lifestyle and goals.

MAKE IT WORK FOR YOU

I promise that you'll easily be able to make this eating plan work in your busy schedule and stick with it for life. It's so simple to follow that you can do so whether you like to cook at home or prefer to eat out. In the Recipe list on page 149 in the Resources for Her section, you'll find delicious recipes I developed with my team that are easy and quick to prepare. When you're dining out, remember the guidelines outlined in this chapter. You can easily find something to fit this eating plan, whether you're eating Mexican, Chinese, or Italian. Wherever you're dining, always make sure that you're eating on plan.

START TODAY!

To help you track your meals and stick with the eating plan, I've included in the Resources for Her section an Eating Planner log for you to copy and fill out every day (see page 143). For a preview, see the handwritten sample on page 31. The log has space for your meals, snacks, water, and supplements. It also has time slots so you make sure that you eat every three hours. It's easy to forget when to eat or whether you've had enough water for the day. Use this log to make sure that you stick to your eating plan and to your three-hour eating times.

(10) BODY AT HOME™ STAR   Michelle Weissinger

Height: 5'3" | **Age:** 28 | **Lost:** 10 pounds (Plus restored 2 pounds of lean muscle)

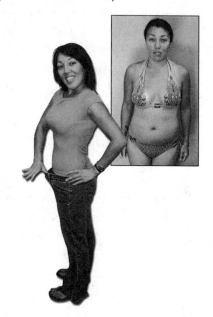

"Before starting I had run two marathons, but I didn't *look* like I was in great shape. I was running 20 to 30 miles a week, but I wasn't happy with my body.

"Once I started Body at Home™, I learned to make better use of my workout time. My morning dog walks now involve hills and power walking, which jump-start my morning and burn additional calories."

Michelle's Secrets to Success

· Set a routine early and stick to it.

· Plan and prepare meals/snacks the night before.

· To see whether boredom or stress or hunger is driving you to the fridge, head outside for a walk when you're tempted to eat.

EATING PLANNER (SAMPLE)

This plan will ensure leaner muscle and a higher metabolism.

Breakfast>time 7:30

	Description
PROTEIN* (3–5oz)	scrambled eggs
CARBS (½ cup or 1 slice of bread)	toast
FRUIT (1 cup)	blueberries
FAT (1 teaspoon)	flax oil on toast

Snack>time 10:30

	Description
WHEY PROTEIN SHAKE (1 scoop)	Jorge's Packs choc. shake

Jorge recommends Jorge's Packs™ for your protein drinks. **>** See list of other recommended snacks at the back of the book.

Lunch>time 1:30

	Description
PROTEIN* (3–5oz)	grilled chicken
CARBS (½ cup or 1 slice of bread)	quinoa
VEGGIES** (2 cups)	zucchini, squash, mushrooms
FAT (1 teaspoon)	Olive oil

Snack>time 4:30

	Description
WHEY PROTEIN SHAKE (1 scoop)	Jorge's Packs vanilla shake

Dinner>time 7:30

	Description
PROTEIN* (3–5oz)	grilled shrimp
VEGGIES** (2–4 cups)	green salad w/basil & tomatoes
FAT (1 teaspoon)	Olive oil

Snack>time 10:30

	Description
WHEY PROTEIN SHAKE (1 scoop)	Jorge's Packs choc. shake

*If you weigh under 150 pounds, eat 3 ounces of protein at every meal; if you weigh over 150 pounds, eat 5 ounces of protein.

**Veggies = nonstarchy vegetables.

Water (eight 8-oz cups) ● ● ● ● ● ● ● ●

Multivitamin ●

Height: 5'6" | **Age:** 28 | **Lost:** 10 pounds (Plus restored 1 pound of lean muscle)

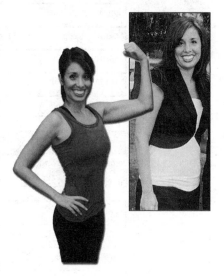

"I have wanted to lose the 'last 5 to 10 pounds' for as long as I can remember. I have been dieting since I was in high school, mostly by trying the latest fad diet. I would get close to my ideal weight, but I could never sustain it because I did it in an unhealthy way. Body at Home™ is the first plan that I knew was healthy, based on a sensible eating plan, and, most importantly, it was something I could adapt easily and make it my own. I know the results I have achieved are maintainable and I look forward to sticking to Jorge's plan for a long time to come! Body at Home™ definitely works and you *will* see results if you stick to it."

Danielle's Secrets to Success

· Do the morning walks every day! It's a great way to have time by yourself or with a loved one.

· Make modifications if you need to so that it works for your life—or you won't stick to it.

· Have a buddy! Doing it with someone else provides a support system and motivation. If you don't have a buddy, try using online friends to keep you accountable.

4 Get Ready to Start

"With a 7-month old, it is not always convenient to get to the gym. I loved being able to work out with just the resistance bands, weights, and ball—I really was able to do the workouts anywhere. I didn't need to go to the gym, and that was key for me. I love how the exercises maximized my effort and time. That was great! This program is exactly what I needed."

—REBECCA PIDGEON, BODY AT HOME™ STAR, LOST 13 POUNDS

In this book, there are two phases for you to experience: the Quick-Start Phase and the Sculpting Phase. You may be tempted to skip around through the plan and try different exercises. But if you want to see the best results, it's critical for you to follow the plan as it was designed.

QUICK-START PHASE

This two-week phase is specifically designed so you can see results right away and drop 10 pounds, which is about one jean size. Remember, you will not need to go to the gym; every single one of your workouts can be done from home, even when you get to the Sculpting Phase.

You will need a few simple tools to get started: a Swiss ball, a set of dumbbells, a mat, a medicine ball, and a set of resistance bands. If you haven't used resistance bands before, you're going to love them. They can challenge your muscles as much as dumbbells but are more compact and easy to store. You can find all of the equipment on the website at BodyatHome.com, or you can pick it up at your local sporting goods store. Look for products made by GoFit™—they are my favorite. Check out page 347 of the Bonus Items section for more information.

SCULPTING PHASE

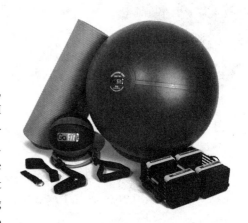

After you complete the first two weeks of the program, you should begin the Sculpting Phase. Now, just because I call it "sculpting" doesn't mean you have to be a super-model or an ultra-fit person to do this part of the program. It simply means that the exercises are going to get a little more challenging, so that you continue to tone and sculpt your muscles as efficiently as possible. If you kept doing the same exercises, your body soon would get used to them and your shape would stay the same. Remember, you're here to create change.

The great thing is even when you begin the Sculpting Phase, you can continue to do the workouts at home. If you want to mix it up and change your environment, feel free to go to the gym, take your workout outside, or partner up and try it at a friend's house. Wherever or whenever you do your workouts, be sure to get uninterrupted time to focus on yourself and your body. Turn off your cell phone and your computer and really commit this time to yourself.

TIME TO WORK OUT

I know that just like my celebrity clients, you have a very busy schedule and have to fit in your workout only *when* you can fit it in, but I have a recommendation for you on the best days to work out: *I highly recommend that you do your workouts on Monday, Wednesday, and Friday.* This way, you have a day of rest between each

How to Start *Right Now*—Even if You Don't Have the Equipment

Great news! If you don't want to wait any longer to begin the program, *you can start right now.* Even if you don't have the recommended equipment for the Quick-Start Phase, I've designed an entirely excuse-free routine. Don't have any dumbbells and bands? You don't need them! Turn to the Weight-Free Routine on page 165 of the Resources for Her section, and you'll find a workout that you can begin right now. All you need is your body's own resistance, a chair, and a mat or towel. The great thing about this routine is that it provides a full-body workout in just 20 minutes, and you can use it in a pinch when you're traveling or stuck at work. Don't rely on this routine for the entire eight weeks, though. Start creating maximum results with the other eight weeks of the program as soon as possible.

workout day, as well as the entire weekend to recuperate so that your body is fresh and energized for your first workout of the week. Plus, you will feel so great getting your week off to such a healthy and invigorating start. *Trust me—it's the best way!* If you absolutely can't work out on these days, be sure to allow at least one day between workouts for essential rest and recovery.

See pages 36 and 37 for useful tracking tools to help you log your progress through the program. You'll see one filled-out example of the Day 1 Workout Log that you will use to record each workout. (For blank versions of the Workout Log for all three workout days that you can copy and use throughout the eight weeks, turn to pages 144–146 in the Resources for Her section.) Next, there is a filled-out example of the 8-Week Workout Chart, a simple but powerful tool that will be a great visual motivator. You should feel good about each workout you track on your way to the new you! (Turn to page 147 of the Resources for Her section for a blank version.)

Before you get started, I want to share four critical secrets to success that will maximize the results you see on this program. Four simple things can make all the difference in how quickly and effectively you see results: form, counting, breathing, and intensity.

The Key to Proper Form

Since the Body at Home™ workouts require you to perform *controlled movements,* you are one step ahead when it comes to achieving proper form. Too often people rush through their exercises and, as a result, compromise their results or, even worse, injure themselves. When you do an exercise incorrectly, you often take the focus off the right muscles. For example, when you're working your triceps, you don't want your back to help you support the weight or press the resistance band. Your triceps won't fully fatigue and you won't see the results you want. Don't cheat yourself out of getting the most from your workouts. Always pay attention to your form.

When you get to the exercises in Chapter 5, you will see that every move has a brief description accompanied by two main photographs of Lacie, my cover fitness model. As you may notice, Lacie is in top shape. She's a busy, working mom who has used the plan to help maintain her toned figure. The key to achieving proper form is to read the descriptions through before you begin your workout and to follow the pointers! The descriptions are short and direct but include some vital information—tips like "Keep your elbows close to your body throughout the exercise" or "Keep your back straight and head up." Although they will help you with each specific exercise, there are some other steps you can take to ensure the most efficient workout possible.

First, I recommend reading through the entire workout before you start each day. This way, you can simply glance at the photographs for a quick reminder while you're doing the exercises. Also, try a "practice run" in which you let your body get familiar with the MTP of each

DAY 1

DATE __3/10__

Start Time __7:00__ Finish Time __7:20__

TOTAL TIME __20 minutes__

Select weights so that by the end of the 4th rep of each exercise you feel an intensity level of 8.

Muscle Group	Exercise	Weight Used	Intensity Level	set 1	set 2
LEGS	Beginning squat	N/A	7	✓	✓
LEGS	Swiss ball squat	10	8	✓	✓
LEGS	Lunge	N/A	7	✓	✓
LEGS	Hamstring curl w/swiss ball	N/A	8	✓	✓

At this point you should be about 6 minutes into your workout.

TRICEPS	Chair dip	N/A	8	✓	✓
TRICEPS	Tricep press-down	5	7	✓	✓
TRICEPS	Dumbell skill crusher	5	6	✓	✓

At this point you should be about 14 minutes into your workout, including 2 minutes of transition time.

ABS	Seated v-up	N/A	7	✓	✓
ABS	Band crunch on ball	5	8	✓	✓
ABS	Up woodchopper on ball	10	8	✓	✓

At this point in your workout you should be at 20 minutes. Congratulations! YOU DID IT!

BONUS CARDIO 20-MINUTE MORNING POWER WALK ●

After my workout I feel __energized__

(e.g., confident, strong)

LARGE · **SMALL** · **ABS**

8-WEEK WORKOUT CHART

Start Date __7/2__   Finish Date __8/26__

Monday	Tuesday	Wednesday	Thursday	Friday	Saturday	Sunday	
DAY 1 WORKOUT 7/2	**DAY 2** DAY OFF	**DAY 3** WORKOUT 7/4	**DAY 4** DAY OFF	**DAY 5** WORKOUT 7/6	**DAY 6** DAY OFF	**DAY 7** DAY OFF	WEEK 1
DAY 8 WORKOUT 7/9	**DAY 9** DAY OFF	**DAY 10** WORKOUT 7/11	**DAY 11** DAY OFF	**DAY 12** WORKOUT 7/13	**DAY 13** DAY OFF	**DAY 14** DAY OFF	WEEK 2
DAY 15 WORKOUT 7/16	**DAY 16** DAY OFF	**DAY 17** WORKOUT 7/18	**DAY 18** DAY OFF	**DAY 19** WORKOUT 7/20	**DAY 20** DAY OFF	**DAY 21** DAY OFF	WEEK 3
DAY 22 WORKOUT 7/23	**DAY 23** DAY OFF	**DAY 24** WORKOUT 7/25	**DAY 25** DAY OFF	**DAY 26** WORKOUT 7/27	**DAY 27** DAY OFF	**DAY 28** DAY OFF	WEEK 4
DAY 29 WORKOUT 7/30	**DAY 30** DAY OFF	**DAY 31** WORKOUT 8/1	**DAY 32** DAY OFF	**DAY 33** WORKOUT 8/3	**DAY 34** DAY OFF	**DAY 35** DAY OFF	WEEK 5
DAY 36 WORKOUT 8/6	**DAY 37** DAY OFF	**DAY 38** WORKOUT 8/8	**DAY 39** DAY OFF	**DAY 40** WORKOUT 8/10	**DAY 41** DAY OFF	**DAY 42** DAY OFF	WEEK 6
DAY 43 WORKOUT 8/13	**DAY 44** DAY OFF	**DAY 45** WORKOUT 8/15	**DAY 46** DAY OFF	**DAY 47** WORKOUT 8/17	**DAY 48** DAY OFF	**DAY 49** DAY OFF	WEEK 7
DAY 50 WORKOUT 8/20	**DAY 51** DAY OFF	**DAY 52** WORKOUT 8/22	**DAY 53** DAY OFF	**DAY 54** WORKOUT 8/24	**DAY 55** DAY OFF	**DAY 56** SUCCESS	WEEK 8

*Please photocopy and place on your refrigerator. As you complete your workouts, cross off the days so you can see your success!

move. You'll pick up the flow and the form of the movements quickly, but don't get frustrated if you feel a little awkward at first. Lastly, you always have your 30-second break between moves to review something if you have to.

Visit BodyatHome.com for videos you can watch to help with proper form.

Counting

Counting is going to be critical to your success. As I shared with you in Chapter 2, you are going to begin each move with a 10-second positive motion, hold for 2 seconds at the MTP, and return to the starting position through another count of 10 seconds. I know it can be tempting to count fast or to shorten the 2-second hold, but timing is the revolutionary core of this plan (adapted from the 12-Second Sequence™), and you really will transform your body if you do it right.

Some of my clients had a great idea to help them with the timing: a metronome. A metronome is a tool often used by musicians to help them keep time, but several of my clients swore by it for keeping time during their workouts. Pick one up at a local music store, or visit Bodyat Home.com for timing videos that will ensure proper counting.

Remember, it's only 20 minutes so it's important to make the most of every second of your workout. Each second your body is working toward the goal of full muscle saturation, and each second you're closer to achieving your best body ever.

Feel the Difference

Several of my clients who followed the 12-Second Sequence™ program, which requires gym time, have asked me if the Body at Home™ program will still create results for them. And my answer is "Absolutely!" This program is strategically designed to focus on women's trouble zones. Using the Body Priority, you will give special attention to those areas that frustrate you most: your belly, butt, hips, and thighs. Plus, I've incorporated resistance bands, which will create a new and unique challenge for your muscles. Remember, continuing to challenge your muscles is critical to accomplishing results—just like us, they get bored sometimes!

If you notice that some of the Body at Home™ moves seem similar to the moves in my other program; that's because when it comes down to the basic *paths of motion* that your muscles follow, there are really only a few directions they can go. So a squat will always follow the same path, as will a curl, a press, and so forth. The difference lies in the Body Priority, a strategy that prioritizes the order in which you do the moves based on what's most important to you. It's like the way letters come together to spell a word—the sequencing can make all the difference in the world. For example, spell L-I-V-E, and you've got an optimistic, positive, affirmative word (think of Lance Armstrong's signature motto "Live Strong"). Flip the letters around and you've got E-V-I-L, which couldn't have a more opposite message. Bottom line: This fundamental difference in how the workouts are designed will create the most effective and precise results for you.

Breathing Right

A lot of people have a tendency to forget to breathe when they work out, and that's a big mistake! Oxygen is essential fuel for your muscles and can help keep you energized throughout your workout. It combines with glycogen and fat to produce energy and keep you going strong. To ensure you maintain proper breathing with your Body at Home™ workouts, I recommend a technique called *feathered breathing*. You need to maintain a continuous, steady stream of oxygen throughout each of your four reps, and feathered breathing helps you accomplish this. It is a rhythmic breathing pattern that prevents you from holding your breath during exercise, and it ensures that you provide your muscles with plenty of oxygen. All you do is take a deep breath in before beginning your exercise, then exhale in small short bursts until you have expelled all of the air out of your lungs. Then repeat. Maintaining this breathing pattern throughout your workout will keep your body and your mind fresh and fueled with oxygen.

Morning Cardio

If you want to accelerate your results, there's one more thing you have to do. You will elevate your heart rate with your workouts, but incorporating the right kind of cardio into your routine not only will speed up results, but also will be beneficial to your heart.

I want you to take a brisk 20-minute walk every morning—and here's the key—*before breakfast.* Walking for 20 minutes right when you get up in the morning is going to help you burn an additional 150 to 200 calories per day. That means if you walk six mornings a week, you'll burn an additional 1,200 calories per week! This will make a big difference in how quickly you reach your goal.

Recent research confirms that cardio done on an empty stomach is more effective than cardio performed after eating. A study conducted at Kansas State University found that fasting exercisers burned "significantly more fat" than exercisers who ate beforehand. Another study, performed at the University of California, Berkeley, confirmed this finding. The UCB researchers wrote that fat loss increased *only* when study participants "exercised in a fasted state."

In addition to helping you burn fat faster, morning cardio will help you get going in the morning, especially if you can walk outside. You'll feel awake, refreshed, and motivated to eat right and stick to your workout plan.

Intensity

You will see the best results from this program if you achieve the right level of intensity during every exercise and every workout. The right level is different for everyone, but what's important is that you achieve the most challenging workout for *your body.* How will you know you've reached the ideal intensity for you? Well, you start by making sure you have the right weight. If you can lift a weight or press a band beyond four reps, you are not working with a heavy enough weight or with enough resistance. However, if you can complete only two or three reps, your weight is too heavy. I know it sounds simple, but it's critical that you create the right level of intensity for your body. Without creating the right challenge for your muscles, you will not accelerate the development of fat-burning lean muscle tissue. So remember, to ensure the best results, don't cheat. Make the commitment with 100 percent of yourself—you deserve it.

USING YOUR RESISTANCE BANDS

If you've never used bands before, I want to give you a quick overview of how to use them. It's especially important that you know how to properly secure them because this will prevent injury and allow you to receive the maximum benefit from the exercises. Most bands come with basic instructions, but I want to be sure you know specifically how to use them with the Body at Home™ exercises.

In the exercise instructions, you will see a variety of setup directions, such as "Secure the band at head level" or "Secure the band at shoulder level." These positions will help you reach different parts of your muscles. To do this you need a "door anchor" attachment system (which comes with most bands; my picks are available at BodyatHome.com). The door anchor provides a way to secure the bands at various heights. To secure your door anchor properly, insert the attachment through the hinge of your door with the "stopper" portion on the back side of the door and the "loop" side facing you. Adjust the anchor at the desired height; then close the door completely and lock it. Your anchor is now safely secured. Next, slip the band through the loop with the anchor loop centered. Give it a good tug to make sure it's secure and you're ready to work out!

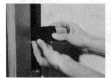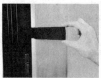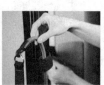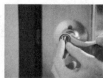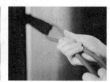

As you begin the workouts in Chapter 5, remember to turn back to these pages if you need a quick review of how to breathe or tips on achieving proper form or the best counting for your success. Body at Home™ is going to create your best body ever; these guidelines will ensure you accomplish this as quickly, effectively, and safely as possible. Now let's get started on the Quick-Start Phase.

(15) BODY AT HOME™ STAR   Veronica Negrete

Height: 5'7" | **Age:** 27 | **Lost:** 15 pounds

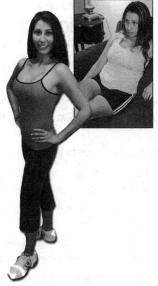

"Before Body at Home™ I tried every new fad diet or diet pills to lose weight. With each attempt, I found myself further and further from my goals and with less self-esteem than I had previously. My self-esteem had dipped so low that I found myself avoiding plans with family and friends.

"This program has completely altered my life *and* my body. I have more self-confidence than I've ever had, and I'm amazed at how quickly I began to see results. This is the easiest program to follow that I've ever been on. The diet is satisfying, and I love that the workouts can be done in the privacy of my own home. Now when I go to my closet, my clothes still don't fit correctly, except now it's because they're too big."

Veronica's Secrets to Success

· Be strict with the diet, especially at the beginning. Drinking alcohol or eating food that is not included in the plan will only set you back.

· If you're just not feeling up to exercising, go for a walk in your neighborhood. Anything is better than missing it altogether!

· Don't be afraid to ask questions. BodyatHome.com is a great resource for anyone who needs a little extra help.

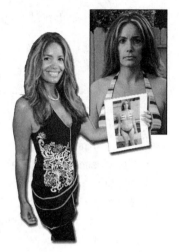

Height: 5'7" | Age: 37 | Lost: 13 pounds

"Before I began the program, I was not at all happy with myself. I had a baby in 2006 and wanted to get back into shape. I did not want to be a frumpy mom. I started the program and began seeing results in just a couple of weeks. This was exactly what I needed. In fact, my husband has lost 16 pounds just by eating the same foods and being on my eating schedule. Not only have I lost 13 pounds, but I also lost 3 inches in my waist, 3½ inches in my hips, and almost 2 inches in my thighs. Thank you so much!"

Rebecca's Secrets to Success

· I would definitely get pictures of what you want to look like so that you can visualize the results. For me, it was looking at pictures of myself in shape and on vacation at my favorite places. That motivated me to want to get back in shape.

· Keeping a food journal is *key* at least for the first four weeks. Write down every single morsel of food. It holds you accountable, and it allows you to see what you're eating and when.

· Find meals and recipes that you like and that fit the plan. Find foods that satisfy you, so you don't feel as though you are missing out. It really helps.

Quick-Start Phase

WEEKS 1 AND 2

20s: INCREASE CONFIDENCE

Body Language Says It All

When you walk into a room, how you stand can create an immediate impression. Stand tall with your shoulders back and chin up and you deliver a message of strength and confidence. Slump over and look down and you deliver a message of insecurity and uncertainty. Not only do your posture and body language impact people's impressions of you; they also create a physical response in your body and can affect how you feel about yourself. When you slump over, you limit the supply of oxygen to your body, which makes your muscles tighten and creates a stressed, deflated feeling. In contrast, a proud, broad, and upright posture increases your lung capacity and allows you to take deep, balanced breaths that distribute oxygen all through your body. Try it for yourself right now: Stand tall with your shoulders back, chest out, and chin up, and walk across the room. You will feel amazing! Correct posture also helps give your organs enough room to function at their best.

30s: MANAGE STRESS

Breathe Deeply

Did I get that report to my boss? Did I call the babysitter? What should we have for dinner? What time is my doctor's appointment? Does all this sound familiar? That's because just about every day is filled with constant questions, planning, and just plain busyness. What happens when you try to manage all of this is you tend to forget to pay attention to the one thing that keeps you going through it all—your breath. When you are under stress, it's easy to hold your breath or take in only short gulps of air at a time. This short supply of oxygen can have a big effect on your body, limiting flow to your muscles, your brain and heart, and your other major organs. Your body may try to give you signs that it needs more air when you sigh or yawn. Help your body—and your mind—by trying this quick and simple breathing exercise that you can do while sitting or lying down: Place your hand on your abdomen so you can feel the movement of your breath. Inhale for a count of 5, and exhale slowly for a count of 10, concentrating on just your breath. Do this for 5 minutes, or even for only a few breaths if that's all you have time for. You'll notice the benefits immediately!

WEEK 1

As you get ready to start week 1, use these tips based on your Life Priority to give you an extra advantage. They are customized to your decade, but I recommend you read every one of them. These tips are jam-packed with valuable information and will give you an extra edge as you face each week.

40s: PREVENT DECLINE

Say No to Salt!

Excess salt can send your blood pressure soaring and increase your risk of heart disease and stroke. Remember, heart disease is the number-one killer of women in the United States, so paying attention to your salt intake isn't just a matter of seasoning. We've all experienced that bloated feeling after a salty meal, but what you may not know is that this water retention does more than make your pants feel a little tight. When salt keeps extra fluid in your body, it puts added stress on your heart because your heart has to work harder to keep your circulation steady. And it's this extra work that makes your blood pressure climb. According to the American Heart Association, you should limit your intake to less than 2,300 milligrams per day, which is about 1 teaspoon. Watch for sneaky salt in processed foods and over-the-counter medications. As an alternative to salt, try some lemon, Mrs. Dash, or fresh herbs for some heart-healthy seasoning.

50s-Plus: REVERSE DECLINE

Get Healthy with Fat!

One of the most important things you can do to immediately improve your health, prevent disease, and reverse aging is to take flaxseed oil. Flax has been shown to prevent cancer and heart disease, improve brain function, increase energy and stamina, and help create radiant, youthful-looking skin. Flaxseed oil is an omega-3 fatty acid and is the best source of naturally occurring chemicals called *lignans.* Lignans may help reduce the incidence of breast and colon cancer by pushing out estrogen that these cancers rely on to start developing. It's important to note, though, that not all flax oils are the same. Flaxseed oil can turn rancid very easily and lose all of its health benefits if it is not stored correctly. Never buy flax oil that is not refrigerated, and look for a label that mentions "high lignans." One of my favorite ways to enjoy flax oil is in the morning over a piece of toast instead of butter, and it's great on popcorn. Try it! You won't be disappointed, I promise.

MONDAY

Chair Beginner Squat

Stand with your feet shoulder-width apart, arms crossed in front of you, knees slightly bent. Feather your breathing as you slowly squat through a count of 10 seconds—keeping your back straight, abs tight, and chest up. Hold for 2 seconds at the MTP (about 2 inches above the chair). Return to starting position through a count of 10 seconds. Without resting, repeat three times.

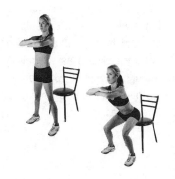

Swiss Ball Squat

Place the ball against a wall and position yourself with the ball supporting your lower back. Hold a pair of dumbbells and keep your arms against your sides. Move your feet forward about 1 foot and stand with them hip-width apart. Feather your breathing as you slowly squat through a count of 10 seconds, never letting your knees drift over your ankles. Hold for 2 seconds at the MTP (when your knees are at about a 90-degree angle). Return to starting position through a count of 10 seconds. Without resting, repeat three times.

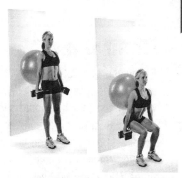

Lunge

Stand in a lunge position with one hand resting on the back of a sturdy chair for balance. Keep your back straight, chest up, and abs tight. Feather your breathing as you drop your back knee toward the ground through a count of 10 seconds. Hold for 2 seconds at the MTP (about 1 inch above the ground). Return to starting position through a count of 10 seconds. Without resting, repeat one more time on this leg and then perform 2 more reps on the other side for a total of 4. (Note: To avoid injury, make sure that your front knee stays aligned with your toes and doesn't bend farther than a 90-degree angle.)

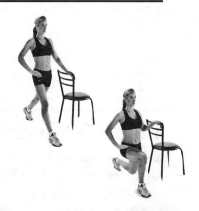

Key

MTP: *Maximum tension point.*

Feather your breathing: *Inhale deeply and exhale in short bursts.*

Timing: *Each exercise should take 90 seconds and be followed by a 30-second rest. The workout should take a total of 20 minutes.*

Hamstring Curl with Swiss Ball

Lie on your back with your arms at your sides, palms flat on the floor. Place your heels on the ball, knees straight but not locked. Tighten your abs and lift your butt and hips off the ground. Feather your breathing and bend your knees as you roll the ball toward your butt with your heels through a count of 10 seconds. Hold for 2 seconds at the MTP. Return to starting position through a count of 10 seconds. Without resting, repeat three times.

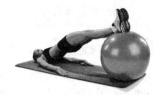

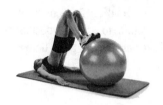

Chair Dip

Sit on the edge of a sturdy chair with your hands behind you, fingers forward and grasping the edge of the chair. Flex your feet so that your weight is on your heels and slide yourself an inch or so away from the chair. Feather your breathing as you lower yourself through a count of 10 seconds. Hold for 2 seconds at the MTP. Push yourself back up to starting position through a count of 10 seconds. Without resting, repeat three times. (Note: The MTP will vary based on your shoulder flexibility—about 1 inch above your most flexible point.)

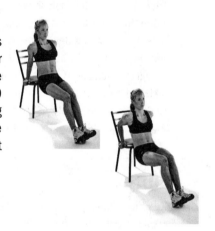

Triceps Press-Down

Secure a resistance band above your head. Grasp the handles so that your hands are shoulder-width apart. Pull your arms down against your sides, elbows bent at just above a 90-degree angle, palms facing down. Feather your breathing as you press down and straighten your arms (but do not lock your elbows). Hold for 2 seconds at the MTP. Resist the weight back to starting position through a count of 10 seconds. Without resting, repeat three times.

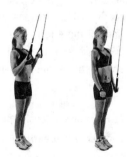

Standing Kickback

Hold a pair of dumbbells, palms facing each other. With your knees slightly bent, bend at the waist as if you were about to tie your shoes; then lift only your chin and chest, creating a slight arch in your back. Raise your elbows as high as possible, keeping them close to your body. Feather your breathing as you extend the weights back (without moving the upper part of the arm) through a count of 10 seconds. Hold and squeeze for 2 seconds at the MTP. Return the weights to starting position through a count of 10 seconds. Without resting, repeat three times.

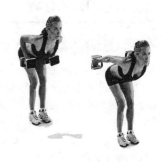

Kneeling Band Crunch

Secure a resistance band above your head and kneel on a mat. Grasp the handles in front of your forehead, palms facing toward you. Keep your abs tight and feather your breathing as you crunch toward the mat through a count of 10 seconds. Hold for 2 seconds at the MTP (about 2 inches from the mat). Resist the band back to starting position through a count of 10 seconds. Without resting, repeat three times.

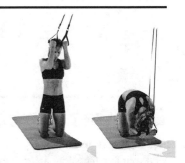

Reverse Crunch

Lie on a mat with your hands by your sides, palms down. Pull your heels up as close to your butt as possible. Raise your heels about 2 inches off the ground. Keep your chin tucked and abs tight. Feather your breathing as you pull your knees toward your chest using your lower abdominals through a count of 10 seconds. Hold and squeeze for 2 seconds at the MTP (when your butt is completely off the ground). Lower your body to starting position through a count of 10 seconds. Without resting, repeat three times.

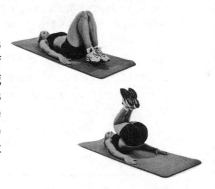

Woodchopper

Secure a resistance band above your head. Stand with your legs about 3 feet apart; keep your chest up, back and arms straight. Feather your breathing as you pull the handles down and across your body by twisting and contracting your obliques through a count of 10 seconds. Hold and squeeze for 2 seconds at the MTP. Resist the band back to starting position through a count of 10 seconds. Without resting, repeat once more on this side and then switch sides and complete 2 more reps for a total of 4.

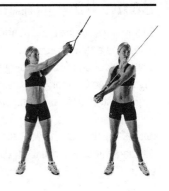

WEDNESDAY

Kneeling Band Pull-Down (Overhand Grip)

Secure a resistance band above your head. Kneel on a mat and grasp the handles with your palms facing forward. Sit back on your heels with your arms fully outstretched; keep your back straight, chest up, and abs tight. Feather your breathing as you pull the handles down toward the top part of your chest through a count of 10 seconds. Hold and squeeze for 2 seconds at the MTP. Resist the band back to starting position through a count of 10 seconds. Without resting, repeat three times.

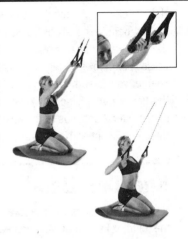

Bent-Over Dumbbell Row (Standard Grip)

Holding a pair of dumbbells, extend your arms, palms facing in. Stand with your feet hip-width apart. Bend at the waist as if you were tying your shoes. Raise your head and chest to create a slight arch in the back. Bend your knees slightly. Feather your breathing as you pull the dumbbells up in a fluid rowing motion through a count of 10 seconds, keeping your elbows close to your body. Hold and squeeze your shoulder blades together for 2 seconds at the MTP. Lower your arms to starting position through a count of 10 seconds. Without resting, repeat three times.

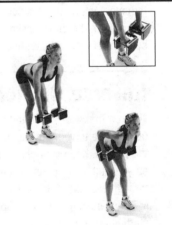

Band Row (Overhand Grip)

Secure a resistance band at about shoulder level. Grasp the handles and hold arms extended at chest height, palms facing down. Take a wide step forward with one foot, keeping your back straight, abs tight, and knees slightly bent. Feather your breathing as you pull the dumbbells toward your chest in a fluid rowing motion through a count of 10 seconds, keeping your elbows close to your body. Hold and squeeze your shoulder blades together at the MTP for 2 seconds. Lower your arms to starting position through a count of 10 seconds. Without resting, repeat three times.

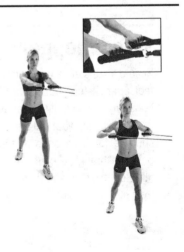

Hyperextension

Lie facedown on the ball with your waist bent and hips supported on the ball, hands resting behind your ears. Feather your breathing as you lift your upper body using the muscles in your lower back, through a count of 10 seconds. Hold for 2 seconds at the MTP. Return to starting position through a count of 10 seconds. Without resting, repeat three times.

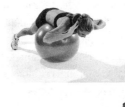

Standing Band Curl

Stand on the center of a resistance band, feet together and knees slightly bent. Grasp the handles, keeping your slightly bent arms by your sides, palms facing forward. Feather your breathing as you curl up through a count of 10 seconds to just past a 90-degree angle. Hold and squeeze for 2 seconds at the MTP. Keep your elbows tight against your body as you lower the handles through a count of 10 seconds. Without resting, repeat three times. (Note: Keep your elbows tight against your sides throughout the exercise.)

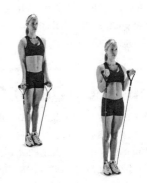

Side Curls on Swiss Ball

Sit on the ball holding a dumbbell in each hand. With your arms down against your sides, palms turned up, and elbows tight against your body, feather your breathing as you curl the weights up through a count of 10 seconds. Hold and squeeze for a count of 2 seconds at the MTP. Lower the weights to starting position through a count of 10 seconds. Without resting, repeat three times.

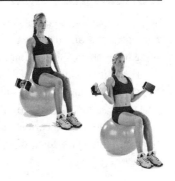

Hammer Curl

Holding a pair of dumbbells, stand with your feet shoulder-width apart, your arms extended slightly in front of your thighs, palms facing each other, and knees slightly bent. Feather your breathing as you curl the weights up through a count of 10 seconds, keeping your palms facing each other. Hold and squeeze for 2 seconds at the MTP. Lower the weights to starting position through a count of 10 seconds. Without resting, repeat three times.

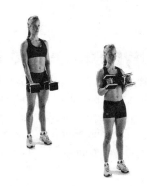

Swiss Ball Crunch

Sit on the ball with your feet on the floor. Walk your feet out until your hips are slightly lower than your knees but your lower and middle back are still firmly supported. Place your hands behind your ears to help support your neck. Feather your breathing and, using your abs only, slowly crunch up through a count of 10 seconds. Hold and squeeze for 2 seconds at the MTP. Lower yourself to starting position through a count of 10 seconds. Without resting, repeat three times.

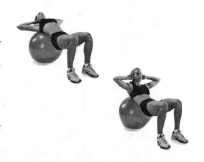

Tuck-Up on Chair

Sit on the front edge of a sturdy chair. Reach behind you and grab the sides of the chair. Extend your legs out and allow your upper body to lean back slightly. Feather your breathing as you slowly draw your knees in and up toward your chest through a count of 10 seconds. Hold and squeeze for 2 seconds at the MTP. Return legs to starting position through a count of 10 seconds. Without resting, repeat three times.

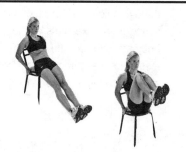

Seated Russian Twist

Sit on the mat with your knees bent, feet together. Keep your chin up off your chest and abs tight as you lean back slightly and cross your feet, lifting them about 2 inches off the mat, engaging your abs. Extend your arms away from your chest with your palms pressed together and turn to one side to begin exercise. Feather your breathing as you slowly rotate your torso as far as possible to the other side through a count of 10 seconds. Hold and squeeze for 2 seconds at the MTP. Rotate back to the other side through a count of 10 seconds. Without resting, repeat three times.

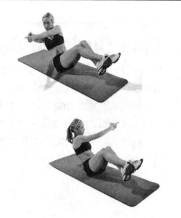

Incline Push-Up

Place your hands in a push-up position against a wall or a set of stairs, so that your upper body is elevated above your feet. Keep your head up, back straight, and abs tight. Feather your breathing as you lower yourself through a count of 10 seconds. Hold for 2 seconds at the MTP. Return to starting position through a count of 10 seconds. Without resting, repeat three times.

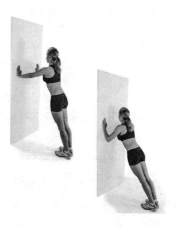

Incline Dumbbell Press

Hold a pair of dumbbells and lie on a ball so that your head and neck are supported. Roll down the ball until your hips drop almost to the ground; do not let your knees go over your ankles. Press the weights up and together, with a slight bend in the elbows, keeping your back straight and abs tight. Feather your breathing as you lower the weights through a count of 10 seconds. Hold for 2 seconds at the MTP. Press the dumbbells up to starting position through a count of 10 seconds. Without resting, repeat three times.

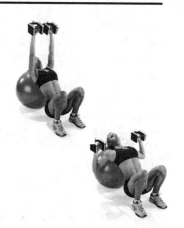

Flat Band Press

Secure a resistance band at about shoulder level. Grasp the handles and hold at chest level, palms facing down. Take a wide step forward with one foot, keeping your back straight, abs tight, and knees slightly bent. Feather your breathing as you press the handles of the band forward through a count of 10 seconds. Hold for 2 seconds at the MTP (just prior to lockout). Return to starting position through a count of 10 seconds. Without resting, repeat three times.

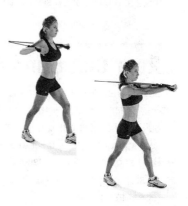

Flat Band Fly

Secure a resistance band at about chest height. Take a wide step forward with one foot, keeping your back straight, abs tight, and knees slightly bent. Grasp the handles with your arms slightly bent at the elbows and stretched in a wide "T" shape, palms facing forward. Feather your breathing as you bring your palms together through a count of 10 seconds. Hold for 2 seconds at the MTP. Return to starting position through a count of 10 seconds. Without resting, repeat three times.

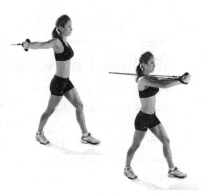

Swiss Ball Shoulder Press

Holding a pair of dumbbells, sit on the ball with your back straight, abs tight, and chin up. Extend the dumbbells up and together directly over your head, palms facing forward. Feather your breathing as you lower the weights through a count of 10 seconds. Hold for 2 seconds at the MTP (when weights are about eye level). Press the dumbbells up to starting position through a count of 10 seconds. Without resting, repeat three times.

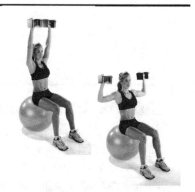

Lateral Band Raise

Stand on top of the center of a resistance band with your feet together, back straight, and abs tight. Grasp the handles so that your arms are straight but not locked, your palms facing inward. Feather your breathing as you raise your arms to a "T" position through a count of 10 seconds. Hold and squeeze for 2 seconds at the MTP. Return to starting position through a count of 10 seconds. Without resting, repeat three times.

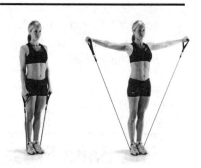

Rear Delt Band Extension

Secure the band at about shoulder level. Grasp the handles and extend your arms in front of you, palms facing in. Feather your breathing as you pull the handles out to a "T" position through a count of 10 seconds, keeping your arms parallel to the floor and a slight bend in your elbows. Hold and squeeze for 2 seconds at the MTP. Resist the band slowly back to starting position through a count of 10 seconds. Without resting, repeat three times.

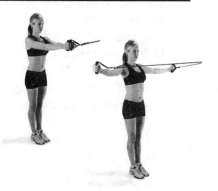

Toe Reach

Lie on your back. Cross your legs, flex your feet, and extend your legs into the air. With your arms extended and chin up off your chest, feather your breathing as you crunch up, reaching toward your toes through a count of 10 seconds. Hold and squeeze for 2 seconds at the MTP. Lower yourself to starting position, keeping your shoulder blades from touching the ground, through a count of 10 seconds. Without resting, repeat three times.

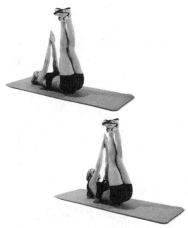

Seated V-Up

Sit on a mat with your arms behind you, elbows bent, and fingertips pointed toward your body. Start with your legs together and extended, knees slightly bent, and heels about 2 inches off the ground. Lean your upper body weight back on your palms slightly. Feather your breathing as you pull your knees into your chest through a count of 10 seconds. Hold and squeeze for 2 seconds at the MTP. Return to starting position through a count of 10 seconds, keeping your abs tight. Without resting, repeat three times.

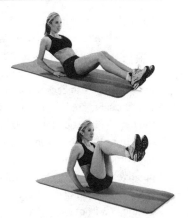

Upward Woodchopper on Swiss Ball

Secure a resistance band at foot level. Sit on the ball and place your feet in front of you about hip-width apart. Grip the handle with both hands, fingers entwined, keeping your chest up and your back and arms straight (do not lock your elbows). Feather your breathing as you pull the handles up and across your body by twisting and contracting your obliques through a count of 10 seconds. Hold and squeeze for 2 seconds at the MTP. Resist the band back to starting position through a count of 10 seconds. Without resting, repeat once more on this side and then switch sides and complete 2 more reps for a total of 4.

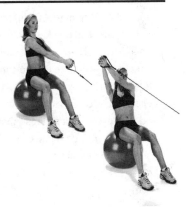

WEEK 2

As you get ready to start week 2, use these tips based on your Life Priority to give you an extra advantage. They are customized to your decade, but I recommend you read every one of them. These tips are jam-packed with valuable information and will give you an extra edge as you face each week.

20s CONFIDENCE

You Are Beautiful

When you think things like "I'm lazy" or "I hate my body" or "I'm never going to get in shape," you're setting yourself up for failure. When you repeat something over and over again, your mind actually begins to accept it as a statement of fact. Your thoughts are incredibly powerful and can set the tone for how you feel about yourself and help determine the choices you make. Creating the right affirmation can be key to achieving a positive and hopeful state of mind. Let's say you want to stop eating carbs at night. Instead of saying, "I will not eat carbs at night," try something positive like "I will make healthy eating choices at night." Or suppose you miss your workout and you keep thinking to yourself, "I'm a loser . . . I can't even get a 20-minute workout in"—it's time to take control of that negative voice in your head. Will yourself into believing you *can* do it: "I am beautiful and strong and I will make choices today that make me feel accomplished and empowered." For a great collection of affirmations, check out my friend Louise L. Hay's *Power Thought Cards* (Hay House, 1999).

30s MANAGE STRESS

Get Organized

If you're like me, you love to shop. I especially love to buy books, which is great, but there's just one problem—I have to find room to keep them all. If you let clutter build up around you, whether it's books or shoes or clothes, you create an unavoidable sense of stress. When you try to find something in your closet or on your desk at work and it's buried in piles of clothes or paper, you are going to add frustration and stress to your life. But guess what? It's simple to take control. Start by purging whatever your problem area may be: Clear out old clothes, books, and unnecessary paperwork. An added benefit is you can take most of your items (minus the paperwork) to an organization such as Goodwill and receive an income-tax deduction. Once you clean out your space, you'll be amazed at how good you feel. Next, of course, you must follow up with a system that keeps you on your new organized, stress-free track. Organize clothes by pants, shirts, and so forth, or by color if that works better for you. I like to keep my books organized by subject. That way if I want to pick something up on sleep, I know exactly what shelf to go to!

40s PREVENT DECLINE

Get Physical

A critical part of prevention is making sure you're getting the right tests and screenings for your age. You may know that once you reach age 40, you should get a mammogram each year, but there are several other tests and checkups you should add to your health-care calendar. According to the National Women's Health Resource Center, you should get a pap smear every two to three years if you've had three normal ones in a row; but if you have a history of risk factors, continue getting one every year. You should have your blood pressure checked every two years to help measure your risk of hypertension, and your cholesterol should be screened every five years (unless there is a history of high cholesterol in your family or you are at risk for cardiovascular disease, in which case your cholesterol should be checked more frequently). If you are overweight and in your forties, ask for a blood glucose test to determine your risk for diabetes. Keep your senses sharp by seeing an eye doctor every two to four years and your dentist every six months. Remember, these are only general guidelines. They could vary based on your personal health and family history so check with your doctor.

50s REVERSE DECLINE

Join a Dance Group

Few things can make you feel as happy as dancing to one of your favorite songs. Add a social setting into the mix and you've got a sure-fire recipe for a good mood. One study revealed the effect of 16 weeks of salsa classes on a group of women. After the four months of classes, the number of women who said they felt depressed went down from 46 percent to 27 percent. Plus, the number of participants who reported feeling lonely dropped from 35 percent to 19 percent. Social interaction can help lower stress hormones, which not only makes you feel calm and happy but also helps keep your immune system strong. On top of mood elevation, dance can burn between 200 and 400 calories in 30 minutes. As you age you also face the threat of a declining sense of balance and weakened bones, a potentially dangerous combination because it can lead to life-threatening bone breaks. Dance helps maintain or improve your sense of balance *and* strengthens your bones. So what are you waiting for? Get moving!

MONDAY

Chair Beginner Squat

Stand with your feet shoulder-width apart, arms crossed in front of you, knees slightly bent. Feather your breathing as you slowly squat through a count of 10 seconds—keeping your back straight, abs tight, and chest up. Hold for 2 seconds at the MTP (about 2 inches above the chair). Return to starting position through a count of 10 seconds. Without resting, repeat three times.

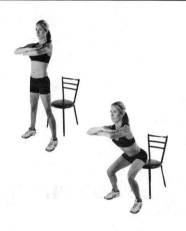

Plié Squat

Holding a dumbbell in each hand, stand with your feet about two times wider than shoulder-width apart, toes turned out to the sides and knees aligned over the toes. Feather your breathing as you squat through a count of 10 seconds. Hold for 2 seconds at the MTP. Push through your heels to return to starting position through a count of 10 seconds. Without resting, repeat three times.

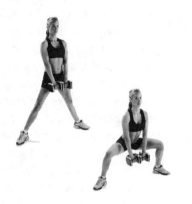

Lunge

Stand in a lunge position with one hand resting on the back of a sturdy chair for balance. Keep your back straight, chest up, and abs tight. Feather your breathing as you drop your back knee toward the ground through a count of 10 seconds. Hold for 2 seconds at the MTP (about 1 inch above the ground). Return to starting position through a count of 10 seconds. Without resting, repeat one more time on this leg; then perform 2 more reps on the other side for a total of 4. (Note: To avoid injury, make sure that your front knee stays aligned with your toes and doesn't bend beyond a 90-degree angle.)

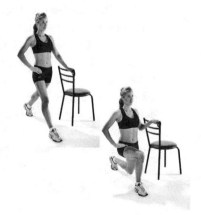

Glute Kickback

Kneel on a mat on all fours with your knees hip-width apart. Lift your leg and bend it to a 90-degree angle. Press the heel of your foot toward the ceiling through a count of 10 seconds. Hold and squeeze for 2 seconds at the MTP. Lower your leg to starting position through a count of 10 seconds. Without resting, repeat one more time on this leg and then switch sides and complete 2 more reps on the other side for a total of 4.

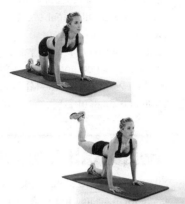

Dumbbell Skull Crusher

Hold a pair of dumbbells and lie on the ball so that your head and neck are supported. Elevate your hips slightly and keep your abs tight. Extend the dumbbells straight up with your palms facing each other, and tilt your arms toward your head slightly. Feather your breathing as you bend your elbows and lower the weights through a count of 10 seconds. Hold for 2 seconds at the MTP (about 1 inch above your forehead). Raise the dumbbells to starting position through a count of 10 seconds. Without resting, repeat three times.

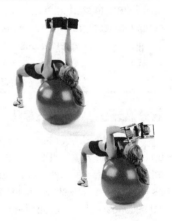

Overhead Triceps Extension

Grasp a dumbbell using the "diamond grip." Sit on the ball with your chest up, back straight, feet shoulder-width apart. Extend your arms with your elbows slightly bent, keeping your biceps tight against your head. Feather your breathing as you lower the dumbbell through a count of 10 seconds. Hold for 2 seconds at the MTP (when your elbows are at about a 90-degree angle). Press the weight up to starting position through a count of 10 seconds. Without resting, repeat three times.

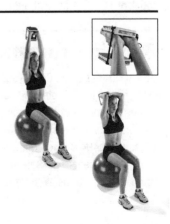

Triceps Press-Down

Secure a resistance band above your head. Grasp the handles, keeping your hands about 1 foot apart. Pull your arms down against your sides, elbows bent at just above a 90-degree angle, palms facing down. Feather your breathing as you press the handles down and straighten your arms (but do not lock your elbows) through a count of 10 seconds. Hold for 2 seconds at the MTP. Resist the band back to starting position through a count of 10 seconds. Without resting, repeat three times.

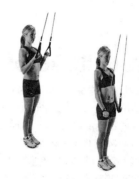

Swiss Ball Crunch with Elevated Feet

Sit on a ball that's about 2 feet away from a wall. Walk your feet out and place them against the wall. Lie down and place your hands behind your ears. Feather your breathing as you crunch up through a count of 10 seconds, using only your abs. Hold and squeeze for 2 seconds at the MTP. Return to starting position through a count of 10 seconds. Without resting, repeat three times. (Note: Keep in mind that the range of motion is significantly smaller on this exercise, so be sure to adjust your pace.)

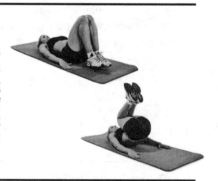

Reverse Crunch

Lie on a mat with your hands by your sides, palms down. Pull your heels up as close to your butt as possible. Raise your heels up about 2 inches off the ground. Keep your chin up and abs tight. Feather your breathing as you pull your knees up using the lower abdominals through a count of 10 seconds. Hold and squeeze for 2 seconds at the MTP (when your butt is just off the ground). Lower your body to starting position through a count of 10 seconds. Without resting, repeat three times.

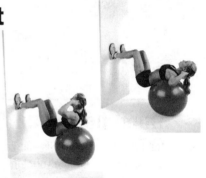

Bicycle Crunch

Lie flat on your back. Place your hands behind your head and raise your legs off the ground, bending your right knee, keeping your chin up and abs tight throughout the exercise. Bring your left elbow to your right knee and feather your breathing as you rotate to the other side for a count of 10 seconds. Hold and squeeze for 2 seconds at the MTP (where your right elbow meets your left knee). Twist to starting position through a count of 10 seconds. Without resting, repeat three times.

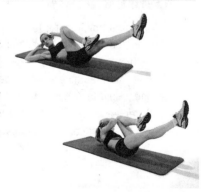

WEDNESDAY

Kneeling Band Pull-Down (Close Grip)

Secure a resistance band above your head. Kneel on a mat and grasp the handles with your palms facing each other. Sit back onto your heels with your arms fully outstretched; keep your back straight, chest up, and abs tight. Feather your breathing as you pull the handles toward the top part of your chest through a count of 10 seconds. Hold and squeeze for 2 seconds at the MTP. Resist the band to starting position through a count of 10 seconds. Without resting, repeat three times.

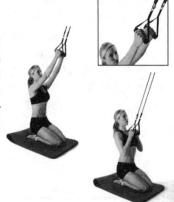

Dumbbell Pull-Over

Grasp a dumbbell using the "diamond grip." Lie on the ball with your head and neck supported. Keep your hips up and abs tight throughout the exercise. Extend the weight over your chest without locking your elbows. Feather your breathing as you lower the weight behind your head through a count of 10 seconds. Hold for 2 seconds at the MTP. Raise the weight to starting position through a count of 10 seconds. Without resting, repeat three times. (Note: The MTP will vary based on your shoulder flexibility. Hold at your most flexible point.)

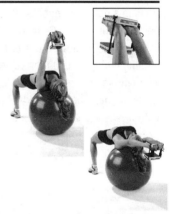

Bent-Over Dumbbell Row (Overhand Grip)

Holding a pair of dumbbells, extend your arms, palms facing toward your body. Stand with your feet hip-width apart. Bend at the waist as if tying your shoes. Raise your head and chest to create a slight arch in your back and bend your knees slightly. Feather your breathing as you pull the dumbbells up in a fluid rowing motion through a count of 10 seconds, keeping your elbows close to your body. Hold and squeeze your shoulder blades together for 2 seconds at the MTP. Lower your arms to starting position through a count of 10 seconds. Without resting, repeat three times.

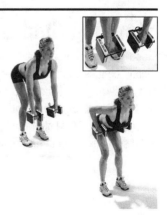

Superman

Lie flat on your stomach with your body completely extended, arms parallel to one another, and legs straight. Keeping your chin up, feather your breathing as you simultaneously lift your arms and your legs through a count of 10 seconds. Hold and squeeze for 2 seconds at the MTP. Return to starting position through a count of 10 seconds. Without resting, repeat 3 more times. (Note: The range of motion is short on this exercise, so be sure to adjust accordingly.)

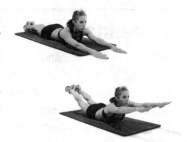

Dumbbell Preacher Curl

Holding a pair of dumbbells, rest your chest on the ball. Knees should be on the floor with a 6- to 8-inch gap between your arms. Bend your elbows to a 90-degree angle. Feather your breathing as you lower the weights through a count of 10 seconds until your arms are extended but your elbows are not locked. Hold and squeeze for 2 seconds at the MTP. Raise the dumbbells to starting position through a count of 10 seconds. Without resting, repeat three times.

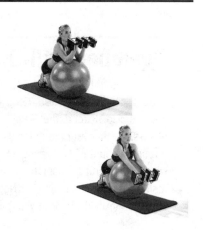

Standing Side Curl

Stand on the center of a resistance band, feet together, and knees slightly bent. Grasp the handles, arms by your sides, palms turned up, and elbows tight against your body. Feather your breathing as you curl the band up through a count of 10 seconds. Hold and squeeze for 2 seconds at the MTP. Lower the band to starting position through a count of 10 seconds. Without resting, repeat three times.

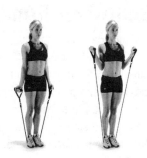

Band Concentration Curl

Secure a resistance band above your head. Grasp the handle with one hand, extending your arm, palm facing up. Keeping a slight bend in your knees, feather your breathing as you curl through a count of 10 seconds to just past a 90-degree angle. Hold and squeeze for 2 seconds at the MTP. Resist the band back to starting position through a count of 10 seconds. Without resting, repeat once more on this side and then switch sides and complete 2 more reps for a total of 4.

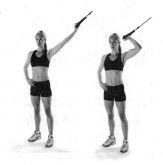

Medicine Ball Pull-Over

Lie on a mat and bring your knees, ankles crossed, up to a 90-degree angle. Grasp a medicine ball and extend it over your head; keep a slight bend in your elbows. Keep your abs tight and feather your breathing as you raise the ball over your head and crunch up through a count of 10 seconds. Hold for 2 seconds at the MTP. Lower the ball to starting position through a count of 10 seconds. Without resting, repeat three times.

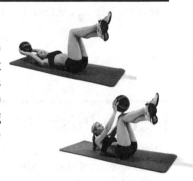

Tuck-Up on Chair

Sit on the front edge of a sturdy chair. Reach behind you and grab the sides of the chair. Extend your legs out and allow your upper body to lean back slightly. Feather your breathing as you slowly draw your knees in and up toward your chest through a count of 10 seconds. Hold and squeeze for 2 seconds at the MTP. Return legs to starting position through a count of 10 seconds. Without resting, repeat three times.

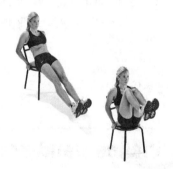

Swiss Ball Woodchopper

Secure a resistance band above your head. Sit on the ball and grasp the handles with both hands, feet on the ground, chest up, back and arms straight. Feather your breathing as you pull the handles down and across your body by twisting and contracting your obliques through a count of 10 seconds. Hold and squeeze for 2 seconds at the MTP. Resist the band back to starting position through a count of 10 seconds. Without resting, repeat once more on this side and then switch position and complete 2 more reps for a total of 4.

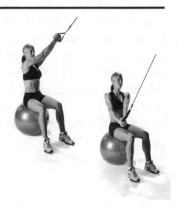

FRIDAY

Flat Dumbbell Press

Holding a pair of dumbbells, lie on a ball so that it comfortably supports your shoulder blades. Extend your arms in front of you, palms facing away from you, pressing the weights together. Feather your breathing as you lower the weights through a count of 10 seconds. Hold for 2 seconds at the MTP (about 1 inch higher than chest level). Press the dumbbells up and together back to starting position through a count of 10 seconds. Without resting, repeat three times.

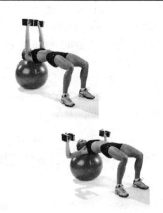

Incline Push-Up

Place your hands in a push-up position against a wall or a set of stairs, so that your upper body is elevated above your feet. Keep your head up, back straight, and abs tight. Feather your breathing as you lower yourself through a count of 10 seconds. Hold for 2 seconds at the MTP. Return to starting position through a count of 10 seconds. Without resting, repeat three times.

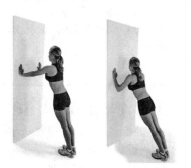

Incline Band Press

Secure a resistance band at about waist height. Grasp the handles and hold at chest height, elbows bent, palms facing down. Take a wide step forward with one foot, keeping your back straight, abs tight, and knees slightly bent. Feather your breathing as you press the handles of the band forward and up through a count of 10 seconds. At the top of the motion, your hands should be in line with your eyes. Hold for 2 seconds at the MTP (when your arms are straight but not locked). Return to starting position through a count of 10 seconds. Without resting, repeat three times.

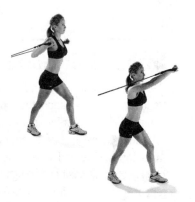

Incline Dumbbell Fly

Holding a pair of dumbbells, lie on a ball supporting your head and neck. Roll down the ball until your hips drop almost to the ground. Extend the dumbbells over your chest, palms facing each other, elbows slightly bent. Feather your breathing as you lower the weights down and out through a count of 10 seconds. Hold for 2 seconds at the MTP. Raise the weights to starting position in a "bear hug" type motion through a count of 10 seconds. Without resting, repeat three times.

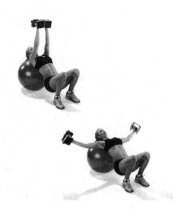

Kneeling Band Press

Kneel on the center of the band with your mat under you for padding. Grasp the handles and raise the band up until your elbows are at about a 90-degree angle (the band should rest on the back of your arms). Feather your breathing as you press the band up through a count of 10 seconds, keeping your elbows slightly bent at the top of the movement. Hold for 2 seconds at the MTP. Return to starting position through a count of 10 seconds. Without resting, repeat three times.

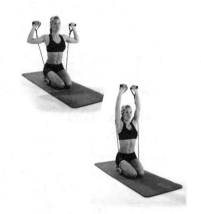

Chicken Wings

Holding a pair of dumbbells, stand with your feet a few inches apart, knees slightly bent. Bend your elbows, holding the dumbbells in front of you at a 45-degree angle. Keep the forearms tight and feather your breathing as you raise your elbows out and up through a count of 10 seconds. Hold and squeeze for 2 seconds at the MTP. Return to starting position through a count of 10 seconds. Without resting, repeat three times. (Note: Be sure to relax your neck and avoid shrugging your shoulders during this movement.)

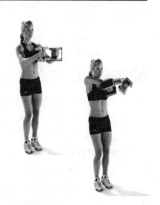

Bent-Over Dumbbell Row (Overhand Grip)

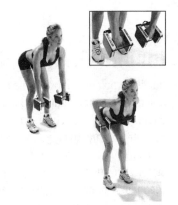

Holding a pair of dumbbells, extend your arms, palms facing toward your body. Stand with your feet hip-width apart. Bend at the waist as if tying your shoes. Raise your head and chest to create a slight arch in the back. Bend your knees slightly. Feather your breathing as you pull the dumbbells up in a fluid rowing motion through a count of 10 seconds, keeping your elbows close to your body. Hold and squeeze your shoulder blades together for 2 seconds at the MTP. Lower your arms to starting position through a count of 10 seconds. Without resting, repeat three times.

Tuck-Up on Chair

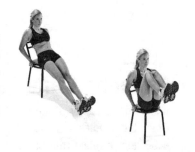

Sit on the front edge of a sturdy chair. Reach your hands behind you and grab the sides of the chair. Extend your legs out and allow your upper body to recline back slightly. Feather your breathing as you slowly draw your knees in and up toward your chest through a count of 10 seconds. Hold and squeeze for 2 seconds at the MTP. Return legs to starting position through a count of 10 seconds. Without resting, repeat three times.

Toe Reach

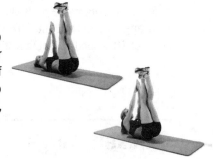

Lie on your back. Cross your legs, flex your feet, and extend your legs into the air. With your arms extended and chin up off your chest, feather your breathing as you crunch up, reaching toward your toes through a count of 10 seconds. Hold and squeeze for 2 seconds at the MTP. Lower yourself to starting position, keeping your shoulder blades from touching the ground, through a count of 10 seconds. Without resting, repeat three times.

Russian Twist on Swiss Ball

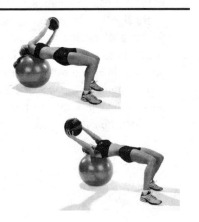

Holding a medicine ball, lie down on the ball with your knees bent, feet about shoulder-width apart. Extend your arms away from your chest with your palms toward each other, and turn to one side to begin the exercise. Feather your breathing as you slowly rotate your torso as far as possible to the other side through a count of 10 seconds, keeping your arms straight. Hold and squeeze for 2 seconds at the MTP. Rotate back to the other side through a count of 10 seconds. Without resting, repeat three times.

6 Sculpting Phase

WEEKS 3 THROUGH 8

20s CONFIDENCE

See Yourself Sexy

Visualization is a powerful way to see yourself living the life you've dreamed of, whether it's getting the job you want or making a new friend. You may not know it, but you practice visualization all the time. Whenever you see cute clothes and you imagine yourself in them, you are performing visualization. My good friend and mentor Tony Robbins says that with visualization you can actually transform your beliefs and expand your reality. Let's try it with your future career. To truly visualize yourself in your dream job, it helps to be in a relaxed, calm, and clear-headed state. Close your eyes and take a deep breath in, followed by a cleansing exhale. Don't just visualize yourself in any job; think about how you'll *feel* when have the career you've always wanted. Imagine yourself helping heal sick people as a doctor or nurse, or maybe running a meeting as a powerful executive, or working with wild animals. Whatever you want to be, create images of yourself in your future profession. Think of how confident you are and how assured you feel when people treat you as a valuable part of a team. You can apply visualization to any area of your life. Remember to aim high because the sky's the limit!

30s MANAGE STRESS

Yoga to Relieve Stress

Yoga is good for more than stretching and exercise. It is also a great way to relieve stress! Yoga's stress-relieving power comes from its deep controlled breathing, which slows your heart rate, stabilizes blood pressure, and can allow you to achieve a meditative-like state. The stretching and relaxing components help your muscles elongate, which eases stress and tension throughout your whole body—think of it as the unwrapping of a tightly wound rubber band. Some studies have even shown that yoga can significantly reduce symptoms of PMS by increasing levels of the hormone allopregnanolone. I enjoy a type of yoga called bikram yoga, also known as "hot yoga." It's the only type of yoga that's truly helped me relieve stress. Bikram yoga is done in a room with a temperature of about 105 degrees, so it's a little more intense than something like a Vinyasa yoga, which is traditional flow yoga. During bikram, the heat allows your muscles to really loosen up and become more flexible. And I can tell you, you will sweat *a lot*! This is fantastic for releasing toxins. Just be sure to drink plenty of water.

WEEK 3

As you get ready to start week 3, use these tips based on your Life Priority to give you an extra advantage. They are customized to your decade, but I recommend you read every one of them. These tips are jam-packed with valuable information and will give you an extra edge as you face each week.

40s PREVENT DECLINE

Eat More Oatmeal

The number-one killer of women in the United States is cardiovascular disease. That's why it's so important for you to take all the precautions you can to lower your risk of developing this life-threatening disease. It's important to maintain your "good" cholesterol levels, which aid in many of the body's metabolic processes and actually can reduce the risk of heart attacks. However, as your estrogen levels begin to drop as you get older, you may naturally experience a drop in "good" cholesterol and an increase in the "bad" cholesterol. High amounts of "bad" cholesterol form plaque, which can narrow the arteries and make them less flexible, creating a condition called *atherosclerosis.* One great way to keep cholesterol levels safe is to eat oatmeal. Oatmeal contains beta-glucan, a soluble fiber that has been shown to lower cholesterol. Also, oatmeal is a healthy carb that provides a great start to your day!

50s REVERSE DECLINE

Copper

Copper is for more than making pennies or jewelry. Copper is key in many important body functions. Copper is responsible for healthy-looking hair and skin; it helps the body produce the skin pigment melanin, which gives your hair, skin, and eyes their color. Copper also helps the body produce collagen and elastin, which keep the skin tight, healthy, and youthful looking. Copper works with iron to produce hemoglobin, which you may remember from biology class helps the blood carry oxygen throughout the body. Copper has been shown to be effective in treating and preventing arthritis and osteoporosis. Too much copper, however, can be toxic. Copper is a *trace mineral* so your body needs only a very small amount. To ensure that a natural amount of copper is absorbed into the body, you may want to consume foods rich in copper such as turnips, spinach, avocados, carrots, oats, papaya, nuts, shellfish, and salmon. Before you use a copper supplement, I recommend consulting your doctor to determine if you have a copper deficiency.

MONDAY

Lunge

Stand in a lunge position with one hand resting on the back of a sturdy chair for balance. Keep your back straight, chest up, and abs tight. Feather your breathing as you drop your back knee toward the ground through a count of 10 seconds. Hold for 2 seconds at the MTP (about 1 inch above the ground). Return to starting position through a count of 10 seconds. Without resting, repeat one more time on this leg and then perform 2 more reps on the other side for a total of 4. (Note: To avoid injury, make sure that your front knee stays aligned with your toes and doesn't bend beyond a 90-degree angle.)

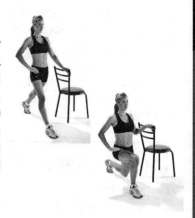

Band Squat

Stand on the center of the band, feet together. Pull the band up to your shoulders, palms facing in. Feather your breathing as you slowly squat through a count of 10 seconds. Hold for 2 seconds at the MTP (where you're about 2 inches above an imaginary chair). Return to starting position through a count of 10 seconds. Without resting, repeat three times.

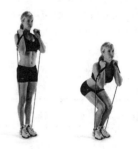

Balance Squat

Stand with feet shoulder-width apart. Grasp a bar or support at about hip level. Feather your breathing as you bend your knees and allow your body to fall backwards, letting your heels come off the floor, through a count of 10 seconds. Hold and squeeze your quads for 2 seconds at the MTP. Return to the starting position through a count of 10 seconds. Without resting, repeat three times.

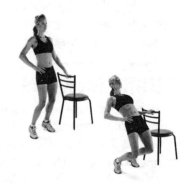

Hamstring Curl with Swiss Ball

Lie on your back with your arms at your sides, palms flat on the floor. Place your and heels on the ball, knees straight but not locked. Tighten your abs and lift your butt and hips off the ground. Feather your breathing and bend your knees as you roll the ball toward your butt with your heels through a count of 10 seconds. Hold for 2 seconds at the MTP. Return to starting position through a count of 10 seconds. Without resting, repeat three times.

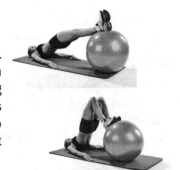

Incline Diamond Push-Up

Place your hands in a push-up position against a wall or a set of stairs; then shift your hands into the center to form a "diamond." Be sure that your upper body is elevated above your feet. Keep your head up, back straight, and abs tight. Feather your breathing as you lower yourself through a count of 10 seconds. Hold for 2 seconds at the MTP. Return to starting position through a count of 10 seconds. Without resting, repeat three times.

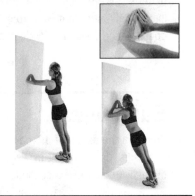

Band Skull Crusher

Secure a resistance band at about foot level. Grasp the handles so that your palms face up, and lie on the ball so that your head and neck are supported. Keep your hips up and abs tight throughout the exercise. Drop your arms back about 2 inches to starting position. Feather your breathing as you extend the band through a count of 10 seconds. Hold for 2 seconds at the MTP (just before your arms become completely straight). Return to starting position through a count of 10 seconds. Without resting, repeat three times.

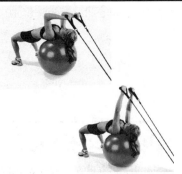

Band Kickback

Stand on the center of the band, feet together. Grasp the handles with your palms facing forward. With your knees slightly bent, bend at the waist as if you were about to tie your shoes; then lift only your chin and chest, creating a slight arch in your back. Raise your elbows up as high as possible, while keeping them close to your body. Feather your breathing as you extend the band back and out (without moving the upper part of the arm) through a count of 10 seconds. Hold and squeeze for 2 seconds at the MTP. Resist the band back to starting position through a count of 10 seconds. Without resting, repeat three times.

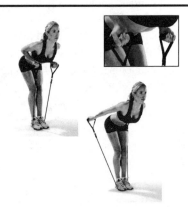

Double Crunch

Lie on a mat with your knees bent and hands behind your head. Raise your feet about 2 inches off the ground. Feather your breathing as you simultaneously crunch and raise your knees up through a count of 10 seconds. Hold and squeeze for 2 seconds at the MTP. Return to starting position through a count of 10 seconds. Keep your feet elevated as you transition into the next rep. Without resting, repeat three times.

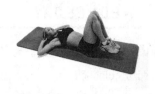

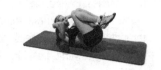

Swiss Ball Ab Roll

Kneel on a mat with your feet resting on the ground behind you. Extend your arms on top of a ball, making fists with your hands. Feather your breathing as you roll forward (using the ball for balance) through a count of 10 seconds, keeping your back straight, head up, and abs tight. Hold for 2 seconds at the MTP (when you're fully extended). Return to starting position through a count of 10 seconds. Without resting, repeat three times.

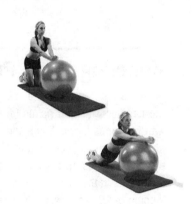

Upward Woodchopper on Swiss Ball

Secure a resistance band at foot level. Sit on the ball and place your feet in front of you about hip-width apart. Grip the handle with both hands, fingers entwined, keeping your chest up and your back and arms straight (do not lock your elbows). Feather your breathing as you pull the handles up and across your body by twisting and contracting your obliques through a count of 10 seconds. Hold and squeeze for 2 seconds at the MTP. Resist the weight back to starting position through a count of 10 seconds. Without resting, repeat once more on this side and then switch sides and complete 2 more reps for a total of 4.

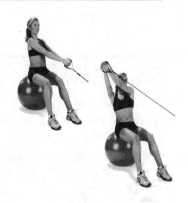

Dumbbell Pull-Over

Grasp a dumbbell using the "diamond grip." Lie on the ball with your head and neck supported. Keep your hips up and abs tight throughout the exercise. Extend the weight over your chest with a slight bend in the elbows. Feather your breathing as you lower the weight behind your head through a count of 10 seconds. Hold for 2 seconds at the MTP. Raise the weight to starting position through a count of 10 seconds. Without resting, repeat three times. (Note: The MTP will vary based on your shoulder flexibility. Hold at your most flexible point.)

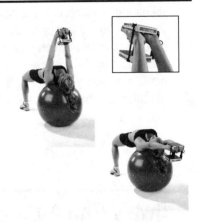

Kneeling Band Pull-Down (Close Grip)

Secure a resistance band above your head. Kneel on a mat and grasp the handles with your palms facing each other. Sit back on your heels with your arms fully outstretched; keep your back straight, chest up, and abs tight. Feather your breathing as you pull the handles toward the top part of your chest through a count of 10 seconds. Hold and squeeze for 2 seconds at the MTP. Resist the band back to starting position through a count of 10 seconds. Without resting, repeat three times.

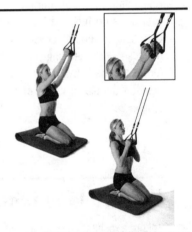

Band Row (Standard Grip)

Secure a resistance band at about waist level. Grasp the handles and hold arms extended at chest height, palms facing in. Take a wide step forward with one foot, keeping your back straight, abs tight, and knees slightly bent. Feather your breathing as you pull the handles toward your chest in a fluid rowing motion through a count of 10 seconds, keeping your elbows close to your body. Hold and squeeze your shoulder blades together for 2 seconds at the MTP. Resist the band back to starting position through a count of 10 seconds. Without resting, repeat three times.

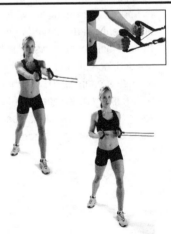

Reverse Hyperextension

Lie facedown on a ball. Roll yourself forward until the ball is under your hips and your upper body is angled toward the floor. Place your palms about 6 inches wider than shoulder-width apart on the floor. With legs together, feather your breathing as you raise your heels toward the ceiling using your lower back and hamstrings through a count of 10 seconds. Hold and squeeze for 2 seconds at the MTP. With straight legs, lower to starting position through a count of 10 seconds, about 2 inches from the ground. Without resting, repeat three times.

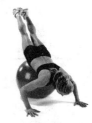

Band Preacher Curl

Secure a resistance band at foot level. Lean over the ball with your knees on the floor and grasp the handles, hands about 1 foot apart, palms facing up. Feather your breathing as you curl the band up through a count of 10 seconds. Hold and squeeze for 2 seconds at the MTP. Resist the band down through a count of 10 seconds. Without resting, repeat three times. (Note: The preacher curl is the only curl in which you shouldn't allow your arm to extend fully. Keep your arm slightly bent at the bottom of the motion.)

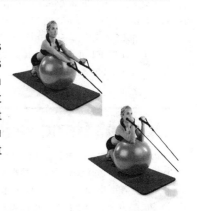

Dumbbell Curl on Swiss Ball

Hold a pair of dumbbells and sit on the ball, arms by your sides with your palms facing away from you. Feather your breathing as you curl the dumbbells through a count of 10 seconds to just past a 90-degree angle. Hold and squeeze for 2 seconds at the MTP. Keep your elbows tight against your body as you lower the weights through a count of 10 seconds. Without resting, repeat three times. (Note: Keep your elbows tight against your sides throughout the exercise.)

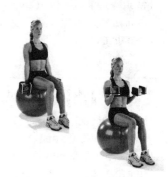

Hammer Curl

Holding a pair of dumbbells, stand with your feet shoulder-width apart, your arms extended slightly in front of your thighs, palms facing each other, knees slightly bent. Feather your breathing as you curl the weights through a count of 10 seconds, keeping your palms facing each other. Hold and squeeze for 2 seconds at the MTP. Lower the weights to starting position through a count of 10 seconds. Without resting, repeat three times.

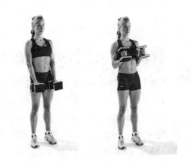

Seated V-Up

Sit on a mat with your arms behind you, elbows bent, and fingertips pointed toward your body. Start with your legs together and extended, knees slightly bent, and heels about 2 inches off the ground. Lean your upper body weight back on your palms slightly. Feather your breathing as you pull your knees into your chest through a count of 10 seconds. Hold and squeeze for 2 seconds at the MTP. Return to starting position through a count of 10 seconds, keeping your abs tight. Without resting, repeat three times.

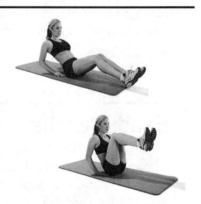

Upright Band Crunch on Swiss Ball

Secure the resistance band above your head. Stand with the ball between you and a wall supporting your middle to upper back. Grasp the handles behind the back of your head, palms facing back. Walk your feet in front of you about 1 foot, keeping your knees slightly bent. Feather your breathing as you crunch your abs in and up as you bring your elbows toward your knees. Hold and squeeze for 2 seconds at the MTP. Return to starting position through a count of 10 seconds. Without resting, repeat three times.

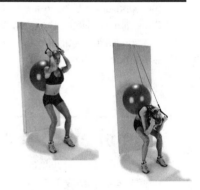

Lying Oblique Twist

Lie on your back with your arms outstretched, palms facing down. Raise your knees to a 90-degree angle, and drop your knees down to one side. Feather your breathing as you lift and rotate your knees to the other side through a count of 10 seconds. Hold and squeeze for 2 seconds at the MTP (about a few inches from the ground). Then rotate to the other side through a count of 10 seconds. Without resting, repeat three times.

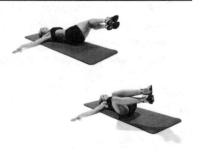

FRIDAY

Push-Up on Knees

Kneel on a mat on all fours with your feet crossed and lifted slightly up off the ground. Your hands should be wider than shoulder-width apart with your fingers and wrists pointing forward. Feather your breathing as you lower your chest toward the floor through a count of 10 seconds. Hold for 2 seconds at the MTP. Push your body back to starting position through a count of 10 seconds, keeping your elbows slightly bent at the top of the move. Without resting, repeat three times.

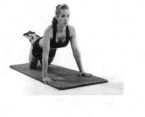
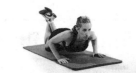

Flat Band Press

Secure a resistance band at about shoulder level. Grasp the handles and hold at chest level, palms facing down. Take a wide step forward with one foot, keeping your back straight, abs tight, and knees slightly bent. Feather your breathing as you press the handles of the band forward through a count of 10 seconds. Hold for 2 seconds at the MTP (just prior to lockout). Return to starting position through a count of 10 seconds. Without resting, repeat three times.

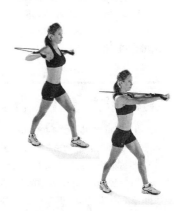

Flat Dumbbell Press

Holding a pair of dumbbells, lie on a ball so that it comfortably supports your shoulder blades. Extend your arms in front of you, palms facing away from you, pressing the weights together. Feather your breathing as you lower the weights through a count of 10 seconds. Hold for 2 seconds at the MTP (about 1 inch higher than chest level). Press the dumbbells up and together back to starting position through a count of 10 seconds. Without resting, repeat three times.

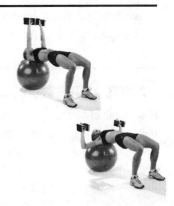

Upward Band Fly

Secure a resistance band at about waist level. Step one foot out in front of the other about 2 feet, your knees slightly bent, back straight, and abs tight. Grasp the handles with your arms extended behind you, palms angled down, with a slight bend in your elbows. Feather your breathing as you bring your palms up and together through a count of 10 seconds. Hold for 2 seconds at the MTP. Return to starting position through a count of 10 seconds. Without resting, repeat three times.

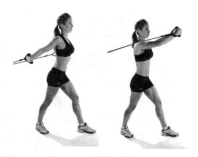

Standing Dumbbell Press

Holding a pair of dumbbells, take a wide step forward with one foot, keeping your back straight, abs tight, and knees slightly bent. Extend the weights up and together directly over your head, palms facing forward. Feather your breathing as you lower the weights through a count of 10 seconds. Hold for 2 seconds at the MTP (chin level). Press the dumbbells up to starting position through a count of 10 seconds. Without resting, repeat three times.

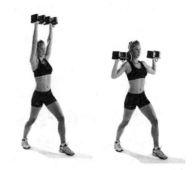

Upright Band Row

Stand in the center of a resistance band with your feet together and knees slightly bent. Grasp the handles of the band with your arms in front of you, elbows slightly bent, palms facing your body. Feather your breathing as you draw the handles up toward your chin through a count of 10 seconds. Hold for 2 seconds at the MTP (just below your chin). Return to starting position through a count of 10 seconds. Without resting, repeat three times. (Note: You should not feel a strain in your neck. If you do, relax your neck muscles and focus the exertion in your shoulder area.)

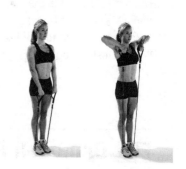

Front Delt Raise on Swiss Ball

Hold a pair of dumbbells and stand with a ball against a sturdy wall, the ball between your shoulder blades and your body slightly angled back. Feather your breathing as you raise the dumbbells up, elbows slightly bent, for a count of 10 seconds. Hold for 2 seconds at the MTP (about eye level). Lower the weights to starting position through a count of 10 seconds. Without resting, repeat three times.

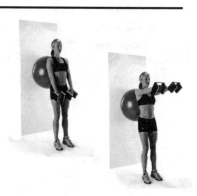

Swiss Ball Crunch with Elevated Feet

Sit on a ball that's about 2 feet away from a wall. Walk your feet out and place them against the wall. Lie down and place your hands behind your ears. Feather your breathing as you crunch up through a count of 10 seconds, using only your abs. Hold and squeeze for 2 seconds at the MTP. Return to starting position through a count of 10 seconds. Without resting, repeat three times. (Note: Keep in mind that the range of motion is significantly smaller on this exercise, so be sure to adjust your pace.)

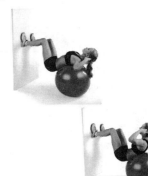

Band Tuck-Up on Chair

Secure a resistance band at foot level. Sit on a sturdy chair and reach your hands behind you to grab the sides. Place your feet in the handles of the band, extend your legs out, and allow your upper body to lean back slightly. Feather your breathing as you draw your knees in and up toward your chin through a count of 10 seconds. Hold and squeeze for 2 seconds at the MTP. Return to starting position through a count of 10 seconds. Without resting, repeat three times.

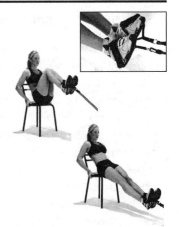

Bicycle Crunch

Lie flat on your back. Place your hands behind your head and raise your legs off the ground, bending your right knee, keeping your chin up and abs tight throughout the exercise. Bring your left elbow to your right knee and feather your breathing as you rotate to the other side for a count of 10 seconds. Hold and squeeze for 2 seconds at the MTP (where your right elbow meets your left knee). Twist to starting position through a count of 10 seconds. Without resting, repeat three times.

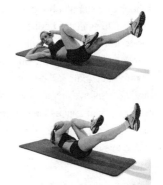

WEEK 4

As you get ready to start week 4, use these tips based on your Life Priority to give you an extra advantage. They are customized to your decade, but I recommend you read every one of them. These tips are jam-packed with valuable information and will give you an extra edge as you face each week.

20s CONFIDENCE

A Little Help from Your Friends

Studies have shown that people may be more influenced by their friends and family than they realize. One study revealed that if your friends are overweight, you are 57 percent more likely to be overweight too. It's not hard to figure out why. If you're with a friend debating about whether or not to go to the gym and your friend's answer is always "I don't want to," it's easier for you to say no too; you enable each other's bad decisions. On the flip side, if you have people in your life who are motivated to get fit and eat right, you'll be more inspired to do the same. The same can be said for any other aspect of your life, whether it's school, drugs or alcohol, or career choices. Take the time to evaluate your support group and think about how your friends influence you. Do your friends empower you and push you forward toward your goals? Or do they hold you back? Having a positive, inspiring support system is crucial to your success in life. So remember to take stock of your surroundings and make sure you're in a group that will propel you forward.

30s MANAGE STRESS

Manage Stress with Magnesium

You probably only remember magnesium as a mineral name tossed around in your high school science classes. What you may not know is that it has a long list of important jobs to do when it comes to keeping your body in tip-top shape. It plays a critical role in heart health, bone formation, and nervous system function, to name a few. Magnesium also helps your muscles relax by opening them up to a proper supply of oxygen. If you're not getting enough magnesium in your diet, you could be putting your body at risk, and perpetuating stress. You see, when you're stressed, your body releases stress hormones, which drain the magnesium from your body. Since this mineral is critical to muscle function and blood flow, when it's depleted your body feels tight and anxious, creating a vicious cycle of stress. Eat magnesium-rich foods such as whole grains, tofu, almonds, and cashews to prevent deficiency. Also, take a magnesium supplement during times of heavy stress to help yourself stay balanced.

40s PREVENT DECLINE

Stock Up on Antioxidants

Oxidation helps us get energy from food, but too much of it can create *free radicals,* nasty little chemicals that travel through the body and beat up on our cells. Free radicals can wear down your immune system and your organs, deteriorate bone and tissue, and advance visible signs of aging. How can you stop them? First, try to limit your intake of things that speed up oxidation, such as cigarettes, alcohol, and pollution. Next, make sure you are sending in enough antioxidants to protect your body from the destructive effects of free radicals. Aim to get your antioxidants by including a nice rainbow of fruits and vegetables from the produce section in your diet. You'll get beta-carotene mostly from orange foods like carrots, cantaloupe, and mangoes; lutein from green, leafy vegetables like kale and spinach; and anthocyanins, which produce deep reds and blue-purples, from blueberries, eggplant, grapes, cherries, and cranberries.

50s REVERSE DECLINE

Use B12 to Prevent Memory Loss

Memory loss is normal as we age, right? Not necessarily. Older people who have a deficiency in vitamin B12 are at a high risk for developing pernicious anemia. Symptoms of this condition include forgetfulness, nerve damage, and loss of the ability to concentrate. In fact, many people diagnosed with senility may actually be suffering from a deficiency of B12. Now, I know you may be thinking, "Jorge, I'm in my fifties or sixties, not eighties!"—but stocking up on B12 vitamins now and as you get older could help prevent frustrating memory issues as you age. Most of us cannot absorb enough B12 through diet alone, so I recommend you take a B12 or B-complex daily supplement to keep yourself feeling good and keep your memory sharp as you get older. A deficiency in B12 can also put you at higher risk for a heart attack, so getting the appropriate amount is good for your head and your heart.

Split Squat with Swiss Ball

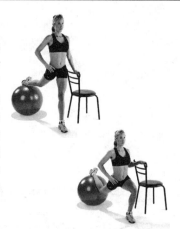

Stand about 3 feet in front of a ball. Place one foot on the ball with the top of your shoe lightly touching it. Hold on to the back of a sturdy chair for support. With your back straight, chest up, and abs tight, feather your breathing as you bend your front knee, lowering yourself toward the ground through a count of 10 seconds. Make sure your front knee doesn't extend beyond your toe. Hold for 2 seconds at the MTP (when there is about a 90-degree bend in the front knee). Return to starting position through a count of 10 seconds. Without resting, repeat once more on this side and then switch sides and perform 2 more reps for a total of 4.

Plié Squat

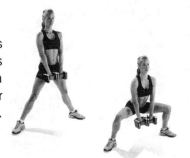

Holding a dumbbell in each hand, stand with your feet about two times wider than shoulder-width apart, toes turned out to the sides, and knees aligned over the toes. Feather your breathing as you squat through a count of 10 seconds. Hold for 2 seconds at the MTP. Push through your heels to return to starting position through a count of 10 seconds. Without resting, repeat three times.

Lateral Squat

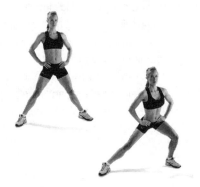

Take a stance about 1 foot wider than shoulder-width on each side. Feather your breathing as you squat toward one leg, keeping your chest high (do not twist or lean forward) and the opposite leg straight, through a count of 10 seconds. Hold for 2 seconds at the MTP. Return to starting position through a count of 10 seconds. Without resting, perform 2 reps on each side for a total of 4.

Glute Kickback

Kneel on a mat on all fours with your knees hip-width apart. Lift your leg and bend it to a 90-degree angle. Press the heel of your foot toward the ceiling through a count of 10 seconds. Hold and squeeze for 2 seconds at the MTP. Lower your leg to starting position through a count of 10 seconds. Without resting, repeat once more on this leg and then switch sides and complete 2 more reps for a total of 4.

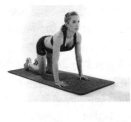
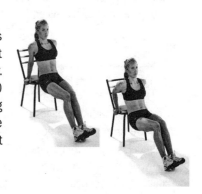

Chair Dip

Sit on the edge of a sturdy chair with your hands behind you, fingers forward, grasping the edge of the chair. Flex your feet so that your weight is on your heels and slide yourself an inch or so away from the chair. Feather your breathing as you lower yourself through a count of 10 seconds. Hold for 2 seconds at the MTP. Push yourself up to starting position through a count of 10 seconds. Without resting, repeat three times. (Note: The MTP will vary based on your shoulder flexibility—about 1 inch above your most flexible point.)

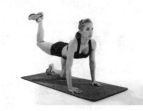

Overhead Triceps Extension

Grasp a dumbbell using the "diamond grip." Sit on the ball with your chest up, back straight, feet shoulder-width apart. Extend your arms, with your elbows slightly bent, keeping your biceps tight against your head. Feather your breathing as you lower the dumbbell through a count of 10 seconds. Hold for 2 seconds at the MTP (when your elbows are at about a 90-degree angle). Press the weight up to starting position through a count of 10 seconds. Without resting, repeat three times.

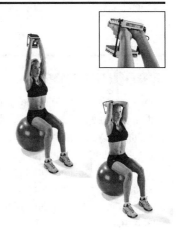

Triceps Press-Down

Secure a resistance band above your head. Grasp the handles, keeping your hands about 1 foot apart. Pull your arms down against your sides, elbows bent at just above a 90-degree angle, palms facing down. Feather your breathing as you press the handles down and straighten your arms (but do not lock your elbows) through a count of 10 seconds. Hold for 2 seconds at the MTP. Resist the weight back to starting position through a count of 10 seconds. Without resting, repeat three times.

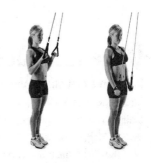

Medicine Ball Pull-Over

Lie on a mat and bring your knees, ankles crossed, up to a 90-degree angle. Grasp a medicine ball and extend it over your head; keep a slight bend in your elbows. Keep your abs tight and feather your breathing as you raise the ball over your head and crunch up through a count of 10 seconds. Hold for 2 seconds at the MTP. Lower the ball to starting position through a count of 10 seconds. Without resting, repeat three times.

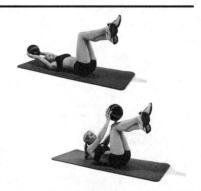

Reverse Crunch

Lie on a mat with your hands by your sides, palms down. Pull your heels up as close to your butt as possible. Raise your heels about 2 inches off the ground. Keep your chin tucked and abs tight. Feather your breathing as you pull your knees toward your chest, using your lower abdominals, through a count of 10 seconds. Hold and squeeze for 2 seconds at the MTP (when your butt is completely off the ground). Lower your body to starting position through a count of 10 seconds. Without resting, repeat three times.

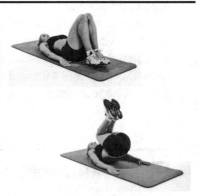

Woodchopper

Secure a resistance band above your head. Stand with your legs about 3 feet apart; keep your chest up, back and arms straight. Feather your breathing as you pull the handles down and across your body by twisting and contracting your obliques through a count of 10 seconds. Hold and squeeze for 2 seconds at the MTP. Resist the band back to starting position through a count of 10 seconds. Without resting, repeat once more on this side and then switch sides and complete 2 more reps for a total of 4.

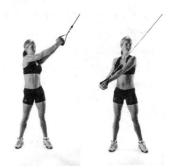

Dumbbell Pull-Over

Grasp a dumbbell using the "diamond grip." Lie on the ball with your head and neck supported. Keep your hips up and abs tight throughout the exercise. Extend the weight over your chest without locking your elbows. Feather your breathing as you lower the weight behind your head through a count of 10 seconds. Hold for 2 seconds at the MTP. Raise the weight to starting position through a count of 10 seconds. Without resting, repeat three times. (Note: The MTP will vary based on your shoulder flexibility. Hold at your most flexible point.)

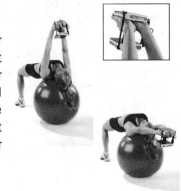

Bird Dog

Kneel on all fours with your knees hip-width apart. Keep your head up and abs tight throughout the exercise. Feather your breathing as you simultaneously lift and extend your left arm and your right leg through a count of 10 seconds. Hold and squeeze for 2 seconds at the MTP (when your arm and thigh are approximately parallel to the floor). Return to starting position through a count of 10 seconds. Without resting, repeat once more on this side and then switch sides and complete 2 more reps for a total of 4.

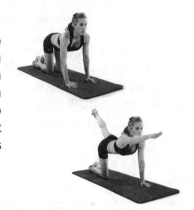

Dumbbell Row on Swiss Ball

Holding a pair of dumbbells, lie on a ball so that the middle of your waist is centered on it. Raise your head and chest, creating a slight arch in the back. Feather your breathing as you pull the dumbbells up and back toward your hips in a rowing motion through a count of 10 seconds. Hold and squeeze the shoulder blades together for 2 seconds at the MTP. Return to starting position through a count of 10 seconds. Without resting, repeat three times.

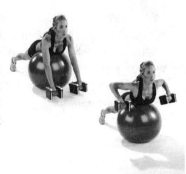

Dumbbell Dead Lift

Stand holding a dumbbell in each hand, with your feet about 6 to 8 inches apart. Bend over at the waist as if you were about to tie your shoes. Lift your chin and chest creating a slight arch in your back. Feather your breathing as you lift your upper body through a count of 10 seconds, driving through your heels and using your lower back and hamstrings, keeping your knees slightly bent. Hold for 2 seconds at the MTP (when you are standing). Return to starting position through a count of 10 seconds. Without resting, repeat three times.

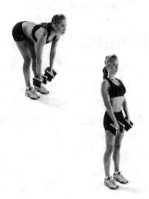

Incline Curl

Hold a pair of dumbbells and stand with a ball against a sturdy wall, the ball between your shoulder blades and the top of your hips. Bend your knees slightly. Keep your abs tight and chest up. Feather your breathing as you curl the weights up through a count of 10 seconds. Hold and squeeze for 2 seconds at the MTP. Lower the weights to starting position through a count of 10 seconds, until your arms are completely straight (but not locked). Without resting, repeat three times. (Note: As you perform the exercise, be sure to not let your elbows move away from the sides of your body.)

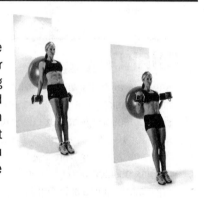

Side Curls on Swiss Ball

Hold a pair of dumbbells and sit on the ball. With your arms down against your sides, palms turned up, and elbows tight against your body, feather your breathing as you curl the weights up through a count of 10 seconds. Hold and squeeze for a count of 2 seconds at the MTP. Lower the weights to starting position through a count of 10 seconds. Without resting, repeat three times.

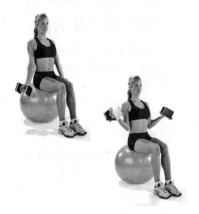

Reverse Band Curl

Stand on the center of a resistance band, feet together, and knees slightly bent. Grasp the handles with your arms by your sides, your palms facing your body, and your elbows slightly bent. Feather your breathing as you curl the handles up through a count of 10 seconds to just past a 90-degree angle. Hold and squeeze for 2 seconds at the MTP. Keep your elbows tight against your body as you lower the handles through a count of 10 seconds. Without resting, repeat three times.

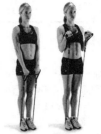
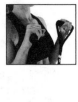

Jackknife

Stand about 3 feet in front of a ball and place your palms on the ground, hands a bit wider than shoulder-width apart. From here, put one foot on the ball slightly below mid-shin level. Once level, place the other foot on the ball keeping your head forward, spine straight, and abs tight. Slowly pull your knees up toward your chin through a count of 10 seconds, as you concentrate on keeping stability by squeezing your abs tight. Hold and squeeze for 2 seconds at the MTP. Return to starting position through a count of 10 seconds. Without resting, repeat three times.

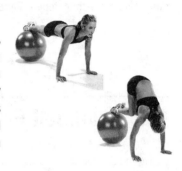

Kneeling Band Crunch

Secure a resistance band above your head and kneel on a mat. Grasp the handles in front of your forehead, palms facing toward you. Keep your abs tight and feather your breathing as you crunch toward the mat through a count of 10 seconds. Hold for 2 seconds at the MTP (about 2 inches from the mat). Resist the band back to starting position through a count of 10 seconds. Without resting, repeat three times.

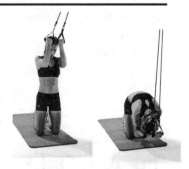

Oblique Twist on Swiss Ball

Lie on the ball holding a medicine ball just under your chin. Walk your feet forward until your hips are slightly lower than your chest. Keep your abs tight and chin up. Turn your upper body to one side to begin the exercise. Slowly twist your torso to the other side through a count of 10 seconds. Hold and squeeze for 2 seconds at the MTP. Then twist to the other side through a count of 10 seconds. Without resting, repeat three times.

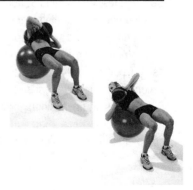

FRIDAY

Chair Push-Up

Place two sturdy chairs in front of you and rest your hands on the seats, slightly wider than shoulder-width apart, arms extended. Feather your breathing as you lower your chest toward the chairs through a count of 10 seconds, keeping your back straight and abs tight. Hold for 2 seconds at the MTP. Push your body back to starting position through a count of 10 seconds, keeping your elbows slightly bent at the top of the move. Without resting, repeat three times.

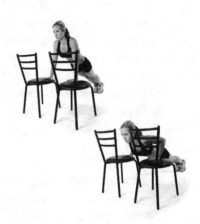

Flat Dumbbell Press

Holding a pair of dumbbells, lie on a ball so that it comfortably supports your shoulder blades. Extend your arms in front of you, palms facing away from you, pressing the weights together. Feather your breathing as you lower the weights through a count of 10 seconds. Hold for 2 seconds at the MTP (about 1 inch higher than chest level). Press the dumbbells up and together, back to starting position, through a count of 10 seconds. Without resting, repeat three times.

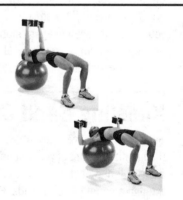

One-Arm Flat Band Press

Secure a resistance band at about shoulder level. Grasp the handle with your left hand (place the other on your hip) and hold at chest level, palm facing down. Take a wide step forward with your left foot, keeping your back straight, abs tight, and knees slightly bent. Feather your breathing as you punch the handle of the band forward through a count of 10 seconds. Hold for 2 seconds at the MTP (just prior to locking your elbow). Return to starting position through a count of 10 seconds. Without resting, repeat once more on this side and then switch sides and complete 2 more reps for a total of 4.

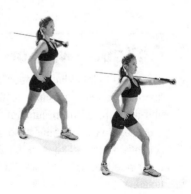

Incline Dumbbell Fly

Holding a pair of dumbbells, lie on a ball with your head and neck supported. Roll down the ball until your hips drop almost to the ground. Extend the dumbbells over your chest, palms facing each other, elbows slightly bent. Feather your breathing as you lower the weights down and out through a count of 10 seconds. Hold for 2 seconds at the MTP. Raise the weights back to starting position in a "bear hug" type motion through a count of 10 seconds. Without resting, repeat three times.

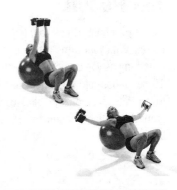

V Push-Up

Plant feet hip-width apart. Bend forward at the hips to place hands on the floor about 3 feet in front of your toes. Keep abs drawn in, head tucked as if you're holding an orange between your chin and chest (you should look like an upside-down "V" from the side). With hands slightly in front of your shoulders, feather your breathing as you bend your elbows and lower your chest and shoulders toward the floor through a count of 10 seconds. Hold for 2 seconds at the MTP. Push back to starting position through a count of 10 seconds. Without resting, repeat three times.

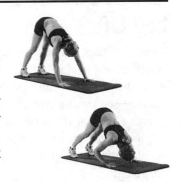

Reverse Lateral Raise

Holding a pair of dumbbells, sit on a ball with your back straight and your abs tight. Extend your arms over your head with a slight bend in your elbows, palms facing each other. Feather your breathing as you lower the weights down and out to your sides for a count of 10 seconds, keeping palms up during the entire movement. Hold for 2 seconds at the MTP (your arms should be parallel to the ground). Return to starting position through a count of 10 seconds. Without resting, repeat three times.

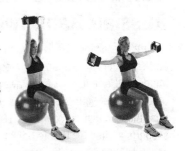

L-Raise

Hold a pair of dumbbells and take a wide step forward with your left foot, keeping your back straight, abs tight, and knees slightly bent. With your arms against your sides and elbows slightly bent, feather your breathing as you raise the weights up through a count of 10 seconds, your left arm extended in front of you and your right out to the side. Hold and squeeze for 2 seconds at the MTP ("L" position). Lower the weights to starting position through a count of 10 seconds. Without resting, repeat once more on this side and then switch sides and complete 2 more reps for a total of 4.

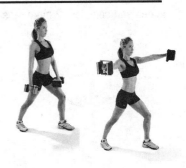

Toe Reach

Lie on your back. Cross your legs, flex your feet, and extend your legs into the air. With your arms extended and chin up off your chest, feather your breathing as you crunch up, reaching toward your toes through a count of 10 seconds. Hold and squeeze for 2 seconds at the MTP. Lower yourself to starting position, keeping your shoulder blades from touching the ground, through a count of 10 seconds. Without resting, repeat three times.

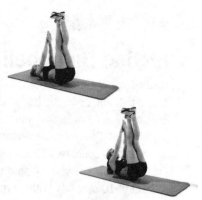

Leg Lift

Lie on your back with your palms down, hands underneath your butt. Crunch up and hold your upper abs tight so that your shoulder blades are off the ground. Lift your legs about 6 inches off the ground. Keep your abs tight and chin up and feather your breathing as you lift your legs through a count of 10 seconds. Hold and squeeze for 2 seconds at the MTP (when your feet are about 2 feet off the ground). Lower your legs to starting position through a count of 10 seconds. Without resting, repeat three times.

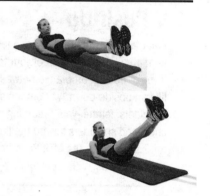

Russian Band Twist on Swiss Ball

Secure a resistance band at head level. Lie on the ball so that your head and shoulders are supported, hips elevated. Hold the handles with both hands and extend your arms away from your chest, palms toward each other. Feather your breathing as you slowly rotate your torso as far as possible through a count of 10 seconds. Hold and squeeze for 2 seconds at the MTP. Rotate back to the other side through a count of 10 seconds. Without resting, repeat once more on this side and then switch sides and complete 2 more reps for a total of 4.

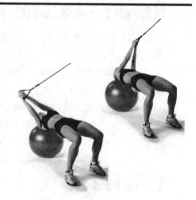

WEEK 5

As you get ready to start week 5, use these tips based on your Life Priority to give you an extra advantage. They are customized to your decade, but I recommend you read every one of them. These tips are jam-packed with valuable information and will give you an extra edge as you face each week.

20s CONFIDENCE

Power Collage

One of my favorite things to do is look for visual motivators in magazines and keep a collection of them to help inspire myself. Such motivators are pictures torn out of books or magazines or printed from the computer to give a visual representation of my goal. Collect images of anything that will inspire *you,* such as a great outfit you'd like to wear or pictures of a tropical place you'd like to visit. Then sit down with these pictures, some scissors, glue, and construction paper or poster board, and get ready to create some motivation you can hang on your wall. Once you have all the images glued on your paper, be sure to hang it where you'll see it every day—maybe on the back of your closet door or even on your refrigerator with magnets. Take the time to look at it daily and imagine yourself realizing these goals. This is a very powerful way to train your mind.

30s MANAGE STRESS

Get a Massage

Getting a massage can be much more than just a pleasurable treat. It's a fantastic way to relieve stress and anxiety. We all know what a tight feeling we get when stress begins to pile up and our muscles feel as if they are being tied into knots. You feel stress in your neck, chest, and back, and it can even lead to severe headaches. A good massage can take care of all that stress and tension because it triggers your body to release natural painkillers and endorphins, which have a euphoric effect on your body. Massage therapy also helps your body's lymphatic system drain toxins from your body and boost your immune system. Check your local listings for massage therapy or healing arts schools. They often offer massages by students for much less than spas or health clubs charge. I recommend you try to incorporate massages into your regular self-care routine—you won't be sorry!

40s PREVENT DECLINE

The 8-Hour Requirement

Sleep your way to heath and beauty. Could it really be that easy? Just sleep more? Yes! As simple as it may sound, it is estimated that up to 40 million Americans suffer from over 70 different sleep disorders. Sleep is essential. It directly affects our health, mood, and appearance, so you would think we would get more of it. However, it's common for most Americans to sleep 6 hours or less a night. It's vital that you understand how important a good night's sleep is to your overall well-being. Eight hours of "quality" sleep should be your goal. That may sound next to impossible, so here are a few tips for getting more sleep:

- *Plan your sleep.* I know from experience that if you don't plan your sleep you will not get enough of it. Calculate what time you need to be in bed to get a full 8 hours, and be sure to include the time it takes you to actually fall asleep.
- *Stick to a regular exercise program.* You're reading this book, so that probably means you're following the Body at Home™ plan. Studies have shown that people who exercise regularly get better sleep.
- *Avoid mid-afternoon caffeine.* I'm not suggesting that you give up your morning cup of coffee, but that should really be it! Consuming caffeine in the afternoon can cause your sleep to suffer since caffeine can take hours to wear off. And if you're getting better sleep at night, you might be surprised to find that you do not feel the need to drink caffeine at all.

50s REVERSE DECLINE

Calcium for Bone Health and More

As we get older it is vital to keep our bones strong! Falls later in life that lead to broken bones can be life threatening. There's no better time than now to make sure you preserve your bone density and help prevent broken bones years down the road. During menopause the production of the hormone estrogen declines rapidly, contributing to calcium deficiencies, which can put you at risk for osteoporosis and weak bones. Calcium makes bones strong, so women should simply consume more calcium, right? Well, you may not be getting enough calcium from your diet alone. That's why it's critical for you to take a calcium supplement. Studies have shown that women who consistently take a calcium supplement increase their bone density. Denser bones will decrease your risk of breaks and fractures. Plus, calcium has been linked to decreased hypertension. One study revealed that a supplement of 1,200 milligrams a day could decrease the chances of developing high blood pressure as you get older.

MONDAY

Dumbbell Squat

Hold a pair of dumbbells and stand with your feet shoulder-width apart. Feather your breathing as you slowly squat through a count of 10 seconds, keeping your back straight, abs tight, and chest up. Hold for 2 seconds at the MTP (where you're about 2 inches above an imaginary chair), never letting your knees extend over your ankles. Return to starting position through a count of 10 seconds. Without resting, repeat three times.

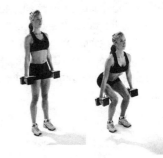

Swiss Ball Squat

Place the ball against a wall and position yourself with the ball supporting your lower back. Hold a pair of dumbbells and keep your arms against your sides. Move your feet forward about 1 foot, hip-width apart, and stand. Feather your breathing as you slowly squat through a count of 10 seconds, never letting your knees extend over your ankles. Hold for 2 seconds at the MTP (when your knees are at about a 90-degree angle). Return to starting position through a count of 10 seconds. Without resting, repeat three times.

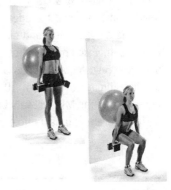

Lunge

Stand in a lunge position with one hand resting on the back of a sturdy chair for balance. Keep your back straight, chest up, and abs tight. Feather your breathing as you drop your back knee toward the ground through a count of 10 seconds. Hold for 2 seconds at the MTP (about 1 inch above the ground). Return to starting position through a count of 10 seconds. Without resting, repeat one more time on this leg and then switch sides and perform 2 more reps for a total of 4. (Note: To avoid injury, make sure that your front knee stays aligned with your toes and doesn't bend beyond a 90-degree angle.)

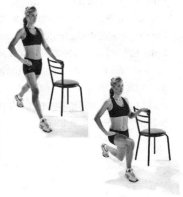

Hamstring Curl with Swiss Ball

Lie on your back with your arms at your sides, palms flat on the floor. Place your heels on the ball, knees straight but not locked. Tighten your abs and lift your butt and hips off the ground. Feather your breathing and bend your knees as you roll the ball toward your butt with your heels through a count of 10 seconds. Hold for 2 seconds at the MTP. Return to starting position through a count of 10 seconds. Without resting, repeat three times.

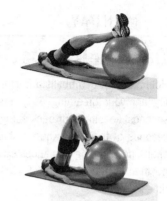

Chair Dip

Sit on the edge of a sturdy chair with your hands behind you, fingers forward and grasping the edge of the chair. Flex your feet so that your weight is on your heels and slide yourself an inch or so away from the chair. Feather your breathing as you lower yourself through a count of 10 seconds. Hold for 2 seconds at the MTP. Push yourself up to starting position through a count of 10 seconds. Without resting, repeat three times. (Note: The MTP will vary based on your shoulder flexibility—about 1 inch above your most flexible point.)

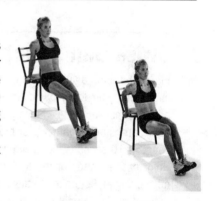

Dumbbell Skull Crusher

Hold a pair of dumbbells and lie on the ball so that your head and neck are supported. Elevate your hips slightly and keep your abs tight. Extend the dumbbells straight up with your palms facing each other, and tilt your arms toward your head slightly. Feather your breathing as you bend your elbows and lower the weights through a count of 10 seconds. Hold for 2 seconds at the MTP (about 1 inch above your forehead). Raise dumbbells to starting position through a count of 10 seconds. Without resting, repeat three times.

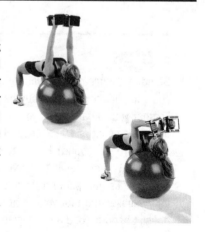

Standing Kickback

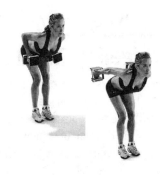

Hold a pair of dumbbells, palms facing each other. With your knees slightly bent, bend at the waist as if you were about to tie your shoes; then lift only your chin and chest, creating a slight arch in your back. Raise your elbows as high as possible, keeping them close to your body. Feather your breathing as you extend the weights back (without moving the upper part of the arm) through a count of 10 seconds. Hold and squeeze for 2 seconds at the MTP. Return the weights to starting position through a count of 10 seconds. Without resting, repeat three times.

Jackknife

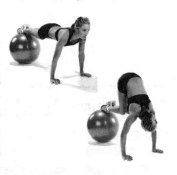

Stand about 3 feet in front of the ball and place your palms on the ground, hands shoulder-width apart. Put one foot on the ball slightly below mid-shin level. Once level, place the other foot on the ball keeping your head forward, spine straight, and abs tight. Slowly pull your knees up to your chin through a count of 10 seconds as you concentrate on keeping stability by squeezing your abs tight. Hold and squeeze for 2 seconds at the MTP. Return to starting position through a count of 10 seconds. Without resting, repeat three times.

Kneeling Band Crunch

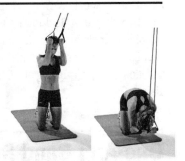

Secure a resistance band above your head and kneel on a mat. Grasp the handles in front of your forehead, palms facing toward you. Keep your abs tight and feather your breathing as you crunch toward the mat through a count of 10 seconds. Hold for 2 seconds at the MTP (about 2 inches from the mat). Resist the band back to starting position through a count of 10 seconds. Without resting, repeat three times.

Russian Twist on Swiss Ball

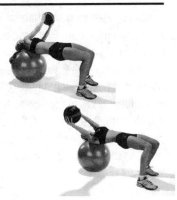

Sit on the ball with your knees bent, feet about shoulder-width apart. Keep your chin up and abs tight as you lean back slightly, engaging your abs. Holding a medicine ball, extend your arms away from your chest with your palms toward each other and turn to one side to begin exercise. Feather your breathing as you slowly rotate your torso as far as possible to the other side through a count of 10 seconds, keeping your arms straight. Hold and squeeze for 2 seconds at the MTP. Rotate back to the other side through a count of 10 seconds. Without resting, repeat three times.

WEDNESDAY

Kneeling Band Pull-Down (Overhand Grip)

Secure a resistance band above your head. Kneel on a mat and grasp the handles with your palms facing forward. Sit back on your heels with your arms fully outstretched; keep your back straight, chest up, and abs tight. Feather your breathing as you pull the handles down toward the top part of your chest through a count of 10 seconds. Hold and squeeze for 2 seconds at the MTP. Resist the band back to starting position through a count of 10 seconds. Without resting, repeat three times.

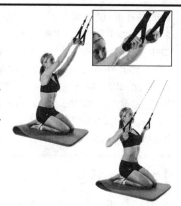

Bent-Over Dumbbell Row (Standard Grip)

Holding a pair of dumbbells, extend your arms, palms facing in. Stand with your feet hip-width apart. Bend at the waist as if you were tying your shoes. Raise your head and chest to create a slight arch in the back. Bend your knees slightly. Feather your breathing as you pull the dumbbells up in a fluid rowing motion through a count of 10 seconds, keeping your elbows close to your body. Hold and squeeze your shoulder blades together for 2 seconds at the MTP. Lower your arms to starting position through a count of 10 seconds. Without resting, repeat three times.

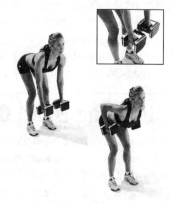

One-Arm Band Row

Secure a resistance band about chest high. Grasp the handle with your left hand and extend your arm, palm facing in. Take a wide step forward with your right foot, keeping your back straight, abs tight, and knees slightly bent. Feather your breathing as you pull the handle toward your chest in a fluid rowing motion through a count of 10 seconds, keeping your elbow close to your body. Hold and squeeze your shoulder blades together for 2 seconds at the MTP. Resist the band back to starting position through a count of 10 seconds. Without resting, repeat once more on this side and then switch sides and complete 2 more reps for a total of 4.

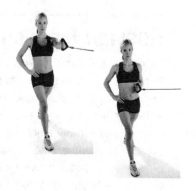

Hyperextension

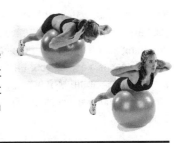

Lie facedown on the ball with your waist bent and hips supported on the ball, hands resting behind your ears. Feather your breathing as you lift your upper body, using the muscles in your lower back, through a count of 10 seconds. Hold for 2 seconds at the MTP. Return to starting position through a count of 10 seconds. Without resting, repeat three times.

Band Preacher Curl

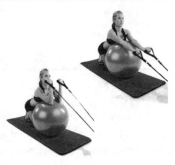

Secure a resistance band at foot level. Lean over the ball with your knees on the floor and grasp the handles, hands about 1 foot apart, palms facing up. Feather your breathing as you curl the band up through a count of 10 seconds. Hold and squeeze for 2 seconds at the MTP. Resist the band down through a count of 10 seconds. Without resting, repeat three times. (Note: The preacher curl is the only curl during which you shouldn't allow your arm to extend fully. Keep your arm slightly bent at the bottom of the motion.)

Dumbbell Curl on Swiss Ball

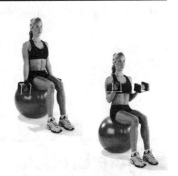

Hold a pair of dumbbells and sit on the ball, arms by your sides with your palms facing away from you. Feather your breathing as you curl the dumbbells through a count of 10 seconds to just past a 90-degree angle. Hold and squeeze for 2 seconds at the MTP. Keep your elbows tight against your body as you lower the weights through a count of 10 seconds. Without resting, repeat three times. (Note: Keep your elbows tight against your sides throughout the exercise.)

Reverse Band Curl

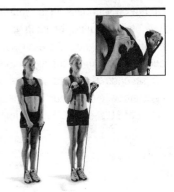

Stand on the center of a resistance band, feet together, and knees slightly bent. Grasp the handles with your arms by your sides, your palms facing back, and your elbows slightly bent. Feather your breathing as you curl the handles up through a count of 10 seconds to just past a 90-degree angle. Hold and squeeze for 2 seconds at the MTP. Keep your elbows tight against your body as you lower the handles through a count of 10 seconds. Without resting, repeat three times. (Note: Keep your elbows tight against your sides throughout the exercise.)

Swiss Ball Ab Roll

Kneel on a mat with your feet resting on the ground behind you. Extend your arms on top of a ball, making fists with your hands. Feather your breathing as you roll forward (using the ball for balance) through a count of 10 seconds, keeping your back straight, head up, and abs tight. Hold for 2 seconds at the MTP (when you're fully extended). Return to starting position through a count of 10 seconds. Without resting, repeat three times.

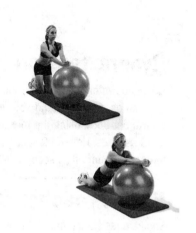

Leg Lift

Lie on your back with your palms down, hands underneath your butt. Crunch up and hold your upper abs tight so that your shoulder blades are off the ground. Lift your legs about 6 inches off the ground. Keep your abs tight and chin up and feather your breathing as you lift your legs through a count of 10 seconds. Hold and squeeze for 2 seconds at the MTP (when your feet are about 2 feet off the ground). Lower your legs to starting position through a count of 10 seconds. Without resting, repeat three times.

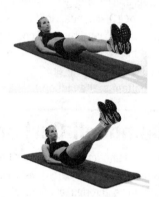

Bicycle Crunch

Lie flat on your back. Place your hands behind your head and raise your legs off the ground, bending your right knee, keeping your chin up and abs tight throughout the exercise. Bring your left elbow to your right knee and feather your breathing as you rotate to the other side for a count of 10 seconds. Hold and squeeze for 2 seconds at the MTP (where your right elbow meets your left knee). Twist to starting position through a count of 10 seconds. Without resting, repeat three times.

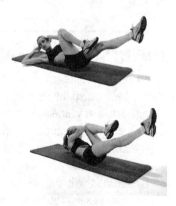

FRIDAY

Flat Dumbbell Press

Holding a pair of dumbbells, lie on a ball so that it comfortably supports your shoulder blades. Extend your arms in front of you, palms facing away from you, pressing the weights together. Feather your breathing as you lower the weights through a count of 10 seconds. Hold for 2 seconds at the MTP (about 1 inch higher than chest level). Press the dumbbells up and together back to starting position through a count of 10 seconds. Without resting, repeat three times.

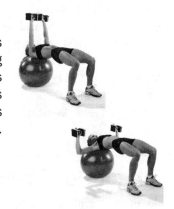

Flat Band Press

Secure a resistance band at about shoulder level. Grasp the handles and hold at chest level, palms facing down. Take a wide step forward with one foot, keeping your back straight, abs tight, and knees slightly bent. Feather your breathing as you press the handles of the band forward through a count of 10 seconds. Hold for 2 seconds at the MTP (just prior to lockout). Return to starting position through a count of 10 seconds. Without resting, repeat three times.

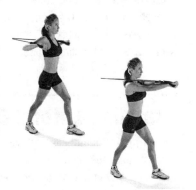

Incline Dumbbell Press

Hold a pair of dumbbells and lie on a ball so that your head and neck are supported. Roll down the ball until your hips drop almost to the ground; do not let your knees go over your ankles. Press the weights up and together, with a slight bend in the elbows, keeping your back straight and abs tight. Feather your breathing as you lower the weights through a count of 10 seconds. Hold for 2 seconds at the MTP. Press the dumbbells up to starting position through a count of 10 seconds. Without resting, repeat three times.

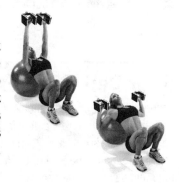

Push-Up on Knees

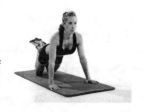

Kneel on a mat on all fours with your feet crossed and lifted slightly off the ground. Your hands should be wider than shoulder-width apart with your fingers and wrists pointing forward. Feather your breathing as you lower your chest toward the floor through a count of 10 seconds. Hold for 2 seconds at the MTP. Push your body back to starting position through a count of 10 seconds, keeping your elbows slightly bent at the top of the move. Without resting, repeat three times.

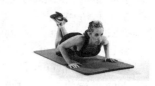

Upright Dumbbell Row

Hold a pair of dumbbells, palms facing your body, your arms extended slightly in front of your thighs. Stand upright with your back straight and abs tight. Feather your breathing as you raise the dumbbells to your chin through a count of 10 seconds. Hold and squeeze for 2 seconds at the MTP. Lower the weights to starting position through a count of 10 seconds. Without resting, repeat three times.

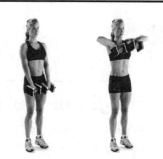

Standing Lateral Dumbbell Raise

Hold a pair of dumbbells and stand with your feet together, your back straight, and abs tight. Extend your arms against your sides, keeping them straight but not locked, and feather your breathing as you raise the weights through a count of 10 seconds. Hold and squeeze for 2 seconds at the MTP ("T" position). Lower the weights to starting position through a count of 10 seconds. Without resting, repeat three times.

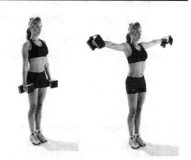

Rear Delt Band Extension

Secure the band at about shoulder level. Grasp the handles and extend your arms in front of you, palms facing in. Feather your breathing as you pull the handles out to a "T" position through a count of 10 seconds, keeping your arms parallel to the floor and a slight bend in your elbows. Hold and squeeze for 2 seconds at the MTP. Resist the band slowly back to starting position through a count of 10 seconds. Without resting, repeat three times.

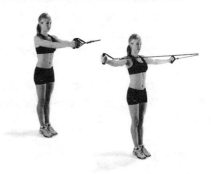

Swiss Ball Crunch with Elevated Feet

Sit on a ball that's about 2 feet away from a wall. Walk your feet out and place them against the wall. Lie down and place your hands behind your ears. Feather your breathing as you crunch up through a count of 10 seconds, using only your abs. Hold and squeeze for 2 seconds at the MTP. Return to starting position through a count of 10 seconds. Without resting, repeat three times. (Note: Keep in mind that the range of motion is significantly smaller on this exercise, so be sure to adjust your pace.)

Reverse Crunch

Lie on a mat with your hands by your sides, palms down. Pull your heels up as close to your butt as possible. Raise your heels about 2 inches off the ground. Keep your chin tucked and abs tight. Feather your breathing as you pull your knees toward your chest, using your lower abdominals, through a count of 10 seconds. Hold and squeeze for 2 seconds at the MTP (when your butt is completely off the ground). Lower your body to starting position through a count of 10 seconds. Without resting, repeat three times.

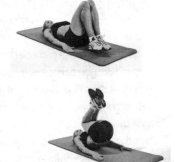

Seated Medicine Ball Twist

Hold a medicine ball just below your chin, about chest level, and sit on the mat with your knees bent, feet crossed. Keep your chin up and abs tight as you lean back slightly and lift your feet from the mat, engaging your abs. Turn to one side to begin exercise. Feather your breathing as you slowly rotate your torso to the other side through a count of 10 seconds. Hold and squeeze for 2 seconds at the MTP (when you've reached the farthest point in the twist). Rotate back to the other side through a count of 10 seconds. Without resting, repeat three times.

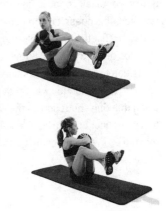

WEEK 6

As you get ready to start week 6, use these tips based on your Life Priority to give you an extra advantage. They are customized to your decade, but I recommend you read every one of them. These tips are jam-packed with valuable information and will give you an extra edge as you face each week.

20s CONFIDENCE

They Make the Woman

The clothing choices you make send a message. Everything from color to fit to style can leave a lasting impression. If you wear UGGS to a job interview, chances are—unless it's for a position like ski instructor—a potential employer isn't going to take you seriously. If your pants are too big or your shirt is wrinkled, you're saying to those around you, "I don't really care that much about this," or, even worse, "I'm lazy and unmotivated." On top of that, you don't feel your best when your clothes are sloppy or fit poorly. There's a saying in sports: "You've got to look good to play good." And the same can be said in the rest of life. If you want to perform your best, you've got to take pride in how you present yourself. This doesn't mean you can't let loose and wear that tiger-print halter top and sexy stilettos out to the clubs. But whenever you're in a position to leave an impression with someone, keep in mind what you want that person to walk away thinking about you. In the world of work, if you want your boss to be able to imagine you moving up in the company, you've got to look professional.

30s MANAGE STRESS

Meditate for a Clear Mind

Doing nothing can sometimes be the best way to relieve stress. Meditation has been used for centuries by many cultures to achieve peace of mind, and even a state of enlightenment. Meditating restores your inner balance and helps release stress. It relaxes the muscles, lowers the heart rate, and raises endorphin levels. It works best when done consistently—every now and then won't be as effective. I generally do it about three times a week and find this effective. First, take off your shoes and get into some loose-fitting clothing. Find a room that is dim and quiet, or maybe you'll want to have a little light music playing in the background. Next, take a comfortable position. Some people prefer the traditional position with legs crossed, but just lying back in your favorite comfortable chair might be better. Now, begin to take a few deep breaths to relax and slow down. Breathe in deeply through your nose and exhale just as deeply from your mouth. Then, instead of trying to "clear" your mind (which for most of us is very difficult to accomplish), visualize an image or an event that brings you joy and focus on that. Continue breathing in through your nose and contract your abs as you exhale. Give yourself about 15 to 20 minutes to "de-stress." Trust me, you will feel a world of difference.

40s PREVENT DECLINE

More Vitamin D

According to my good friend Dr. Mehmet Oz, vitamin D deficiency affects over half of all Americans—and most of them don't even know it! Vitamin D—the "sunshine vitamin"—has been shown to help prevent diseases such as cancer, diabetes, and multiple sclerosis. Plus, it helps prevent muscle loss and protects your bones by helping boost your body's ability to absorb calcium. The problem is most of us live in regions where we don't get enough natural sunlight year round, or we've followed doctor's orders and stayed out of the sun for our skin's sake. While this may be good for your skin, it's potentially putting you at risk for a number of other health problems. Another thing that can prevent your body from properly absorbing vitamin D: being overweight. One research study linked obesity and vitamin D deficiency—another reason to be at your healthy weight. Try getting 10 minutes a day of sunlight and make sure your diet has some quality vitamin D sources such as salmon, tuna, and milk. A quick blood test at your doctor's office will show you where you stand with this critical vitamin.

50s REVERSE DECLINE

Use Wheatgrass to Rejuvenate

One of the greatest preventions against cancer and other diseases may be right beneath your feet. Several studies suggest that wheatgrass may improve the digestive system *and* prevent cancer, diabetes, heart disease, and constipation. Plus, it can detoxify heavy metals from the bloodstream, cleanse the liver, and promote general well-being. Wheatgrass is rich in folic acid and consists mostly of the plant molecule chlorophyll, which is what makes plants green. Chlorophyll has a structure similar to that of our own blood cells and is the part of the wheatgrass that can get into the bloodstream and help clean it up. Wheatgrass also acts as a natural deodorizer, reversing the odor caused by long-term tobacco use. It is commonly sold in 2-ounce "shots" at health-food stores or nationwide at Jamba Juice stores. Even if you're doubtful about the lasting benefits of wheatgrass, there's no denying that it's a good source of vitamins and minerals. So fill up your shot glass, and here's to good health!

MONDAY

Band Squat

Stand on the center of the band, feet together. Pull the band up to your shoulders, palms facing in. Feather your breathing as you slowly squat through a count of 10 seconds. Hold for 2 seconds at the MTP (where you're about 2 inches above an imaginary chair). Return to starting position through a count of 10 seconds. Without resting, repeat three times.

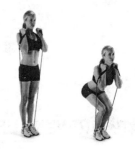

Swiss Ball Squat

Place the ball against a wall and position yourself with the ball supporting your lower back. Hold a pair of dumbbells and keep your arms against your sides. Move your feet forward about 1 foot, hip-width apart, and stand. Feather your breathing as you slowly squat through a count of 10 seconds, never letting your knees extend over your ankles. Hold for 2 seconds at the MTP (when your knees are at about a 90-degree angle). Return to starting position through a count of 10 seconds. Without resting, repeat three times.

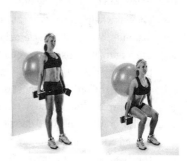

Split Squat

Stand about 3 feet in front of a chair. Place your rear foot on the chair with the top of your shoe lightly touching the chair. With your back straight, chest up, and abs tight, feather your breathing as you bend your front knee, lowering yourself toward the ground through a count of 10 seconds. Hold for 2 seconds at the MTP (when there is about a 90-degree bend in the front knee). Return to starting position through a count of 10 seconds. Without resting, repeat once more on this side and then switch sides and perform 2 more reps for a total of 4.

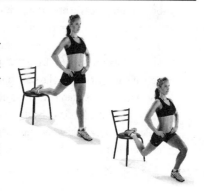

Standing Glute Kickback <small>(with Ankle Cuff)</small>

Secure the band at foot level and attach it to your leg using the ankle cuff. Place a chair in front of you for support, keeping your back straight and head up. Keep your knee slightly bent and feather your breathing as you extend your leg back through a count of 10 seconds, contracting the muscles in your glutes. Hold and squeeze for 2 seconds at the MTP. Return to starting position through a count of 10 seconds. Without resting, repeat once more and then switch sides and perform 2 more reps for a total of 4.

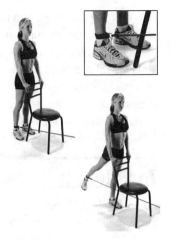

Overhead Triceps Extension

Grasp a dumbbell using the "diamond grip." Sit on the ball with your chest up, back straight, feet shoulder-width apart. Extend your arms with your elbows slightly bent, keeping your biceps tight against your head. Feather your breathing as you lower the dumbbell through a count of 10 seconds. Hold for 2 seconds at the MTP (when your elbows are at about a 90-degree angle). Press the weight up to starting position through a count of 10 seconds. Without resting, repeat three times.

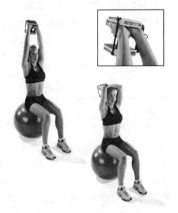

Triceps Press-Down <small>(Reverse Grip)</small>

Secure a resistance band above your head. Grasp the handles with your palms facing up, hands shoulder-width apart. Pull your arms down against your sides, elbows bent at just above a 90-degree angle, palms facing up. Feather your breathing as you pull the handles down and straighten your arms (but do not lock your elbows) through a count of 10. Hold for 2 seconds at the MTP. Resist the band back to starting position through a count of 10 seconds. Without resting, repeat three times.

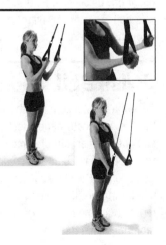

Dumbbell Skull Crusher

Hold a pair of dumbbells and lie on the ball so that your head and neck are supported. Elevate your hips slightly and keep your abs tight. Extend the dumbbells straight up with your palms facing each other, and tilt your arms toward your head slightly. Feather your breathing as you bend your elbows and lower the weights through a count of 10 seconds. Hold for 2 seconds at the MTP (about 1 inch above your forehead). Raise dumbbells to starting position through a count of 10 seconds. Without resting, repeat three times.

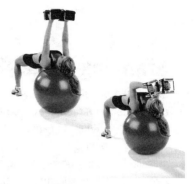

Toe Reach

Lie on your back. Cross your legs, flex your feet, and extend your legs into the air. With your arms extended and chin up off your chest, feather your breathing as you crunch up, reaching toward your toes through a count of 10 seconds. Hold and squeeze for 2 seconds at the MTP. Lower yourself to starting position, keeping your shoulder blades from touching the ground, through a count of 10 seconds. Without resting, repeat three times.

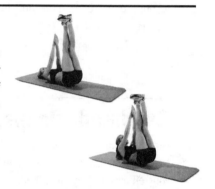

Reverse Crunch

Lie on a mat with your hands by your sides, palms down. Pull your heels up as close to your butt as possible. Raise your heels about 2 inches off the ground. Keep your chin tucked and abs tight. Feather your breathing as you pull your knees toward your chest, using your lower abdominals, through a count of 10 seconds. Hold and squeeze for 2 seconds at the MTP (when your butt is completely off the ground). Lower your body to starting position through a count of 10 seconds. Without resting, repeat three times.

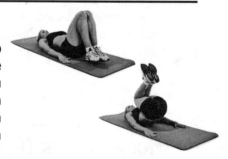

Swiss Ball Woodchopper

Secure a resistance band above your head. Sit on the ball and grasp the handles with both hands, feet on the ground, chest up, back and arms straight. Feather your breathing as you pull the handles down and across your body by twisting and contracting your obliques through a count of 10 seconds. Hold and squeeze for 2 seconds at the MTP. Resist the band to starting position through a count of 10 seconds. Without resting, repeat once more on this side and then switch position and complete 2 more reps for a total of 4.

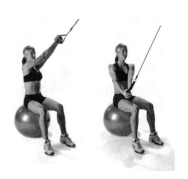

WEDNESDAY

Kneeling Band Pull-Down (Close Grip)

Secure a resistance band above your head. Kneel on a mat and grasp the handles with your palms facing each other. Sit back on your heels with your arms fully outstretched; keep your back straight, chest up, and abs tight. Feather your breathing as you pull the handles toward the top part of your chest through a count of 10 seconds. Hold and squeeze for 2 seconds at the MTP. Resist the band back to starting position through a count of 10 seconds. Without resting, repeat three times.

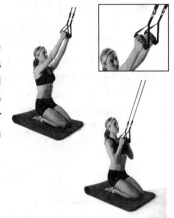

Dumbbell Row on Swiss Ball

Holding a pair of dumbbells, lie on a ball so that the middle of your waist is centered on it. Raise your head and chest, creating a slight arch in the back. Feather your breathing as you pull the dumbbells up and back toward your hips in a rowing motion through a count of 10 seconds. Hold and squeeze the shoulder blades together for 2 seconds at the MTP. Return to starting position through a count of 10 seconds. Without resting, repeat three times.

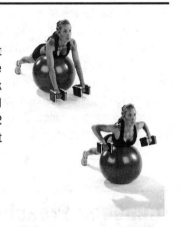

Band Row (Overhand Grip)

Secure a resistance band at about shoulder level. Grasp the handles and hold arms extended at chest height, palms facing down. Take a wide step forward with one foot, keeping your back straight, abs tight, and knees slightly bent. Feather your breathing as you pull the dumbbells toward your chest in a fluid rowing motion through a count of 10 seconds, keeping your elbows close to your body. Hold and squeeze your shoulder blades together for 2 seconds at the MTP. Lower your arms to starting position through a count of 10 seconds. Without resting, repeat three times.

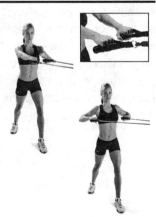

Reverse Hyperextension

Lie facedown on a ball. Roll yourself forward until the ball is under your hips and your upper body is angled toward the floor. Place your palms about 6 inches wider than shoulder-width apart on the floor. With legs together, feather your breathing as you raise your heels toward the ceiling, using your lower back and hamstrings, through a count of 10 seconds. Hold and squeeze for 2 seconds at the MTP. With straight legs, lower to starting position through a count of 10 seconds, about 2 inches from the ground. Without resting, repeat three times.

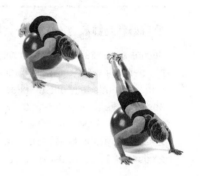

Standing Band Curl

Stand on the center of a resistance band, feet together and knees slightly bent. Grasp the handles, keeping your slightly bent arms by your sides, palms facing forward. Feather your breathing as you curl up through a count of 10 seconds to just past a 90-degree angle. Hold and squeeze for 2 seconds at the MTP. Keep your elbows tight against your body as you lower the handles through a count of 10 seconds. Without resting, repeat three times. (Note: Keep your elbows tight against your sides throughout the exercise.)

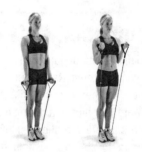

Dumbbell Preacher Curl

Holding a pair of dumbbells, rest your chest on the ball. Knees should be on the floor with a 6- to 8-inch gap between your arms. Bend your elbows to a 90-degree angle. Feather your breathing as you lower the weights through a count of 10 seconds until your arms are extended but your elbows are not locked. Hold and squeeze for 2 seconds at the MTP. Raise the dumbbells to starting position through a count of 10 seconds. Without resting, repeat three times.

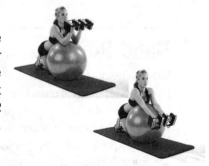

Band Concentration Curl

Secure a resistance band above your head. Grasp the handle with one hand, extending your arm, palm facing up. Keeping a slight bend in your knees, feather your breathing as you curl through a count of 10 seconds to just past a 90-degree angle. Hold and squeeze for 2 seconds at the MTP. Resist the band to starting position through a count of 10 seconds. Without resting, repeat once more on this side and then switch sides and complete 2 more reps for a total of 4.

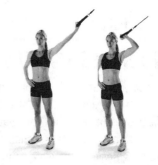

Reverse Crunch

Lie on a mat with your hands by your sides, palms down. Pull your heels up as close to your butt as possible. Raise your heels about 2 inches off the ground. Keep your chin tucked and abs tight. Feather your breathing as you pull your knees toward your chest, using your lower abdominals, through a count of 10 seconds. Hold and squeeze for 2 seconds at the MTP (when your butt is completely off the ground). Lower your body to starting position through a count of 10 seconds. Without resting, repeat three times.

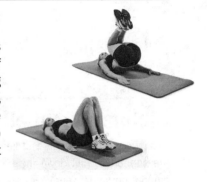

Kneeling Band Crunch

Secure a resistance band above your head and kneel on a mat. Grasp the handles in front of your forehead, palms facing toward you. Keep your abs tight and feather your breathing as you crunch toward the mat through a count of 10 seconds. Hold for 2 seconds at the MTP (about 2 inches from the mat). Resist the band back to starting position through a count of 10 seconds. Without resting, repeat three times.

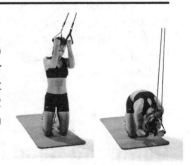

Seated Medicine Ball Twist

Hold a medicine ball just below your chin, about chest level, and sit on the mat with your knees bent, feet crossed. Keep your chin up and abs tight as you lean back slightly and lift your feet from the mat, engaging your abs. Turn to one side to begin exercise. Feather your breathing as you slowly rotate your torso to the other side through a count of 10 seconds. Hold and squeeze for 2 seconds at the MTP (when you've reached the farthest point in the twist). Rotate back to the other side through a count of 10 seconds. Without resting, repeat three times.

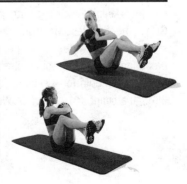

FRIDAY

Incline Push-Up

Place your hands in a push-up position against a wall or a set of stairs, so that your upper body is elevated above your feet. Keep your head up, back straight, and abs tight. Feather your breathing as you lower yourself through a count of 10 seconds. Hold for 2 seconds at the MTP. Return to starting position through a count of 10 seconds. Without resting, repeat three times.

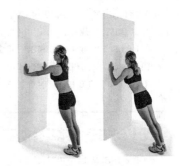

Incline Dumbbell Press

Hold a pair of dumbbells and lie on a ball so that your head and neck are supported. Roll down the ball until your hips drop almost to the ground; do not let your knees go over your ankles. Press the weights up and together, with a slight bend in the elbows, keeping your back straight and abs tight. Feather your breathing as you lower the weights through a count of 10 seconds. Hold for 2 seconds at the MTP. Press the dumbbells up to starting position through a count of 10 seconds. Without resting, repeat three times.

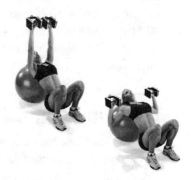

Downward Band Fly

Secure a resistance band above your head. Take a wide step forward with one foot, keeping your back straight, abs tight, and knees slightly bent. Grasp the handles with your arms slightly bent at the elbows and stretched in a wide "T" shape, palms facing forward. Feather your breathing as you bring your palms down and together through a count of 10 seconds. Hold for 2 seconds at the MTP. Return to starting position through a count of 10 seconds. Without resting, repeat three times.

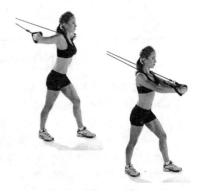

Upward Band Fly

Secure a resistance band at about waist level. Take a wide step forward with one foot, keeping your back straight, abs tight, and knees slightly bent. Grasp the handles with your arms extended behind you, palms angled down, with a slight bend in your elbows. Feather your breathing as you bring your palms up and together through a count of 10 seconds. Hold for 2 seconds at the MTP. Return to starting position through a count of 10 seconds. Without resting, repeat three times.

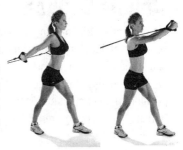

Chicken Wings

Holding a pair of dumbbells, stand with your legs hip-width apart, knees slightly bent. Bend your elbows, holding the dumbbells in front of you at a 45-degree angle. Keep the forearms tight and feather your breathing as you raise your elbows out and up through a count of 10 seconds. Hold and squeeze for 2 seconds at the MTP. Return to starting position through a count of 10 seconds. Without resting, repeat three times. (Note: Be sure to relax your neck and avoid shrugging your shoulders during this movement.)

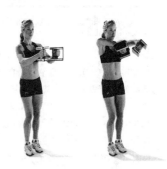

Bent-Over Rear Delt Raise

Hold a pair of dumbbells, palms facing each other. Bend at the waist as if you were about to tie your shoes; then lift only your chin and chest, creating a slight arch in your back. Feather your breathing as you raise the weights out and up to your sides through a count of 10 seconds. Hold and squeeze for 2 seconds at the MTP. Lower the weights to starting position through a count of 10 seconds. Without resting, repeat three times.

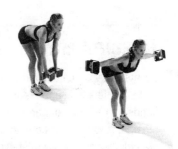

Upright Dumbbell Row

Hold a pair of dumbbells, palms facing your body, your arms extended slightly in front of your thighs. Stand upright with your back straight and abs tight. Feather your breathing as you raise the dumbbells to your chin through a count of 10 seconds. Hold and squeeze for 2 seconds at the MTP. Lower the weights to starting position through a count of 10 seconds. Without resting, repeat three times.

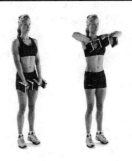

Double Crunch

Lie on a mat with your knees bent and hands behind your head. Raise your feet about 2 inches off the ground. Feather your breathing as you simultaneously crunch and raise your knees up through a count of 10 seconds. Hold and squeeze for 2 seconds at the MTP. Return to starting position through a count of 10 seconds. Keep your feet elevated as you transition into the next rep. Without resting, repeat three times.

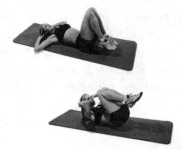

Leg Lift

Lie on your back with your palms down, hands underneath your butt. Crunch up and hold your upper abs tight so that your shoulder blades are off the ground. Lift your legs about 6 inches off the ground. Keep your abs tight and chin up and feather your breathing as you lift your legs through a count of 10 seconds. Hold and squeeze for 2 seconds at the MTP (when your feet are about 2 feet off the ground). Lower your legs to starting position through a count of 10 seconds. Without resting, repeat three times.

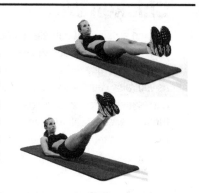

Russian Band Twist on Swiss Ball

Secure a resistance band at head level. Lie on the ball so that your head and shoulders are supported, hips elevated. Hold the handles with both hands and extend your arms away from your chest, palms toward each other. Turn your upper body to one side to begin exercise. Feather your breathing as you slowly rotate your torso as far as possible to the other side through a count of 10 seconds. Hold and squeeze for 2 seconds at the MTP. Rotate back to the other side through a count of 10 seconds. Without resting, repeat once more on this side and then switch sides and complete 2 more reps for a total of 4.

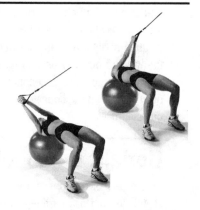

WEEK 7

As you get ready to start week 7, use these tips based on your Life Priority to give you an extra advantage. They are customized to your decade, but I recommend you read every one of them. These tips are jam-packed with valuable information and will give you an extra edge as you face each week.

20s CONFIDENCE

Skin Care

When you're in your twenties, you're lucky to have fresh-looking, wrinkle-free skin. But guess what? All those nights of not enough sleep and days of poor eating will catch up with you! That's why it's important to take some simple steps today to keep your skin clear and free from things like sun damage and scars. Having clear skin can also help increase your confidence, so even if you have a few blemishes now, treating your skin right will create immediate rewards. Start by making sure you wear sunscreen every day, regardless of the weather; skin-care experts recommend at least SPF 15 or higher. Also, never go to sleep with your makeup still on. Doing so can clog pores and prevent the beneficial effects of sleep from working their magic on your skin. My friend and makeup empress extraordinaire, Bobbi Brown, reminds us that hydration is important too. She says (as I do) to shoot for about eight 8-ounce glasses a day, or more depending on your body weight (see Chapter 3 for details). Try herbal teas instead of coffee to mix it up a bit—some studies have shown the polyphenols in green tea could be beneficial in preventing skin cancer.

30s MANAGE STRESS

Use Natural Herbs

Let's face it, no matter what we do there will always be some level of stress in our lives. While there really isn't a way to "cure" stress, you can learn how to manage it. Stress is a mental and physical reaction we have to events that disrupt our personal balance in some way, and it can wreak havoc on your health if you're not careful. Before you run to the pharmacist for help, I recommend you try a more natural solution. Certain herbs have been used for centuries to help ease the effects of stress. Here are a few that I recommend and use. I also recommend that you consult your doctor if you currently take any medications or supplements.

- *Valerian:* A very mild sedative, traditionally used to treat mild anxiety. It is usually taken about an hour before you go to bed.
- *Kava:* Great for stress and anxiety.
- *St. John's wort:* Used for centuries in many countries to reduce anxiety and to treat depression.
- *Chamomile:* Most often consumed as a tea. I usually have it after dinner since it aids in digestion and helps me fall asleep.
- *Skullcap:* A mild sedative that is great for relaxing. You can find it as a tea or in pill or liquid extract form.

40s PREVENT DECLINE

Swap Meat for Soy

To help prevent an increase in your LDL, otherwise known as "bad" cholesterol, explore soy as an alternative to animal protein. Reducing your intake of saturated fats such as those found in fatty cuts of meat will also help lower your risk of developing some types of cancers. Getting more soy does not mean putting more soy sauce on your rice. It means taking a great dish like the Beef Tenderloin Salad with Garlic Vinaigrette on page 160 and replacing the beef with tofu or tempeh. Soy comes in many forms, but tofu or tempeh would be the easiest to use in place of meat. Also try soy nuts as a snack or use soy milk in your morning cereal. What's soy's secret? For one, it has soluble fiber, which helps clean cholesterol out of your body. Soy also has been shown to reduce symptoms of perimenopause, such as hot flashes, and it is thought to be one of the main reasons why women in Japan and some other countries experience a less difficult transition from perimenopause into menopause.

50s REVERSE DECLINE

Consume More Fiber

Fiber consumption is absolutely critical to your health, and many women don't consume nearly enough of it! Consuming 25 to 30 grams of fiber each day can drastically reduce the risk of certain diseases, such as colon cancer, breast cancer, and heart disease. Fiber keeps things moving along regularly—it speeds up the passage of food through the colon. This keeps harmful elements in certain foods from affecting the colon and can prevent colon cancer. Consuming more fiber also has fantastic weight-loss benefits because it can eliminate "false belly fat" and it helps reduce appetite. Another benefit is a lower blood cholesterol level, which reduces your risk for developing heart disease. Be sure to choose you fiber sources wisely. A delicious-looking whole-grain muffin might be full of fiber, but it might also be full of fat and sugar. Be aware of where your fiber is coming from.

Plié Squat

Secure a resistance band at head level. Lie on the ball so that your head and shoulders are supported, hips elevated. Hold the handles with both hands and extend your arms away from your chest, palms toward each other. Turn your upper body to one side to begin exercise. Feather your breathing as you slowly rotate your torso as far as possible to the other side through a count of 10 seconds. Hold and squeeze for 2 seconds at the MTP. Rotate back to the other side through a count of 10 seconds. Without resting, repeat once more on this side and then switch sides and complete 2 more reps for a total of 4.

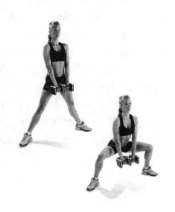

Dumbbell Squat

Hold a pair of dumbbells and stand with your feet shoulder-width apart. Feather your breathing as you slowly squat through a count of 10 seconds, keeping your back straight, abs tight, and chest up. Hold for 2 seconds at the MTP (where you're about 2 inches above an imaginary chair), never letting your knees extend over your ankles. Return to starting position through a count of 10 seconds. Without resting, repeat three times.

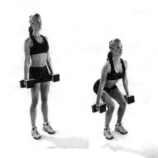

Lateral Squat

Take a stance about 1 foot wider than shoulder-width on each side. Feather your breathing as you squat toward one leg, keeping your chest high (do not twist or lean forward) and the opposite leg straight, through a count of 10 seconds. Hold for 2 seconds at the MTP. Return to starting position through a count of 10 seconds. Without resting, perform 2 reps on each side for a total of 4.

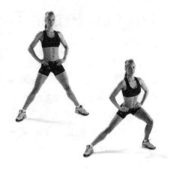

Swiss Ball Squat

Place the ball against a wall and position yourself with the ball supporting your lower back. Hold a pair of dumbbells and keep your arms against your sides. Move your feet forward about 1 foot, hip-width apart, and stand. Feather your breathing as you slowly squat through a count of 10 seconds, never letting your knees extend over your ankles. Hold for 2 seconds at the MTP (when your knees are at about a 90-degree angle). Return to starting position through a count of 10 seconds. Without resting, repeat three times.

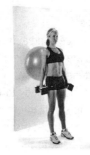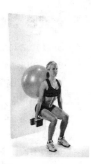

Incline Diamond Push-Up

Place your hands in a push-up position against a wall or a set of stairs; then shift your hands into the center to form a "diamond." Be sure that your upper body is elevated above your feet. Keep your head up, back straight, and abs tight. Feather your breathing as you lower yourself through a count of 10 seconds. Hold for 2 seconds at the MTP. Return to starting position through a count of 10 seconds. Without resting, repeat three times.

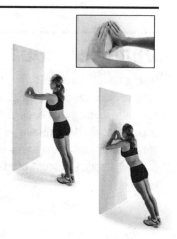

Triceps Press-Down

Secure a resistance band above your head. Grasp the handles, keeping your hands about 1 foot apart. Pull your arms down against your sides, elbows bent at just above a 90-degree angle, palms facing down. Feather your breathing as you press the handles down and straighten your arms (but do not lock your elbows) through a count of 10 seconds. Hold for 2 seconds at the MTP. Resist the band back to starting position through a count of 10 seconds. Without resting, repeat three times.

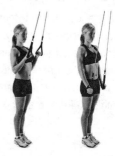

Standing Kickback

Hold a pair of dumbbells, palms facing each other. With your knees slightly bent, bend at the waist as if you were about to tie your shoes; then lift only your chin and chest, creating a slight arch in your back. Raise your elbows as high as possible, keeping them close to your body. Feather your breathing as you extend the weights back (without moving the upper part of the arm) through a count of 10 seconds. Hold and squeeze for 2 seconds at the MTP. Return the weights to starting position through a count of 10 seconds. Without resting, repeat three times.

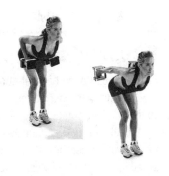

Seated V-Up

Sit on a mat with your arms behind you, elbows bent, and fingertips pointed toward your body. Start with your legs together and extended, knees slightly bent, and heels about 2 inches off the ground. Lean your upper body weight back on your palms slightly. Feather your breathing as you pull your knees into your chest through a count of 10 seconds. Hold and squeeze for 2 seconds at the MTP. Return to starting position through a count of 10 seconds, keeping your abs tight. Without resting, repeat three times.

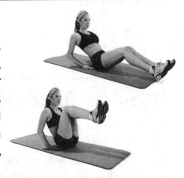

Swiss Ball Crunch with Elevated Feet

Sit on a ball that's about 2 feet away from a wall. Walk your feet out and place them against the wall. Lie down and place your hands behind your ears. Feather your breathing as you crunch up through a count of 10 seconds, using only your abs. Hold and squeeze for 2 seconds at the MTP. Return to starting position through a count of 10 seconds. Without resting, repeat three times. (Note: Keep in mind that the range of motion is significantly smaller on this exercise, so be sure to adjust your pace.)

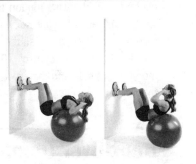

Bicycle Crunch

Lie flat on your back. Place your hands behind your head and raise your legs off the ground, bending your right knee, keeping your chin up and abs tight throughout the exercise. Bring your left elbow to your right knee and feather your breathing as you rotate to the other side for a count of 10 seconds. Hold and squeeze for 2 seconds at the MTP (where your right elbow meets your left knee). Twist to starting position through a count of 10 seconds. Without resting, repeat three times.

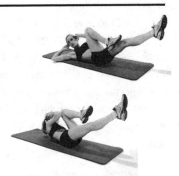

WEDNESDAY

Kneeling Band Pull-Down (Overhand)

Secure a resistance band at about head level. Kneel on a mat and grasp the handles with your palms facing down. Sit back on your heels with your arms fully outstretched; keep your back straight, chest up, and abs tight. Feather your breathing as you pull the handles down toward the top part of your chest through a count of 10 seconds. Hold and squeeze for 2 seconds at the MTP. Resist the band back to starting position through a count of 10 seconds. Without resting, repeat three times.

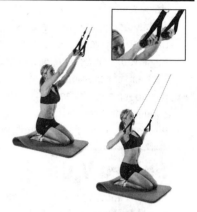

One-Arm Band Row

Secure a resistance band about chest high. Grasp the handle with your left hand and extend your arm, palm facing in. Take a wide step forward with your right foot, keeping your back straight, abs tight, and knees slightly bent. Feather your breathing as you pull the handle toward your chest in a fluid rowing motion through a count of 10 seconds, keeping your elbow close to your body. Hold and squeeze your shoulder blades together for 2 seconds at the MTP. Resist the band back to starting position through a count of 10 seconds. Without resting, repeat once more on this side and then switch sides and complete 2 more reps for a total of 4.

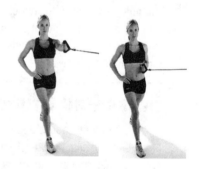

Bent-Over Dumbbell Row (Underhand Grip)

Holding a pair of dumbbells, extend your arms, palms facing forward. Stand with your feet hip-width apart. Bend at the waist as if you were tying your shoes. Raise your head and chest to create a slight arch in the back. Bend your knees slightly. Feather your breathing as you pull the dumbbells up in a fluid rowing motion through a count of 10 seconds, keeping your elbows close to your body. Hold and squeeze your shoulder blades together for 2 seconds at the MTP. Lower your arms to starting position through a count of 10 seconds. Without resting, repeat three times.

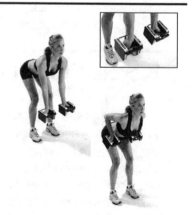

Dumbbell Dead Lift

Stand holding a dumbbell in each hand with your feet about 6 to 8 inches apart. Bend over at the waist as if you were about to tie your shoes. Lift your chin and chest creating a slight arch in your back. Feather your breathing as you lift your upper body through a count of 10 seconds, driving through your heels and using your lower back and hamstrings, keeping your knees slightly bent. Hold for 2 seconds at the MTP (when you are standing). Return to starting position through a count of 10 seconds. Without resting, repeat three times.

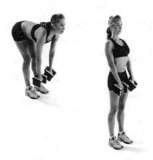

Side Curls on Swiss Ball

Hold a pair of dumbbells and sit on the ball. With your arms down against your sides, palms turned up, and elbows tight against your body, feather your breathing as you curl the weights up through a count of 10 seconds. Hold and squeeze for 2 seconds at the MTP. Lower the weights to starting position through a count of 10 seconds. Without resting, repeat three times.

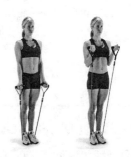

Standing Band Curl

Stand on the center of a resistance band, feet together and knees slightly bent. Grasp the handles, keeping your slightly bent arms by your sides, palms facing forward. Feather your breathing as you curl up through a count of 10 seconds to just past a 90-degree angle. Hold and squeeze for 2 seconds at the MTP. Keep your elbows tight against your body as you lower the handles through a count of 10 seconds. Without resting, repeat three times. (Note: Keep your elbows tight against your sides throughout the exercise.)

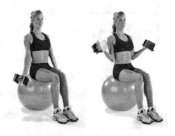

Hammer Curl

Holding a pair of dumbbells, stand with your feet shoulder-width apart, your arms extended slightly in front of your thighs, palms facing each other, knees slightly bent. Feather your breathing as you curl the weight through a count of 10 seconds, keeping your palms facing each other. Hold and squeeze for 2 seconds at the MTP. Lower the weight to starting position through a count of 10 seconds. Without resting, repeat three times.

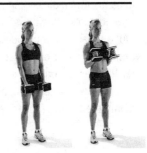

Medicine Ball Pull-Over

Lie on a mat and bring your knees up to a 90-degree angle, feet crossed. Grasp a medicine ball and extend it over your head, keeping a slight bend in your elbows. Keep your abs tight and feather your breathing as you raise the ball over your head and crunch up through a count of 10 seconds. Hold for 2 seconds at the MTP. Lower the ball to starting position through a count of 10 seconds. Without resting, repeat three times.

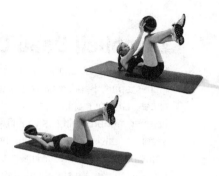

Jackknife

Stand about 3 feet in front of the ball and place your palms on the ground, hands shoulder-width apart. Put one foot on the ball slightly below mid-shin level. Once level, place the other foot on the ball keeping your head forward, spine straight, and abs tight. Slowly pull your knees up to your chin through a count of 10 seconds as you concentrate on keeping stability by squeezing your abs tight. Hold and squeeze for 2 seconds at the MTP. Return to starting position through a count of 10 seconds. Without resting, repeat three times.

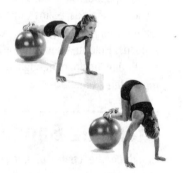

Upward Woodchopper on Swiss Ball

Secure a resistance band at foot level. Sit on the ball and place your feet in front of you about hip-width apart. Grip the handle with both hands, fingers entwined, keeping your chest up and your back and arms straight (do not lock your elbows). Feather your breathing as you pull the handles up and across your body by twisting and contracting your obliques through a count of 10 seconds. Hold and squeeze for 2 seconds at the MTP. Resist the band to starting position through a count of 10 seconds. Without resting, repeat once more on this side and then switch sides and complete 2 more reps for a total of 4.

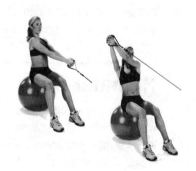

FRIDAY

Incline Dumbbell Press

Hold a pair of dumbbells and lie on a ball so that your head and neck are supported. Roll down the ball until your hips drop almost to the ground; do not let your knees go over your ankles. Press the weights up and together, with a slight bend in the elbows, keeping your back straight and abs tight. Feather your breathing as you lower the weights through a count of 10 seconds. Hold for 2 seconds at the MTP. Press the dumbbells up to starting position through a count of 10 seconds. Without resting, repeat three times.

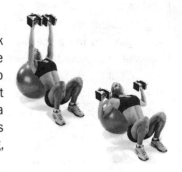

Incline Band Press

Secure a resistance band at about waist height. Grasp the handles and hold at chest height, elbows bent, palms facing down. Take a wide step forward with one foot, keeping your back straight, abs tight, and knees slightly bent. Feather your breathing as you press the handles of the band forward and up through a count of 10 seconds. At the top of the motion, your hands should be in line with your eyes. Hold for 2 seconds at the MTP (when your arms are straight but not locked). Return to starting position through a count of 10 seconds. Without resting, repeat three times.

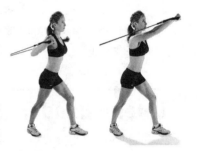

Flat Band Press

Secure a resistance band at about shoulder level. Grasp the handles and hold at chest level, palms facing down. Take a wide step forward with one foot, keeping your back straight, abs tight, and knees slightly bent. Feather your breathing as you press the handles of the band forward through a count of 10 seconds. Hold for 2 seconds at the MTP (just prior to lockout). Return to starting position through a count of 10 seconds. Without resting, repeat three times.

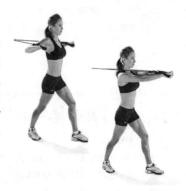

Push-Up on Knees

Kneel on a mat on all fours with your feet crossed and lifted slightly off the ground. Your hands should be wider than shoulder-width apart with your fingers and wrists pointing forward. Feather your breathing as you lower your chest toward the floor through a count of 10 seconds. Hold for 2 seconds at the MTP. Push your body back to starting position through a count of 10 seconds, keeping your elbows slightly bent at the top of the move. Without resting, repeat three times.

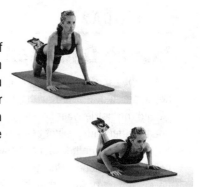

Standing Dumbbell Press

Holding a pair of dumbbells, take a wide step forward with one foot, keeping your back straight, abs tight, and knees slightly bent. Extend the weights up and together directly over your head, palms facing forward. Feather your breathing as you lower the weights through a count of 10 seconds. Hold for 2 seconds at the MTP (chin level). Press the dumbbells up to starting position through a count of 10 seconds. Without resting, repeat three times.

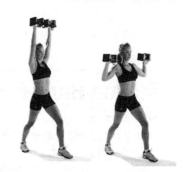

Lateral Band Raise

Stand on top of the center of a resistance band with your feet together, back straight, and abs tight. Grasp the handles so that your arms are straight but not locked, your palms facing inward. Feather your breathing as you raise your arms to a "T" position through a count of 10 seconds. Hold and squeeze for 2 seconds at the MTP. Return to starting position through a count of 10 seconds. Without resting, repeat three times.

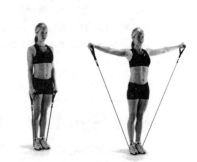

Bent-Over Rear Delt Raise

Hold a pair of dumbbells, palms facing each other. Bend at the waist as if you were about to tie your shoes; then lift only your chin and chest, creating a slight arch in your back. Feather your breathing as you raise the weights out and up to your sides through a count of 10 seconds. Hold and squeeze for 2 seconds at the MTP. Lower the weights to starting position through a count of 10 seconds. Without resting, repeat three times.

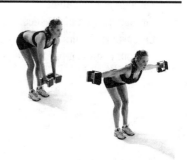

Band Crunch on Swiss Ball

Secure a resistance band at about head level. Hold the handles, palms facing back. Position a ball on the ground between you and the wall. Sit on it; then roll down the ball until your hips drop almost to the ground, never letting your knees go over your ankles. Pull the handles down until they rest against the top of your head. Feather your breathing as you crunch down, pulling your elbows to your knees, through a count of 10 seconds. Hold and squeeze for 2 seconds at the MTP. Lower yourself to starting position through a count of 10 seconds. Without resting, repeat three times.

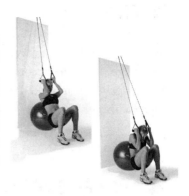

Band Tuck-Up on Chair

Secure a resistance band at foot level. Sit on a sturdy chair and reach your hands behind you to grab the sides. Place your feet in the handles of the band, extend your legs out, and allow your upper body to lean back slightly. Feather your breathing as you draw your knees in and up toward your chin through a count of 10 seconds. Hold and squeeze for 2 seconds at the MTP. Return to starting position through a count of 10 seconds. Without resting, repeat three times.

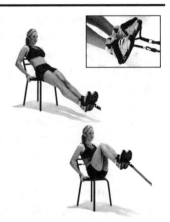

Woodchopper

Secure a resistance band above your head. Stand with your legs about 3 feet apart; keep your chest up, back and arms straight. Feather your breathing as you pull the handles down and across your body by twisting and contracting your obliques through a count of 10 seconds. Hold and squeeze for 2 seconds at the MTP. Resist the weight back to starting position through a count of 10 seconds. Without resting, repeat once more on this side and then switch sides and complete 2 more reps for a total of 4.

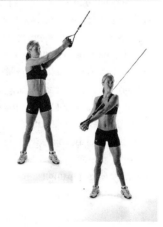

WEEK 8

As you get ready to start week 8, use these tips based on your Life Priority to give you an extra advantage. They are customized to your decade, but I recommend you read every one of them. These tips are jam-packed with valuable information and will give you an extra edge as you face each week.

20s CONFIDENCE

Lessening PMS

PMS can put a cramp in your style—literally. Not only cramps but bloating, cravings, and irritability can make this a very tough time of the month. Luckily, there are some steps you can take to help make PMS a smoother sail. First, try swapping out high-fat foods for lower-fat selections. Instead of a big juicy steak, try a nice grilled piece of salmon. To help relieve bloating, keep your salt intake down and be sure to drink plenty of water to help flush out extra fluids. Be sure to load up on nutrient-rich foods. Vitamin B6, vitamin A, vitamin E, calcium, and magnesium all help relieve PMS symptoms, so look for foods rich in these. Eat more fish, citrus fruits, olive oil, and spinach, to name just a few. For herbal remedies, try valerian root and evening primrose, which have been shown to relieve mood swings and depression that result from PMS. And even though it may be the last thing you feel like doing, get up and exercise! Try getting your 20 minutes of cardio in and you'll notice the stress in your body deflate—because you're moving oxygen through your body and opening those tight muscles. Plus, getting exercise helps regulate your hormone levels.

30s MANAGE STRESS

The Celebrity Secret

One great but simple trick I like to use when I feel stress creeping up is a tension-release exercise. Actors and many public speakers have been using it for years to calm their nerves and get rid of unwanted anxiety, and the best thing is, you can do it anywhere. First, lie flat on your back if possible; if not, a chair will be fine. Then close your eyes and take a few very deep breaths, inhaling for an entire 6-second count and using the same count on your exhale. After a few deep breaths, tense your brow and keep it tense through an inhale count of 6 seconds; then, as you exhale, relax your forehead and imagine that all the stress that was building up is purged from your body with the release of your breath. Working from top to bottom, continue to use this technique with all the muscles in your face, then your neck, and so on, working your way one section at a time down to the tips of your toes. Remember, tense on the inhale and then relax and release your stress on the exhale. Once you have completed this exercise for every section of your body, take one final extra deep inhale and try tensing every muscle in your whole body; then completely relax and breathe out any remaining stress. This simple 5-minute technique is great whenever you need a mental health break.

40s PREVENT DECLINE

Go Organic!

Consider the little extra money you spend on organic foods as an investment in your health. Studies have shown that organic foods have higher levels of *flavonoids*—compounds that have been linked to protecting against cardiovascular disease and age-related diseases such as dementia. Researchers at the University of California, Davis, compared tomatoes grown in organic and nonorganic fields over ten years and discovered surprising results: The organic tomatoes had almost double the amount of flavonoids compared with the regular ones. Another study, done in Wales, found that organic milk contained over 60 percent more omega-3s than conventional milk. Each study suggested that the increase in nutritional benefits was due to natural processes used at organic farms—the organic tomato fields were fertilized with tomato mulch and not pesticides, and cows on the organic farm ate clover instead of synthetic concentrates. Bottom line: You can eat less of organic foods and get *more* disease-fighting benefits—and that's a deal no one should turn down.

50s REVERSE DECLINE

Glucosamine and Chondroitin

As we get older, here come aches and pains in our joints and sometimes the nasty, nagging pain of arthritis. Want a more natural and safer remedy for joint pain than an anti-inflammatory? Try taking the natural supplements glucosamine and chondroitin. These are the molecules that actually make up your cartilage, which is worn down as you age. The deterioration of cartilage is what creates stiff and sore joints and can lead to arthritis. Our bodies naturally produce a certain amount of glucosamine, but as we grow older our ability to produce glucosamine declines and the risk for developing osteoarthritis and other joint problems increases. Studies have shown that a glucosamine and chondroitin supplement is effective in easing osteoarthritis pain, rehabilitating cartilage, and repairing joints damaged from wear and tear. Glucosamine and chondroitin have also been shown to combat the effects of osteoporosis. Again, talk with your doctor before supplementing with this or any other natural remedy.

MONDAY

Split Squat

Stand about 3 feet in front of a chair. Place your rear foot on the chair with the top of your shoe lightly touching the chair. With your back straight, chest up, and abs tight, feather your breathing as you bend your front knee, lowering yourself toward the ground through a count of 10 seconds. Hold for 2 seconds at the MTP (when there is about a 90-degree bend in the front knee). Return to starting position through a count of 10 seconds. Without resting, repeat once more and then switch sides and perform 2 more reps for a total of 4.

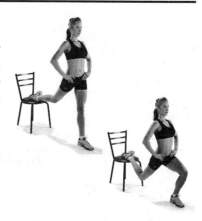

Swiss Ball Squat

Place the ball against a wall and position yourself with the ball supporting your lower back. Hold a pair of dumbbells and keep your arms against your sides. Move your feet forward about 1 foot, hip-width apart, and stand. Feather your breathing as you slowly squat through a count of 10 seconds, never letting your knees over your ankles. Hold for 2 seconds at the MTP (when your knees are at about a 90-degree angle). Return to starting position through a count of 10 seconds. Without resting, repeat three times.

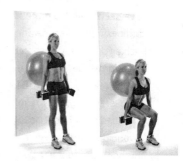

Weighted Lunge

Stand in a lunge position holding a dumbbell in one hand and the other resting on the back of a chair for balance. Keep your back straight, chest up, and abs tight. Feather your breathing as you drop your back knee toward the ground through a count of 10 seconds. Hold for 2 seconds at the MTP (about 1 inch above the ground). Return to starting position through a count of 10 seconds. Without resting, repeat one more time on this leg and then perform 2 more reps on the other side for a total of 4. (Note: To avoid injury, make sure that your front knee stays aligned with your toes and doesn't bend beyond a 90-degree angle.)

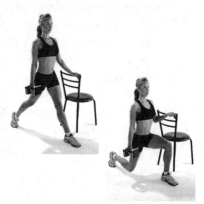

Hamstring Curl with Swiss Ball

Lie on your back with your arms at your sides, palms flat on the floor. Place your heels on the ball, knees straight but not locked. Tighten your abs and lift your butt and hips off the ground. Feather your breathing and bend your knees as you roll the ball toward your butt with your heels through a count of 10 seconds. Hold for 2 seconds at the MTP. Return to starting position through a count of 10 seconds. Without resting, repeat three times.

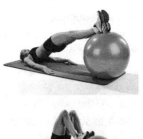

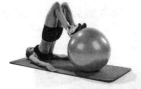

Chair Dip

Sit on the edge of a sturdy chair with your hands behind you, fingers forward, grasping the edge of the chair. Flex your feet so that your weight is on your heels and slide yourself an inch or so away from the chair. Feather your breathing as you lower yourself through a count of 10 seconds. Hold for 2 seconds at the MTP. Push yourself up to starting position through a count of 10 seconds. Without resting, repeat three times. (Note: The MTP will vary based on your shoulder flexibility—about 1 inch above your most flexible point.)

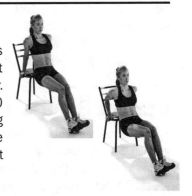

Overhead Triceps Extension

Grasp a dumbbell using the "diamond grip." Sit on the ball with your chest up, back straight, feet shoulder-width apart. Extend your arms with your elbows slightly bent, keeping your biceps tight against your head. Feather your breathing as you lower the dumbbell through a count of 10 seconds. Hold for 2 seconds at the MTP (when your elbows are at about a 90-degree angle). Press the weight up to starting position through a count of 10 seconds. Without resting, repeat three times.

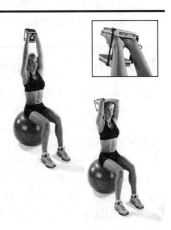

Dumbbell Skull Crusher

Hold a pair of dumbbells and lie on the ball so that your head and neck are supported. Elevate your hips slightly and keep your abs tight. Extend the dumbbells straight up with your palms facing each other, and tilt your arms toward your head slightly. Feather your breathing as you bend your elbows and lower the weights through a count of 10 seconds. Hold for 2 seconds at the MTP (about 1 inch above your forehead). Raise dumbbells to starting position through a count of 10 seconds. Without resting, repeat three times.

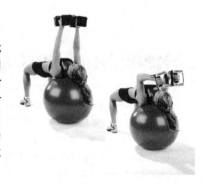

Seated V-Up

Sit on a mat with your arms behind you, elbows bent, and fingertips pointed toward your body. Start with your legs together and extended, knees slightly bent, and heels about 2 inches off the ground. Lean your upper body weight back on your palms slightly. Feather your breathing as you pull your knees into your chest through a count of 10 seconds. Hold and squeeze for 2 seconds at the MTP. Return to starting position through a count of 10 seconds, keeping your abs tight. Without resting, repeat three times.

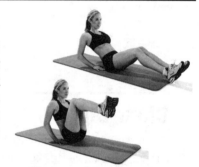

Upright Band Crunch on Swiss Ball

Secure the resistance band above your head. Stand with the ball between you and a wall supporting your middle to upper back. Grasp the handles behind the back of your head, palms facing back. Walk your feet in front of you about 1 foot, keeping your knees slightly bent. Feather your breathing as you crunch your abs in and up as you bring your elbows toward your knees. Hold and squeeze for 2 seconds at the MTP. Return to starting position through a count of 10 seconds. Without resting, repeat three times.

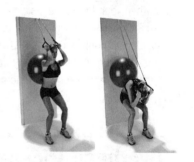

Upward Woodchopper on Swiss Ball

Secure a resistance band at foot level. Sit on the ball and place your feet in front of you about hip width-apart. Grip the handle with both hands, fingers entwined, keeping your chest up and your back and arms straight (do not lock your elbows). Feather your breathing as you pull the handles up and across your body by twisting and contracting your obliques through a count of 10 seconds. Hold and squeeze for 2 seconds at the MTP. Resist the band back to starting position through a count of 10 seconds. Without resting, repeat once more on this side and then switch sides and complete 2 more reps for a total of 4.

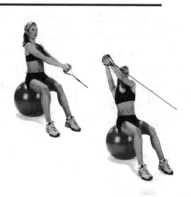

WEDNESDAY

Dumbbell Pull-Over

Grasp a dumbbell using the "diamond grip." Lie on the ball with your head and neck supported. Keep your hips up and abs tight throughout the exercise. Extend the weight over your chest with a slight bend in the elbows. Feather your breathing as you lower the weight behind your head through a count of 10 seconds. Hold for 2 seconds at the MTP. Raise the weight to starting position through a count of 10 seconds. Without resting, repeat three times. (Note: The MTP will vary based on your shoulder flexibility. Hold at your most flexible point.)

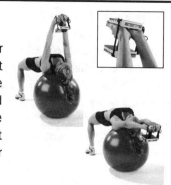

Kneeling Band Pull-Down (Close Grip)

Secure a resistance band above your head. Kneel on a mat and grasp the handles with your palms facing each other. Sit back on your heels with your arms fully outstretched; keep your back straight, chest up, and abs tight. Feather your breathing as you pull the handles toward the top part of your chest through a count of 10 seconds. Hold and squeeze for 2 seconds at the MTP. Resist the band back to starting position through a count of 10 seconds. Without resting, repeat three times.

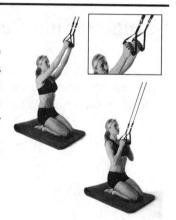

Bent-Over Dumbbell Row (Overhand Grip)

Holding a pair of dumbbells, extend your arms, palms facing toward your body. Stand with your feet hip-width apart. Bend at the waist as if tying your shoes. Raise your head and chest to create a slight arch in your back and bend your knees slightly. Feather your breathing as you pull the dumbbells up in a fluid rowing motion through a count of 10 seconds, keeping your elbows close to your body. Hold and squeeze your shoulder blades together for 2 seconds at the MTP. Lower your arms to starting position through a count of 10 seconds. Without resting, repeat three times.

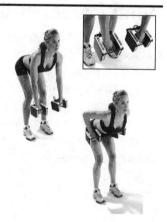

Hyperextension

Holding a pair of dumbbells, extend your arms, palms facing toward your body. Stand with your feet hip-width apart. Bend at the waist as if tying your shoes. Raise your head and chest to create a slight arch in your back and bend your knees slightly. Feather your breathing as you pull the dumbbells up in a fluid rowing motion through a count of 10 seconds, keeping your elbows close to your body. Hold and squeeze your shoulder blades together for 2 seconds at the MTP. Lower your arms to starting position through a count of 10 seconds. Without resting, repeat three times.

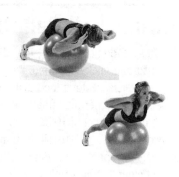

Standing Side Curl

Stand on the center of a resistance band, feet together, and knees slightly bent. Grasp the handles, arms by your sides, palms turned up, and elbows tight against your body. Feather your breathing as you curl the band up through a count of 10 seconds. Hold and squeeze for 2 seconds at the MTP. Lower the band to starting position through a count of 10 seconds. Without resting, repeat three times.

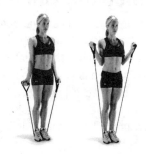

Band Preacher Curl

Secure a resistance band at foot level. Lean over the ball with your knees on the floor and grasp the handles, hands about 1 foot apart, palms facing up. Feather your breathing as you curl the band up through a count of 10 seconds. Hold and squeeze for 2 seconds at the MTP. Resist the band down through a count of 10 seconds. Without resting, repeat three times. (Note: The preacher curl is the only curl in which you shouldn't allow your arm to extend fully. Keep your arm slightly bent at the bottom of the motion.)

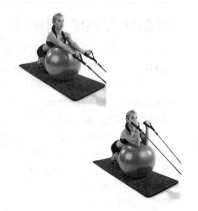

Dumbbell Curl on Swiss Ball

Hold a pair of dumbbells and sit on the ball, arms by your sides with your palms facing away from you. Feather your breathing as you curl the dumbbells through a count of 10 seconds to just past a 90-degree angle. Hold and squeeze for 2 seconds at the MTP. Keep your elbows tight against your body as you lower the weights through a count of 10 seconds. Without resting, repeat three times. (Note: Keep your elbows tight against your sides throughout the exercise.)

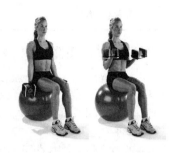

Double Crunch

Lie on a mat with your knees bent and hands behind your head. Raise your feet about 2 inches off the ground. Feather your breathing as you simultaneously crunch and raise your knees through a count of 10 seconds. Hold and squeeze for 2 seconds at the MTP. Return to starting position through a count of 10 seconds. Keep your feet elevated as you transition into the next rep. Without resting, repeat three times.

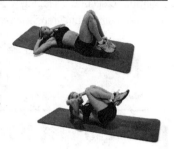

Swiss Ball Crunch

Sit on the ball with your feet on the floor. Walk your feet out until your hips are slightly lower than your knees but your middle and lower back are still firmly supported. Place your hands behind your ears to help support your neck. Feather your breathing and, using your abs only, slowly crunch up through a count of 10 seconds. Hold and squeeze for 2 seconds at the MTP. Lower yourself to starting position through a count of 10 seconds. Without resting, repeat three times.

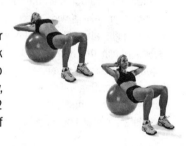

Bicycle Crunch

Lie flat on your back. Place your hands behind your head and raise your legs off the ground, bending your right knee, keeping your chin up and abs tight throughout the exercise. Bring your left elbow to your right knee and feather your breathing as you rotate to the other side for a count of 10 seconds. Hold and squeeze for 2 seconds at the MTP (where your right elbow meets your left knee). Twist to starting position through a count of 10 seconds. Without resting, repeat three times.

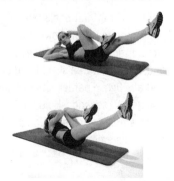

Push-Up on Knees

Kneel on a mat on all fours with your feet crossed and lifted slightly off the ground. Your hands should be wider than shoulder-width apart with your fingers and wrists pointing forward. Feather your breathing as you lower your chest toward the floor through a count of 10 seconds. Hold for 2 seconds at the MTP. Push your body to starting position through a count of 10 seconds, keeping your elbows slightly bent at the top of the move. Without resting, repeat three times.

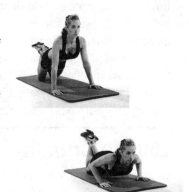

One-Arm Flat Band Press

Secure a resistance band at about shoulder level. Grasp the handle with your left hand (place the other on your hip) and hold at chest level, palm facing down. Take a wide step forward with your left foot, keeping your back straight, abs tight, and knees slightly bent. Feather your breathing as you punch the handle of the band forward through a count of 10 seconds. Hold for 2 seconds at the MTP (just prior to locking your elbow). Return to starting position through a count of 10 seconds. Without resting, repeat once more on this side and then switch sides and complete 2 more reps for a total of 4.

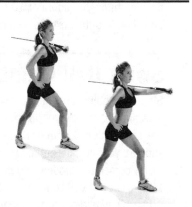

Incline Dumbbell Press

Hold a pair of dumbbells and lie on a ball so that your head and neck are supported. Roll down the ball until your hips drop almost to the ground; do not let your knees go over your ankles. Press the weights up and together, with a slight bend in the elbows, keeping your back straight and abs tight. Feather your breathing as you lower the weights through a count of 10 seconds. Hold for 2 seconds at the MTP. Press the dumbbells up to starting position through a count of 10 seconds. Without resting, repeat three times.

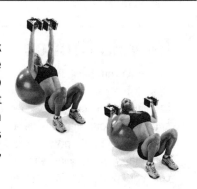

Upward Band Fly

Secure a resistance band at about waist level. Take a wide step forward with one foot, keeping your back straight, abs tight, and knees slightly bent. Grasp the handles with your arms extended behind you, palms angled down, with a slight bend in your elbows. Feather your breathing as you bring your palms up and together through a count of 10 seconds. Hold for 2 seconds at the MTP. Return to starting position through a count of 10 seconds. Without resting, repeat three times.

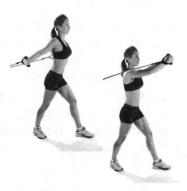

V Push-Up

Plant feet hip-width apart. Bend forward at the hips to place hands on the floor about 3 feet in front of your toes. Keep abs drawn in, head tucked as if you're holding an orange between your chin and chest (you should look like an upside-down "V" from the side). With hands slightly in front of your shoulders, feather your breathing as you bend your elbows and lower your chest and shoulders toward the floor through a count of 10 seconds. Hold for 2 seconds at the MTP. Push back to starting position through a count of 10 seconds. Without resting, repeat three times.

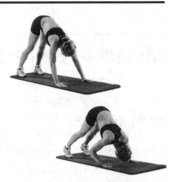

Lateral Raise on Swiss Ball

Hold a pair of dumbbells and sit on a ball, your back straight, your abs tight, and your feet together in front of you. With your arms against your sides and elbows slightly bent, feather your breathing as you raise the weights up through a count of 10 seconds. Hold and squeeze for 2 seconds at the MTP ("T" position). Lower the weights to starting position through a count of 10 seconds. Without resting, repeat three times.

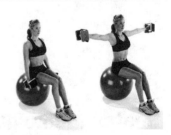

Rear Delt Band Extension

Secure the band at about shoulder level. Grasp the handles and extend your arms in front of you, palms facing in. Feather your breathing as you pull the handles out to a "T" position through a count of 10 seconds, keeping your arms parallel to the floor and a slight bend in your elbows. Hold and squeeze for 2 seconds at the MTP. Resist the band slowly back to starting position through a count of 10 seconds. Without resting, repeat three times.

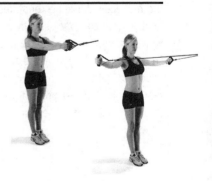

Jackknife

Stand about 3 feet in front of the ball, and place your palms on the ground, hands shoulder-width apart. Place one foot on the ball slightly below mid-shin level. Once level, place the other foot on the ball keeping your head forward, spine straight, and abs tight. Slowly pull your knees up to your chin through a count of 10 seconds, as you concentrate on keeping stability by squeezing your abs tight. Hold and squeeze for 2 seconds at the MTP. Return to starting position through a count of 10 seconds. Without resting, repeat three times.

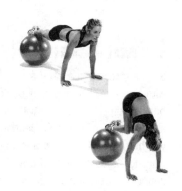

Medicine Ball Pull-Over

Lie on a mat and bring your knees, ankles crossed, up to a 90-degree angle. Grasp a medicine ball and extend it over your head; keep a slight bend in your elbows. Keep your abs tight and feather your breathing as you raise the ball over your head and crunch up through a count of 10 seconds. Hold for 2 seconds at the MTP. Lower the ball to starting position through a count of 10 seconds. Without resting, repeat three times.

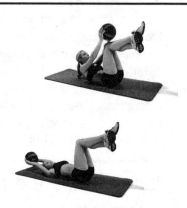

Seated Medicine Ball Twist

Hold a medicine ball just below your chin, about chest level, and sit on the mat with your knees bent, feet crossed. Keep your chin up and abs tight as you lean back slightly and lift your feet from the mat, engaging your abs. Turn to one side to begin exercise. Feather your breathing as you slowly rotate your torso to the other side through a count of 10 seconds. Hold and squeeze for 2 seconds at the MTP (when you've reached the farthest point in the twist). Rotate back to the other side through a count of 10 seconds. Without resting, repeat three times.

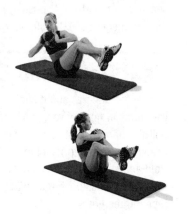

7 Making Your Results Last

"On this program, I learned that small changes add up to a huge difference. For example, I learned that cardio in the morning is better than cardio in the evening and that I can actually eat more often and lose weight. The program was so easy to work into my lifestyle!"

—ALISON ROSS, BODY AT HOME™ STAR, LOST 14 POUNDS

Congratulations! I'm so proud of all the hard work you've done over the last eight weeks. You should be proud of your success too—you deserve it.

So, what do you do now? Well, the most important thing to keep in mind is that the Body at Home™ program is a *lifestyle* change, not something you should stop after two weeks or even eight. Just like your teeth and your car, your body needs consistent maintenance. If you go right back to your old ways of ignoring your health, you risk breaking down—if not right away, at some point in your life! Remember what happened after all those fad diets you tried? The weight, and accompanying frustration and disappointment, came right back—and probably more. The only way to prevent that is to continue with your new lifestyle.

Maintaining this new lifestyle is going to ensure that you continue to create and sculpt lean muscle tissue and burn fat. You'll grant yourself the gift of a long, happy life of health and wellness.

The first thing to consider is whether you've reached your goal or want to lose more weight. If you've reached your goal weight, again, congratulations! The hard part is behind you. Treat yourself to a healthy reward, such as a massage, a manicure or pedicure, or a shopping spree. Buy some new clothes that show off your svelte new figure. Take a day or two off to rest, recuperate, and motivate yourself to continue eating healthfully and exercising.

If you've reached your goal weight, the key for you is maintenance. You don't need to lose more, which means that you can add more calories to your daily intake. As for your workouts, you can decide if you want to start a new 8-Week Challenge. You may start the program from the beginning, or you can mix it up to suit your own preferences. Maybe you preferred the dumbbells to the bands, or vice versa. Maybe you want to challenge yourself even more by going to the gym. Be creative and use the Body at Home™ method to keep your muscles looking firm and toned. This program is flexible enough for anybody, so create the plan that best suits you.

To help get you started, here are a few examples of how you can modify and mix up your routines:

Option 1—Repeat: You can simply repeat the eight-week program. This option will give you enough variety to keep your body adaptive and responsive, and keep you in those new jeans!

Option 2—Odds and Evens: This is a great way to create some variety. Do the odd-numbered workouts in your first four weeks, and then do the even-numbered workouts in your last four weeks, or vice versa. Here is an example of how the program would break down:

WEEK	WORKOUTS
Week 1	Workouts 1, 2, 3
Week 2	Workouts 7, 8, 9
Week 3	Workouts 13, 14, 15
Week 4	Workouts 19, 20, 21
Week 5	Workouts 4, 5, 6
Week 6	Workouts 10, 11, 12
Week 7	Workouts 16, 17, 18
Week 8	Workouts 22, 23, 24

Option 3—Try My 12-Second Sequence™: You can try the eight-week program from my *12-Second Sequence™* book. It has required gym time. It's in a circuit-training format and will provide another option to keep your new lifestyle going—and keep it exciting! Of course, if you want to continue doing all of the workouts at home, follow Option 1 or Option 2.

If you haven't yet reached your goal, I strongly encourage you to start another 8-Week Challenge soon. As I stated above, you should definitely take a short break and reward yourself with a healthy treat. And feel free to mix up the program to suit your personal preferences. But it's important to start a new Challenge soon because having a goal and a time line is crucial to your success. After all, you're still losing weight, and having a goal and a deadline to shoot for will help you stay motivated.

KEY TIPS FOR SUCCESS

I asked some of my most sensational clients for their top tips for long-term success. I think these are great, and I'm sure you'll find that they will help keep you focused.

- *Make new goals.* If you don't set new goals for yourself along the way, it's inevitable that you will lose motivation to continue your healthy new lifestyle. Your goal can be targeted to something specific, like a trip or an event coming up that you really want to look and feel great for. Or you can really take it up a notch and challenge yourself physically. Use Body at Home™ as a springboard into other physical activities. Maybe you want to train for a run or take a new fitness class at the gym that you've never felt ready for. Create goals that will pull you forward, toward a lasting life of health and fitness. And remember to write your goals in your journal or create a power collage that helps you visualize your direction.

- *Stick to eating every three hours.* Even if you've reached your goal weight and can start eating a little more to maintain your weight, you should still eat regularly throughout the day. You'll keep your metabolism at an optimal level, keep your blood sugar steady, and keep your appetite under control.

- *Fortify your support circle.* If you've made it this far, chances are you've found the key that's unlocked your deepest inner motivation. But maybe it wasn't as easy for you as it could be. Perhaps you had to struggle to keep negative influences out of your life—friends who want you to drink or eat a lot with them or family members who don't offer encouragement. I can't emphasize enough how critical your support circle will be to creating *lasting* success. To help yourself continue living the Body at Home™ lifestyle, surround yourself with positive influences. Try encouraging your family and friends to try the program with you, or consider starting a workout group in your local area. Whatever you do, make clear to the people in your life that "This is the new me and I couldn't be happier!"

The most important thing to take with you from this experience is the incredible determination and willpower you showed in completing this program. It wasn't easy, but you did it! The changes that you made affected not only your life but also the lives of your close family and friends. You've taken steps that improved more than your appearance; you've improved the quality and length of your life. You've become an inspiration to those close to you. That's why it's crucial for you to maintain this new lifestyle. Living your best life possible will encourage others to follow your lead.

Congratulations on your new body, your new health, and your new confidence! I wish you all the best as you continue along this awesome adventure.

 BODY AT HOME™ STAR Alison Ross

Height: 5'9" | Age: 23 | Lost: 14 pounds

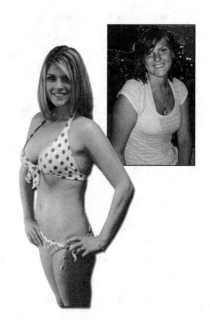

"Before starting Body at Home™ I was frustrated. I worked out all the time, but I just couldn't seem to get my body to where I wanted it to be. This program taught me that small changes in lifestyle could add up to big changes in my body. The program was easy to work into my lifestyle."

Alison's Secrets to Success

· Always keep your goals in the forefront of your mind. If you're thinking about them, you are more likely to follow through.

· Keep a food diary so that you keep yourself accountable and can see exactly how much you are eating.

· Get a pair of pants in the size you want to be, and keep trying them on to give yourself more motivation. Also, keep a pair of pants that became too big on you so that you can really see how far you've come.

8 Frequently Asked Questions

EXERCISE

Will this program make me look big and bulky?

Unlike men, women don't produce the testosterone necessary to create big and bulky muscles. A lot of the professional body-building women you see in magazines and on TV use steroids or other hypertrophy enhancements to dramatically increase the size of their muscles. Moreover, they lift extremely heavy weights. With the Body at Home™ program, you'll lift weights heavy enough to shape and define your muscles but not heavy enough to make you big and bulky.

Will doing even more ab exercises help me flatten my tummy? Can I spot-reduce?

No. There's no such thing as spot reduction. You can't turn fat into muscle. What you can do is burn fat all over your body to uncover the shapely muscle you're building with your strength moves. This plan offers the perfect number of ab moves to get your tummy muscles flat and toned. It also offers just the right amount of cardio to burn fat and reveal those muscles in the least amount of time. Doing additional ab exercises will only cut into your healing time and sabotage your progress.

Do I have to do all the exercises? Can't I just do the ones I like once a week?

This program is designed to help women achieve maximum results in the shortest amount of time. Not completing some of the exercises or missing workouts will slow your progress. In order to burn more calories, you need to increase your metabolism with new lean muscle tissue, and creating new lean muscle tissue requires that you work your entire body. Missing exercises or entire workouts will cause imbalances within your body and fail to create the results you desire.

Can I do cardio at any time of day or does it have to be done in the morning?

As I stated in Chapter 3, brisk walking for 20 minutes before breakfast in the morning will help you burn more calories in less time. Several research studies support the fact that morning cardio on an empty stomach burns more fat, especially belly fat, than cardio done after eating. Plus, you're more likely to take your walk in the morning rather than later in the day when everyday stresses pile up and distract you from your workouts. That's why it's so important to get it out of the way when you wake up.

However, if you live in a neighborhood that isn't conducive to walking, if you don't have access to a treadmill, or if you can't get up early enough, then get your cardio in later in the day. Just be aware that you won't burn as much fat as quickly as you would if you did it in the morning. Take your walk when it works for you. If the only time you can walk is in the evening, do it then. Don't let small details keep you from succeeding. Remember, walking in the morning is best, but if you can't, walk when you can.

Can I exercise more than three times a week and do more cardio to speed up my results?

You can do more cardio in the afternoons to help speed up your results, but you should only do 20 minutes of cardio in the morning before breakfast. Any other cardio should be done after you have nourished your body so you will have the proper energy to push yourself. Adding cardio later in the day will strengthen your heart and burn more calories. Doing more than three workouts a week, however, could impede your results and slow your progress. Your muscles grow and become stronger while they are at rest, so too much resistance training can do more harm than good. If you feel the exercises are not hard enough, you may need to use heavier weights and increase your intensity.

What if I don't feel the burn?

If you're counting correctly throughout your 10-second motions and 2-second holds, you should feel a significant burn when you finish each set. If you aren't feeling that burn, your form or your intensity may not be at the ideal level. To make sure that you get the most out of your workout, make sure that you maintain proper form. You should feel the intensity of each move on the muscle you're working. Don't let surrounding muscles support your movements. When you do a biceps curl, for example, you should feel the full weight of the dumbbell or band on your biceps, not in your back or shoulders. Bad form not only cheats you out of an effective workout but also puts you at risk for debilitating injuries.

Intensity is just as important to getting maximum results as form. Since you're only doing four reps per exercise, it's important to make those reps count. This workout is 20 minutes, three times a week, so giving it your best effort is crucial. You should pick a weight that completely fatigues the muscle after four reps. If you can do only two or three reps, the weight is too heavy. If you can do five or six reps, the weight is too light. Remember, you can create new lean muscle tissue only when you completely fatigue muscles, so correct form and intensity are essential to your success.

EATING

Do I have to drink the whey shakes for my snacks or is there an alternative?

As I mentioned, whey protein shakes are your ideal snacks on the Body at Home™ plan. Whey protein shakes are the best way to feed your muscles what they need to build and repair themselves after your workouts—no other protein source is more bioavailable. However, I understand that you might want another option. So your next best choice is low-fat (2 percent) cottage cheese. One-half cup has only 100 calories, has only 2 grams of fat, and provides over 15 grams of good protein. But remember, you are here to create your best body ever . . . you need to keep it simple and effective. See page 342 for more possible alternatives to whey protein shakes. But try to use the whey shakes first!

Years of yo-yo dieting have wrecked my metabolism. Can this plan help me?

Actually, your metabolism isn't "wrecked." But years of yo-yo dieting probably have cost you lean muscle tissue, which would decrease your metabolism. You see, when you diet, especially when you drastically cut calories, you lose muscle tissue along with fat. That's exactly what the Body at Home™ plan is designed to recover—your lean muscle tissue! As we discussed earlier, muscle burns more calories than any other body tissue burns. So the more muscle you have, the more calories you will burn, and the higher your metabolism will be. That's why resistance training is so important. It is going to sculpt your muscles, burn fat, and increase your metabolism so you burn more calories every day even while you're doing absolutely nothing.

What if I slip up and have a bowl of ice cream or a bag of chips? Or what if I miss one of my workouts? Do I have to start over?

No. Don't beat yourself up when you slip. You're not going to be perfect, and that's okay. Changing your body and becoming a healthier person is a lifelong process. When you eat too much or miss a workout, accept it and vow to do better tomorrow. You don't have to start the program over, and the last thing you should do is call yourself names. These things are going to happen: Maybe it's your birthday and you want a piece of cake, or you're out for Mexican food and you eat too many tortilla chips. It's not the end of the world. It's most important to make this program work in your everyday life; this is the only way you'll sustain your new lifestyle for life.

Before my period, I get intense cravings for junk food and I'm tired and irritable, so I don't want to work out. How can I deal with this and stay on plan?

This plan is actually great for relieving some of the symptoms of PMS. Doctors believe that premenstrual syndrome (PMS) results from hormones—estrogen and progesterone—and the way they interact with some *neurotransmitters*—brain chemicals that regulate mood, appetite, and stress responses. Some of the symptoms of PMS, especially depression, fatigue, and junk-food cravings, can be relieved by consuming a healthy, balanced diet—like the plan I recommend! Also, exercise has been proven to help improve mood, reduce bloating, and increase energy. I know that it's hard to find motivation to work out when you're tired, irritable, and hungry, but remember that staying on the plan will help you feel better and get you through that time.

I cope with stress by eating. What are more positive ways for me to deal with stress?

Craving sugary or fatty foods is a natural response to stress. Comfort foods relieve anxiety and stimulate the release of feel-good hormones in the brain. Unfortunately, many of us are under chronic stress and therefore munch on chocolate, candy, or potato chips way too often. How do you overcome this common habit? One good solution is exercise. Even something as simple as a quick walk around the block can ease anxiety and minimize food cravings. Relaxation is another way to help you cope with stress without consuming calories. Try closing your eyes for 10 minutes, clearing your mind, and breathing slowly and deeply. Finally, if you just can't fight those cravings for junk food—give in. Have a little bit of whatever you're craving, like a square of dark chocolate or a small scoop of ice cream. You won't set your progress back, and you'll be more motivated to continue until the end.

GENERAL

I'm a nursing mother. Can I still do this program? Will it help me lose baby weight?

This program will definitely help you lose baby weight. In fact, I helped my wife return to her pre-baby shape using this program. The walking and strength-training moves are the perfect tools to help you reshape your muscles and burn off that excess fat. Plus, the time commitment is so small with this plan, and because you can do the moves in your own home, it's perfect for new mothers. However, check with your doctor before beginning the eating plan. Since you're nursing, you may need more calories than the plan requires.

I'm over 50, and I've been inactive for most of my life. Is it too late for me to do this program and get in shape?

No! It's never too late to improve your muscle tone and eliminate body fat. In fact, resistance training is particularly important for women as they get older, because it improves strength and bone density and reduces the risk of breaking bones.

I would advise that you talk to your doctor before starting the program to make sure that you're in good health and able to complete the Body at Home™ exercises. Once you get the go-ahead, you're on your way!

Is this program appropriate for my overweight teenage daughter?

Pediatric and adolescent obesity is a serious and growing problem in our culture. I certainly encourage you to help your child get in shape and eat more healthfully. A teenager can definitely do the exercises and the walking with you. However, check with your daughter's doctor before your teen starts the eating plan. The calorie suggestions are appropriate for a teenage girl, but this plan may have more protein than your daughter is used to consuming. Before your daughter starts the program, confirm that the suggested amount of protein would be healthy for your child to consume.

I gained 20 pounds when I went through menopause and it just won't come off. Will this program help me?

Yes! Most women gain weight after menopause, and they gain it in their bellies—you're not alone. This plan will work for you—it will make you stronger, leaner, and more defined—but it might take a little longer than it might have before menopause. Your best defense against middle-age spread is lean muscle tissue. Even if you've gone through menopause, your metabolism is largely regulated by how much muscle you have on your body. The more muscle you have, the more fat you burn. So don't get frustrated or impatient. You will see results.

I'm naturally skinny and don't need to lose fat. Will this program help me become stronger and more toned?

Absolutely! You've got an advantage: Since you don't need to lose fat, you'll see results much more quickly. This program will increase your muscle tone and make you stronger and more fit. It will give you a firm tummy, a rounded backside, knockout legs, and shapely arms. Check with your doctor to be sure you're eating enough calories, though. Since you already have a high metabolism, you may need to consume more than this program recommends.

I've hit a plateau. How can I lose more weight?

At some point in her weight-loss journey, every woman reaches a plateau. It's frustrating to work so hard and see no change on the scale. But don't get discouraged! All you need to do is change your program around a bit. Think about your eating plan. Are you now under 150 pounds? You need to start eating less protein, and therefore fewer calories, at every meal. Try increasing the intensity of your strength training or adding more walking to your routine. To burn more calories, try walking in a hilly neighborhood, if you've been walking on level ground. Also, if you are beyond your first 8-Week Challenge, turn to Chapter 7 and read about how to modify the program to create a new challenge for your body. If you mix up your routine a bit, I promise that you'll reach your goal.

Can my husband follow this plan with me?

Your husband can definitely start this plan with you. If he wants to lose weight, the eating plan is perfect for him. As for the strength training, he might need higher resistance bands—the bands may not provide enough resistance for him—or heavier dumbbells, and he may need to go to the gym. I suggest that he simply turn to the men's version of Body at Home™. The program offers exercises tailored specifically to men's unique fitness needs. In the meantime, he can do the walking and the same strength moves as you, but he may need heavier weights.

(13) BODY AT HOME™ STAR   Michela Dixon

Height: 5'6" | Age: 22 | Lost: 13 pounds

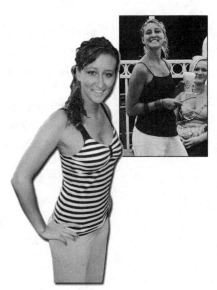

"Body at Home™ has given me back myself. I have been told that I again have the 'spark' that I was missing for a while. I feel strong, proud, and, most important, I feel in control of my life. I know that I will never again be stuck and helpless. I have been given the tools I need to stay healthy, in shape, and looking hot! I love looking at my body now and feel absolutely amazing in a bikini!"

Michela's Secrets to Success

· Once you have committed yourself to getting your dream body, don't cheat. If you do slip, jump right back in.

· Walk in the morning. This is an incredibly vital piece of the plan and it helped me feel great.

· Have milestones along the way. I picked things that weren't always related to the scale, such as fitting into my "skinny jeans."

RESOURCES FOR HER

TOOLS FOR STAYING ON TRACK

The Eating Planner and Workout Logs on the following pages will help keep you organized during the two weeks of the Quick-Start Phase and then during the Sculpting Phase of the plan. You will use the Eating Planner every day so make at least 14 copies of it for the first two weeks. Plus, you will need at least two copies of each Workout Log (Days 1, 2, and 3) to get you through the Quick-Start Phase. Photocopy these charts, three-hole-punch them, and place them in a binder. You can also stay organized throughout your challenge with downloadable logs that you can find at BodyatHome.com.

EATING PLANNER

This plan will ensure leaner muscle and a higher metabolism.

Breakfast>time_____   Description

○ PROTEIN* (3–5oz)	
○ CARBS (½ cup or 1 slice of bread)	
○ FRUIT (1 cup)	
○ FAT (1 teaspoon)	

Snack>time_____   Description

○ WHEY PROTEIN SHAKE (1 scoop)	

Jorge recommends Jorge's Packs™ for your protein drinks. **>** See list of other recommended snacks at the back of the book.

Lunch>time_____   Description

○ PROTEIN* (3–5oz)	
○ CARBS (½ cup or 1 slice of bread)	
○ VEGGIES** (2 cups)	
○ FAT (1 teaspoon)	

Snack>time_____   Description

○ WHEY PROTEIN SHAKE (1 scoop)	

Dinner>time_____   Description

○ PROTEIN* (3–5oz)	
○ VEGGIES** (2–4 cups)	
○ FAT (1 teaspoon)	

Snack>time_____   Description

○ WHEY PROTEIN SHAKE (1 scoop)	

*If you weigh less than 150 pounds, eat 3 ounces of protein at every meal; if you weigh more than 150 pounds, eat 5 ounces of protein.

**Veggies = nonstarchy vegetables.

Water (eight 8-oz cups)   ○ ○ ○ ○ ○ ○ ○ ○

Multivitamin   ○

DAY 1

DATE_____

Start Time_____ Finish Time_____

TOTAL TIME_____

Select weights so that by the end of the 4th rep of each exercise you feel an intensity level of 8.

Muscle Group	Exercise	Weight Used	Intensity Level	set 1	set 2
LEGS					
LEGS					
LEGS					
LEGS					

At this point you should be about 6 minutes into your workout.

TRICEPS					
TRICEPS					
TRICEPS					

At this point you should be about 14 minutes into your workout, including 2 minutes of transition time.

ABS					
ABS					
ABS					

At this point in your workout you should be at 20 minutes. Congratulations! YOU DID IT!

LARGE / **SMALL** / **ABS**

BONUS CARDIO 20-MINUTE MORNING POWER WALK ◯

After my workout I feel _____

(e.g., confident, strong)

DAY 2

DATE_____

Start Time_____ Finish Time_____

TOTAL TIME_____

Select weights so that by the end of the 4th rep of each exercise you feel an intensity level of 8.

	Muscle Group	Exercise	Weight Used	Intensity Level	set 1	set 2
LARGE	BACK					
	BACK					
	BACK					
	BACK					

At this point you should be about 6 minutes into your workout.

SMALL	BICEPS					
	BICEPS					
	BICEPS					

At this point you should be about 14 minutes into your workout, including 2 minutes of transition time.

ABS	ABS					
	ABS					
	ABS					

At this point in your workout you should be at 20 minutes. Congratulations! YOU DID IT!

BONUS CARDIO 20-MINUTE MORNING POWER WALK ◯

After my workout I feel _____

(e.g., confident, strong)

DAY 3

DATE_____

Start Time_____ Finish Time_____

TOTAL TIME_____

Select weights so that by the end of the 4th rep of each exercise you feel an intensity level of 8.

Muscle Group	Exercise	Weight Used	Intensity Level	set 1	set 2
CHEST					
CHEST					
CHEST					
CHEST					

At this point you should be about 6 minutes into your workout.

SHOULDERS					
SHOULDERS					
SHOULDERS					

At this point you should be about 14 minutes into your workout, including 2 minutes of transition time.

ABS					
ABS					
ABS					

At this point in your workout you should be at 20 minutes. Congratulations! YOU DID IT!

LARGE · **SMALL** · **ABS**

BONUS CARDIO 20-MINUTE MORNING POWER WALK ◯

After my workout I feel _____

(e.g., confident, strong)

8-WEEK WORKOUT CHART

Start date_____   **Finish** date_____

Monday	Tuesday	Wednesday	Thursday	Friday	Saturday	Sunday	
DAY 1 WORKOUT 1	**DAY 2** DAY OFF	**DAY 3** WORKOUT 2	**DAY 4** DAY OFF	**DAY 5** WORKOUT 3	**DAY 6** DAY OFF	**DAY 7** DAY OFF	WEEK 1
DAY 8 WORKOUT 1	**DAY 9** DAY OFF	**DAY 10** WORKOUT 2	**DAY 11** DAY OFF	**DAY 12** WORKOUT 3	**DAY 13** DAY OFF	**DAY 14** DAY OFF	WEEK 2
DAY 15 WORKOUT 1	**DAY 16** DAY OFF	**DAY 17** WORKOUT 2	**DAY 18** DAY OFF	**DAY 19** WORKOUT 3	**DAY 20** DAY OFF	**DAY 21** DAY OFF	WEEK 3
DAY 22 WORKOUT 1	**DAY 23** DAY OFF	**DAY 24** WORKOUT 2	**DAY 25** DAY OFF	**DAY 26** WORKOUT 3	**DAY 27** DAY OFF	**DAY 28** DAY OFF	WEEK 4
DAY 29 WORKOUT 1	**DAY 30** DAY OFF	**DAY 31** WORKOUT 2	**DAY 32** DAY OFF	**DAY 33** WORKOUT 3	**DAY 34** DAY OFF	**DAY 35** DAY OFF	WEEK 5
DAY 36 WORKOUT 1	**DAY 37** DAY OFF	**DAY 38** WORKOUT 2	**DAY 39** DAY OFF	**DAY 40** WORKOUT 3	**DAY 41** DAY OFF	**DAY 42** DAY OFF	WEEK 6
DAY 43 WORKOUT 1	**DAY 44** DAY OFF	**DAY 45** WORKOUT 2	**DAY 46** DAY OFF	**DAY 47** WORKOUT 3	**DAY 48** DAY OFF	**DAY 49** DAY OFF	WEEK 7
DAY 50 WORKOUT 1	**DAY 51** DAY OFF	**DAY 52** WORKOUT 2	**DAY 53** DAY OFF	**DAY 54** WORKOUT 3	**DAY 54** DAY OFF	**DAY 56** SUCCESS!	WEEK 8

*Please photocopy and place on your refrigerator. As you complete your workouts, cross off the days so you can see your success!

7-DAY MENU PLANNER

This is a sample planner. The amount of protein you eat will vary based on your weight. Please see page 22 for guidelines.

Day 1
Breakfast: Mixed Berry Smoothie
Snack: ½ cup of low-fat cottage cheese
Lunch: Grilled Ham and Cheese with Tomato Soup
Snack: Whey protein shake
Dinner: Chicken Stuffed with Spinach and Sun-Dried Tomatoes
Snack: Whey protein shake

Day 2
Breakfast: Peaches and Cream Oatmeal
Snack: Whey protein shake
Lunch: Cobb Salad
Snack: ½ cup Muscle Milk 'n Oats™
Dinner: Lemon and Rosemary Chicken Skewers
Snack: Whey protein shake

Day 3
Breakfast: Scrambled Eggs with Leeks and Tarragon
Snack: Whey protein shake
Lunch: Thai Chicken Wraps
Snack: Instone High Protein Pudding™
Dinner: Grilled Shrimp and White Bean Salad
Snack: Whey protein shake

Day 4
Breakfast: Smoked Salmon Crepes with Dill and Crème Fraîche
Snack: Chef Jay Trioplex Protein Cookies™
Lunch: Tuscan Chicken Sandwiches
Snack: Whey protein shake
Dinner: Pork Tenderloin with Sherry Mushroom Sauce
Snack: Whey protein shake

Day 5
Breakfast: Baked Eggs with Mushroom and Spinach
Snack: Whey protein shake
Lunch: Chicken and Grilled Vegetable Quinoa Salad
Snack: Ostrim™ high-protein ostrich snacks
Dinner: Red Snapper Piccata
Snack: Whey protein shake

Day 6
Breakfast: Strawberry Balsamic Parfait
Snack: Muscle Milk® Bar
Lunch: Shrimp and Avocado Salad with Grapefruit Vinaigrette
Snack: Whey protein shake
Dinner: Baked Salmon with Citrus and Herbs
Snack: Whey protein shake

Day 7
Breakfast: Vegetable Frittata
Snack: Schwartz Labs Protein Pancake Mix™
Lunch: Grilled Salmon Caesar Salad
Snack: Whey protein shake
Dinner: Beef Tenderloin Salad with Garlic Vinaigrette
Snack: Whey protein shake

BODY AT HOME™ RECIPES

Breakfast

Baked Eggs with Mushrooms and Spinach

Mixed Berry Smoothie

Peaches and Cream Oatmeal

Scrambled Eggs with Leeks and Tarragon

Smoked Salmon Crepes with Dill and Crème
  Fraîche

Strawberry Balsamic Parfait

Vegetable Frittata

Lunch

Chicken and Grilled Vegetable Quinoa Salad

Cobb Salad

Grilled Ham and Cheese with Tomato Soup

Grilled Salmon Caesar Salad

Shrimp and Avocado Salad with Grapefruit
  Vinaigrette

Thai Chicken Wraps

Tuscan Chicken Sandwiches

Dinner

Baked Salmon with Citrus and Herbs

Beef Tenderloin Salad with Garlic Vinaigrette

Chicken Stuffed with Spinach and Sun-Dried
  Tomatoes

Grilled Shrimp and White Bean Salad

Lemon and Rosemary Chicken Skewers

Pork Tenderloin with Sherry Mushroom Sauce

Red Snapper Piccata

NOTE: Remember to refer to the Bonus Items section (page 341) for the Ideal Foods List and the Fast and Frozen Foods List for additional ideas and suggestions.

Baked Eggs with Mushrooms and Spinach

Serves 4
COOKING TIME: 15 minutes

Cooking spray
2 shallots, diced
2 garlic cloves, minced
Salt and pepper
2 cups sliced mushrooms
2 boxes frozen chopped
 spinach, thawed and
 squeezed dry
12 eggs
2 whole-wheat English
 muffins, halved
4 teaspoons flaxseed oil
Pinch of nutmeg

Preheat the oven to 450°F.

Heat a large nonstick skillet over medium heat and spray with cooking spray. Sauté the shallots and garlic until tender; season with salt and pepper. Add the mushrooms and sauté until they have released their liquid and turn a deep golden brown. Stir in the spinach until incorporated. Remove from the heat. Spray four 8-ounce ramekins with cooking spray. Divide the spinach mixture among the ramekins and carefully break 3 eggs into each. Place the ramekins on a baking sheet and bake until the whites of the eggs are set and the yolks are still runny, 7 to 10 minutes.

Toast the English muffins and drizzle with flaxseed oil. Sprinkle nutmeg over each dish. Serve each person one ramekin and half an English muffin.

Mixed Berry Smoothie

Serves 1
NO COOKING TIME

½ very ripe banana
1 cup frozen mixed berries
¾ cup low-fat plain yogurt
1 scoop vanilla-flavored
 protein powder
1 teaspoon flaxseed oil

Purée all ingredients in a blender until smooth. Serve.

Peaches and Cream Oatmeal

In a medium saucepan over medium heat, bring water to a boil and add the salt. Stir in the oats, peaches, and protein powder and bring the mixture to a boil. Reduce heat to low and simmer, uncovered, stirring occasionally until the oatmeal and peaches are tender, 10 to 15 minutes. Stir in the cream and cinnamon and serve.

Serves 4
COOKING TIME: 10–15 minutes

3½ cups water
½ teaspoon coarse salt
2 cups rolled oats
½ cup diced dried peaches
4 scoops unflavored protein powder
¼ cup light cream
½ teaspoon ground cinnamon

Scrambled Eggs with Leeks and Tarragon

Heat a large nonstick skillet over medium-low heat and spray with cooking spray. Add the leeks and season with salt and pepper. Sauté until tender. Whisk the eggs, egg whites, tarragon, mustard, and salt and pepper to taste. Pour the egg mixture into the skillet and scramble until soft curds form. Fold in the tomatoes and cook until they soften slightly, 1 minute. Remove from heat.

Drizzle the flaxseed oil on the toast. Divide the egg mixture into four portions and serve with toast and apples.

Serves 4
COOKING TIME: 10 minutes

Cooking spray
2 leeks, sliced and well washed
Pinch of salt and freshly ground black pepper
8 eggs
12 egg whites
1½ tablespoons chopped fresh tarragon
1 tablespoon Dijon mustard
2 Roma tomatoes, seeded and diced
4 teaspoons flaxseed oil
2 slices whole-wheat bread, toasted
4 apples

Smoked Salmon Crepes
with Dill and Crème Fraîche

Serves 4
COOKING TIME: 10 minutes

Cooking spray
2 eggs
8 egg whites
2 tablespoons skim milk
4 ounces smoked salmon, diced
2 tablespoons plus 4 small sprigs fresh dill
Salt and freshly ground black pepper
Four 8-inch prepared crepes
2 tablespoons crème fraîche or sour cream
4 oranges

Heat a large nonstick skillet over medium heat and spray with cooking spray. Whisk the eggs, egg whites, and milk in a large bowl and pour into the skillet. Scramble until the eggs look about half cooked and add the salmon and chopped dill. Scramble until soft curds form. Season with salt and pepper.

Heat the crepes in the microwave for 20 to 30 seconds.

In a small bowl, mix the crème fraîche with enough water to make it pourable, about 1 tablespoon. Divide the egg mixture among the crepes and roll into a burrito shape. Drizzle with the crème fraîche mixture and garnish with the dill sprigs. Serve with the oranges.

Strawberry Balsamic Parfait

Serves 4
COOKING TIME: 10 minutes

4 cups quartered and hulled strawberries
1 teaspoon sugar
Freshly ground black pepper to taste
½ cup balsamic vinegar
4 cups 2% cottage cheese
2 tablespoons sliced almonds, toasted
4 teaspoons flaxseed oil
4 slices whole-wheat bread, toasted

Place the strawberries in a medium bowl and toss with the sugar and a few twists of black pepper. Set aside.

Bring the balsamic vinegar to a boil in a small saucepan over medium-high heat. Reduce by half.

Place ½ cup of cottage cheese in each of four tall clear glasses. Top with ½ cup strawberries and drizzle with ½ tablespoon balsamic syrup. Continue layering the cottage cheese and strawberries, finishing with the strawberries and a drizzle of the syrup. Sprinkle each parfait with ½ tablespoon almonds.

Drizzle the flaxseed oil on the toast. Serve each person one parfait and one slice of toast.

Vegetable Frittata

Preheat the broiler.

Beat the eggs and egg whites in a medium bowl. Stir in the chives and feta cheese.

Heat a large nonstick, oven-safe skillet over medium heat and spray with cooking spray. Add the zucchini, onion, and garlic to the skillet and sauté until tender, 5 minutes. Add the spinach and tomato and sauté until the spinach wilts, 1 more minute. Add the egg mixture and stir gently to combine all the ingredients. Cook the mixture, without stirring, until the bottom is set but the top is still runny. Transfer the skillet to the oven and broil until the top of the frittata is browned and it's cooked all the way through.

Drizzle the flaxseed oil on the toast. Slice the frittata into four pieces and serve with the toast.

Serves 4
COOKING TIME: 10 minutes

8 eggs
6 egg whites
2 tablespoons chopped fresh chives
2 ounces feta cheese
Cooking spray
1 zucchini, diced
½ onion, diced
1 garlic clove, minced
1 cup baby spinach
1 tomato, diced
4 teaspoons flaxseed oil
4 slices whole-wheat bread, toasted

Chicken and Grilled Vegetable Quinoa Salad

Serves 4
COOKING TIME: 15 minutes

1 cup uncooked quinoa
Cooking spray
1 red onion, sliced into ½-inch rings, rings kept intact
1 zucchini, sliced lengthwise into ½-inch planks
1 yellow squash, sliced lengthwise into ½-inch planks
2 large Portobello mushroom caps, gills scraped clean
Pinch of salt and freshly ground black pepper
1 pound cooked chicken breast meat, diced
1 7-oz. jar roasted red bell peppers, drained and sliced
1 garlic clove, minced
Juice of ½ lemon, about 2 tablespoons
¼ cup chopped flat-leaf parsley
2 tablespoons extra virgin olive oil or flaxseed oil

Combine the quinoa with 1½ cups water in a medium saucepan and bring to a boil. Reduce heat to low, cover, and simmer until tender, 10 to 15 minutes.

Meanwhile, heat a grill or grill pan over medium heat and spray with cooking spray. Season the onion, zucchini, yellow squash, and mushrooms with salt and pepper and place on the grill. Grill the vegetables until they show distinct grill marks and are tender (approximately 5 minutes). Remove the vegetables from the heat and chop into bite-size pieces.

Drain the quinoa and rinse with cold water to stop the cooking process. Shake off as much water as possible and place the quinoa in a large bowl. Add the chicken, grilled vegetables, peppers, garlic, lemon juice, parsley, and oil. Toss all the ingredients to combine. Season to taste with salt and pepper and serve.

Cobb Salad

Combine the romaine, spinach, turkey, bacon, tomatoes, cucumber, and croutons in a large bowl. Season with salt and pepper and add dressing. Toss to combine. Top with the eggs and avocado. Serve.

Serves 4

NO COOKING TIME; 12-minute prep time

8 cups chopped romaine lettuce

4 cups baby spinach

1 pound cooked turkey breast meat, diced

6 slices turkey bacon, cooked and crumbled

2 cups cherry tomatoes, halved

½ cucumber, sliced

2 cups croutons

Pinch of salt and pepper

¼ cup reduced-fat ranch dressing

2 hard-boiled eggs, sliced

1 avocado, diced

Grilled Ham and Cheese with Tomato Soup

Heat the soup in a medium saucepan over medium heat. Keep warm.

Heat a grill or grill pan over medium heat and spray with cooking spray. Spread the mustard on the bread and layer with the ham, cheese, and spinach. Grill the sandwiches until the bread is toasted and the cheese is melted, 3 to 4 minutes per side. Spray the pan again when you flip the sandwiches.

Serve one sandwich with 1 cup of soup.

Serves 4

COOKING TIME: 10 minutes

4 cups Pacific Foods® Roasted Red Pepper and Tomato Soup

Cooking spray

4 teaspoons Dijon mustard

8 slices reduced-calorie whole-wheat bread

12 ounces turkey ham, thinly sliced

Four 1-ounce slices reduced-fat Swiss cheese

½ cup baby spinach

Grilled Salmon Caesar Salad

Serves 4
COOKING TIME: 10 minutes

Cooking spray
1 pound skinless salmon fillets (preferably wild Alaskan salmon)
Pinch of salt and freshly ground black pepper
12 cups chopped romaine lettuce
2 cups croutons
¼ cup Caesar Dressing (recipe follows)
4 tablespoons grated Parmesan cheese
1 lemon, cut into wedges

Heat a grill or grill pan over medium-high heat and spray with cooking spray. Season the salmon with salt and pepper and place on the grill. Grill the salmon to desired doneness, 3 to 4 minutes per side for medium. Remove from the heat and set aside to prepare the salad.

Toss the lettuce and croutons with the dressing in a large bowl and season with salt and pepper. Divide among four plates and sprinkle with the Parmesan. Top each salad with one salmon fillet and serve with the lemon wedges.

Caesar Dressing

Yields 1 cup

6 ounces light silken tofu
1 teaspoon anchovy paste or Worcestershire sauce
Juice of ½ lemon
2 tablespoons grated Parmesan cheese
1 garlic clove
2 tablespoons extra virgin olive oil
Salt and freshly ground black pepper

Combine the tofu, anchovy paste, lemon juice, cheese, and garlic in a blender. Purée until smooth, and stream in olive oil. Thin the dressing with water to desired consistency. Season to taste with salt and pepper.

Shrimp and Avocado Salad with Grapefruit Vinaigrette

Cut the top and bottom off the grapefruit. Stand the grapefruit vertically and, going around the fruit, slice off the skin and all the white pith. Over a small bowl, cut out the grapefruit segments, and place the segments in a separate salad bowl, reserving the juice in the small bowl. When all the segments are cut out, squeeze the membrane over the small bowl to extract any remaining juice. Discard membrane. Add the vinegar, shallot, honey, salt, and pepper to the grapefruit juice and whisk to combine. Slowly whisk in oil.

Combine the lettuce, shrimp, onion, bell pepper, avocado, basil, and croutons in the bowl with the grapefruit segments. Add dressing and gently toss to coat. Divide among four plates and serve.

Serves 4
COOKING TIME: 10 minutes

1 large grapefruit
1 tablespoon white wine vinegar
1 small shallot, minced
1 teaspoon honey
Pinch of salt and pepper
2 tablespoons olive oil
1 head Bibb or butter lettuce, torn into bite-size pieces
20 ounces precooked medium shrimp, with or without tails
$\frac{1}{4}$ red onion, thinly sliced
1 red bell pepper, thinly sliced
1 ripe avocado, diced
$\frac{1}{4}$ cup fresh basil leaves, cut into ribbons
2 cups croutons

NO COOKING TIME; 15-minute prep time

1 garlic clove, minced

½ teaspoon minced ginger

Juice of 1 lime

½ teaspoon honey

1 tablespoon soy sauce

2 tablespoons peanut oil

1 pound cooked chicken breast meat, shredded

1 red bell pepper, cut into thin strips

2 scallions, sliced

¼ cup chopped fresh cilantro

1 carrot, shredded

4 cups shredded Napa cabbage

Four 98% fat-free Mission® tortillas

Thai Chicken Wraps

In a large bowl, whisk together the garlic, ginger, lime juice, honey, and soy sauce. Slowly stream in the oil, whisking constantly. Add the chicken, bell pepper, scallions, cilantro, carrot, and cabbage and toss to combine. Divide the mixture among the tortillas and roll into a burrito shape. Serve.

Tuscan Chicken Sandwiches

Mix the pesto and the mayonnaise together in a small bowl and spread on each slice of bread. Arrange the chicken, artichoke, tomatoes, onion, and spinach on four slices of bread. Season with salt and pepper and top with remaining slices of bread. Slice the sandwiches in half and serve.

Serves 4

NO COOKING TIME; 10-minute prep time

2 tablespoons reduced-fat pesto

4 tablespoons reduced-fat mayonnaise

20 ounces cooked chicken breast meat, thinly sliced or shredded

2 canned artichoke hearts, thinly sliced

2 Roma tomatoes, thinly sliced

4 thin slices red onion

2 cups baby spinach

8 slices low-calorie whole-wheat bread

Pinch of salt and pepper

Baked Salmon with Citrus and Herbs

Serves 4
COOKING TIME: 10 minutes

Cooking spray
Four 6-ounce salmon fillets
Pinch of salt and freshly
   ground black pepper
1 orange, zested and juiced
1 lemon, zested and juiced
1 lime, zested and juiced
½ red onion, sliced
3 garlic cloves, smashed
2 tablespoons each chopped
   fresh basil, parsley, dill,
   and tarragon
2 tablespoons extra virgin
   olive oil
4 garlic cloves, thinly sliced
2 pounds baby spinach
Pinch of nutmeg

Preheat the oven to 425° F.

Spray a baking dish (large enough to hold all the fish in one layer) with cooking spray. Season the salmon with salt and pepper and place in the dish. Pour the citrus juices over the top and sprinkle with the zests, onion, garlic, and herbs. Drizzle with 1 tablespoon olive oil. Bake the salmon to desired doneness, 6 to 8 minutes for medium.

Meanwhile, heat the remaining tablespoon olive oil in a large nonstick skillet over medium heat. Add the garlic and sauté until golden. Add the spinach in batches and sauté until wilted. Season to taste with salt, pepper, and nutmeg.

Serve each person one salmon fillet and one-quarter of the spinach.

Beef Tenderloin Salad with Garlic Vinaigrette

Serves 4
COOKING TIME: 10 minutes

In a small bowl, whisk the garlic, mustard, and lemon juice with 1 teaspoon water. Whisking constantly, stream in the olive oil. Stir in the parsley and season with salt and pepper. Set the dressing aside.

Heat a grill or grill pan over high heat and spray with cooking spray. Season the beef cubes with salt, pepper, and rosemary. Thread the cubes on skewers (if using wooden skewers, soak them in water for at least 1 hour to prevent them from burning on the grill) and place on the grill. Cook to desired doneness, about 1 minute per side for medium rare. Remove from the heat.

In a large bowl, toss the romaine, arugula, tomatoes, scallions, and bell pepper with the dressing. Divide among four plates. Top each salad with the beef skewers and serve.

2 garlic cloves, minced

1 tablespoon Dijon mustard

1 tablespoon freshly squeezed lemon juice

1 teaspoon water

2 tablespoons extra virgin olive oil

1 tablespoon chopped flat-leaf parsley

Salt and freshly ground black pepper

Cooking spray

1½ pounds beef tenderloin, well trimmed and cut into 1-inch cubes

2 tablespoons chopped rosemary

8 cups chopped romaine lettuce

4 cups arugula

1 pint cherry tomatoes, halved

6 scallions, sliced

1 red or yellow bell pepper, sliced into strips

1 ounce sun-dried tomatoes
(not oil-packed), sliced
into strips

Hot water

1 box frozen chopped
spinach, thawed and
squeezed dry

½ cup basil leaves, sliced
into thin ribbons

2 tablespoons toasted pine
nuts

¼ cup grated Parmesan
cheese

2 garlic cloves, minced

Salt and freshly ground black
pepper

Four 5-ounce chicken breast
halves

Cooking spray

½ cup white wine

½ cup low-sodium chicken
broth

1 teaspoon butter

2 pounds asparagus spears,
trimmed

Chicken Stuffed with Spinach and Sun-Dried Tomatoes

Preheat the oven to 425° F. Place the tomatoes in a small bowl and pour enough hot water over to cover. Soak the tomatoes until plump and softened, 15 minutes. Drain.

Mix together the spinach, tomatoes, half of the basil, pine nuts, Parmesan, and garlic. Season to taste with salt and pepper.

Place one chicken breast half on a cutting board with the thick end pointing toward your dominant hand. Holding a thin, sharp knife horizontally, cut a slit in the thick end, with the tip of the knife pointing toward the thin end. Carefully maneuver the knife to create a pocket inside the breast without cutting all the way through. Repeat with remaining chicken breasts. Using your fingers, stuff the filling inside the chicken breasts and secure with toothpicks. Season the outside of the breasts with salt and pepper.

Heat a large oven-safe, nonstick skillet over medium-high heat and spray with cooking spray. Add the chicken and sear until well browned, 2 minutes. Flip the chicken and place the pan in the oven. Bake until the chicken reaches 165° F in the center, 10 to 15 minutes. Remove the chicken from the pan and tent with foil.

Return the pan to the stovetop over high heat and add the wine and broth. Bring the mixture to a boil and reduce by half. Return the chicken to the pan and coat with sauce. Swirl in the butter and remaining basil.

Meanwhile, bring 2 inches of water to a boil in a large stockpot and add a steamer basket. Place the asparagus in the basket, cover, and reduce heat to low. Steam the asparagus until tender, 6 to 7 minutes.

Serve each person one chicken breast with sauce and one-quarter of the asparagus.

Grilled Shrimp and White Bean Salad

Heat a grill or grill pan over medium-high heat and spray with cooking spray. Season the shrimp with salt and pepper and place on the grill. Cook until the shrimp are opaque throughout, 2 minutes per side.

Combine the greens, beans, basil, and tomatoes in a large bowl. Toss with the olive oil and lemon juice. Divide the salad among four plates. Top with the shrimp and serve.

Serves 4
COOKING TIME: 10 minutes

Cooking spray
1½ pounds large shrimp, peeled and deveined
Salt and freshly ground black pepper
12 cups mixed salad greens
1 can white beans, drained and well rinsed
12 basil leaves, sliced into thin ribbons
1 pint cherry tomatoes
2 tablespoons extra virgin olive oil
Juice of ½ lemon (about 2 tablespoons, or to taste)

Lemon and Rosemary Chicken Skewers

Season the chicken with salt and pepper and place in a large bowl. Add the lemon juice, olive oil, rosemary, and garlic and toss to combine. Cover with plastic wrap and refrigerate for 6 hours or overnight.

Heat a grill or grill pan over medium-high heat and spray with cooking spray. Thread the chicken on metal or wooden skewers (if using wooden skewers, be sure to soak them in water for at least an hour before using so they don't burn on the grill) and place on the grill. Cook until the chicken shows nice grill marks and is cooked through, 3 to 4 minutes per side.

Toss the greens, cucumber, and tomatoes with the dressing in a large bowl. Divide among four salad plates.

Place the skewers on top of the salad and serve.

Serves 4
COOKING TIME: 10 minutes

1½ pounds chicken breast tenders
Salt and freshly ground black pepper
¼ cup freshly squeezed lemon juice
2 tablespoons extra virgin olive oil
2 tablespoons chopped fresh rosemary
4 garlic cloves, roughly chopped
Cooking spray
12 cups mixed salad greens
½ cucumber, sliced
1 cup cherry tomatoes, halved
½ cup reduced-fat vinaigrette

Serves 4

COOKING TIME: 30 minutes

Cooking spray

1½ pounds pork tenderloin, well trimmed

Salt and pepper

1 pound mixed mushrooms (button, Crimini, Portobello, Shiitake, etc.), sliced

1 large shallot, diced

2 garlic cloves, minced

2 sprigs fresh thyme

½ cup dry sherry

1 cup low-sodium chicken broth

2 heads cauliflower, separated into florets

2 tablespoons butter

2 tablespoons skim milk

2 pounds green beans, trimmed

Pork Tenderloin with Sherry Mushroom Sauce

Heat a large oven-safe skillet over medium-high heat and spray with cooking spray. Season the pork with salt and pepper and place in the pan. Sear the pork on all sides to create an even, golden-brown crust. Place the pan in the oven and roast until the pork reaches an internal temperature of 150° F, about 20 minutes. Remove the pork from the skillet and tent with foil to keep warm.

Return the skillet to the stovetop over medium heat and spray again with cooking spray. Add the mushrooms and sauté until they give off most of their liquid and turn deep golden-brown, 10 minutes. Add the shallot, garlic, and thyme and season with salt and pepper. Sauté until the shallot softens, 2 minutes. Add the sherry and chicken broth and raise the heat to high. Boil until the liquid is reduced by half. Reduce the heat to low. Slice the pork into 8 disks and add to the skillet. Turn the pork to coat in the sauce and reheat.

While the pork is roasting, bring a large pot of salted water to a boil. Add the cauliflower and boil until very tender, 6 to 8 minutes. Transfer the cauliflower to a blender or food processor (leave the water in the pot) and purée until smooth. Add the butter and milk and season with salt and pepper.

Bring the water back to a boil and add the green beans. Boil until tender, 3 to 4 minutes. Remove from the water and season with salt and pepper.

Serve each person two slices of pork with sauce, one-quarter of the puréed cauliflower, and one-quarter of the green beans.

Red Snapper Piccata

Heat a large nonstick skillet over medium-high heat and spray with cooking spray. Season the fish with salt and pepper. Carefully place the fish in the skillet and sear until the fillets are about half cooked, 1 to 2 minutes per side. Remove the fillets from the skillet and tent with foil to keep warm.

Add the wine, stock, lemon juice, and capers to the skillet and raise the heat to high. Boil the liquids until reduced by half. Reduce heat to low and return the fillets to the pan. Swirl in the butter and parsley. Simmer until the fish is cooked through, 1 to 2 minutes.

Bring 2 inches of water to a simmer in a large stockpot and add a steamer basket. Add the broccoli and steam until tender, 6 to 8 minutes. Drizzle the broccoli with flaxseed oil and season with salt and pepper.

Serve the fish with the broccoli.

Serves 4
COOKING TIME: 10 minutes

Cooking spray

1½ pounds red snapper fillets

Pinch of salt and freshly ground black pepper

½ cup white wine

½ cup fish stock or bottled clam juice

1 tablespoon lemon juice

¼ cup capers, rinsed

1 tablespoon butter

¼ cup chopped fresh parsley

8 cups broccoli florets

4 teaspoons flaxseed oil

This routine is designed to cut out all excuses. You can do it anywhere at any time with no equipment. So it's perfect if you're traveling or stuck in your office and can't get home to work out. It takes only 20 minutes and will provide you with an intense and effective workout. Use this workout to get started today!

Lunge

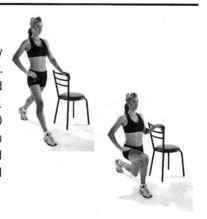

Stand in a lunge position with one hand resting on the back of a sturdy chair for balance. Keep your back straight, chest up, and abs tight. Feather your breathing as you drop your back knee toward the ground through a count of 10 seconds. Hold for 2 seconds at the MTP (about 1 inch above the ground). Return to starting position through a count of 10 seconds. Without resting, repeat one more time on this leg and then perform 2 more reps on the other side for a total of 4. (Note: To avoid injury, make sure that your front knee stays aligned with your toes and doesn't bend farther than a 90-degree angle.)

Balance Squat

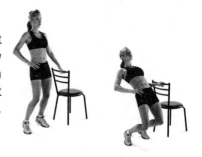

Stand with feet shoulder-width apart. Grasp a sturdy chair for support at about hip level. Feather your breathing as you bend your knees and allow your body to fall backward, letting your heels come off the floor, through a count of 10 seconds. Hold and squeeze your quads for 2 seconds at the MTP. Return to starting position through a count of 10 seconds. Without resting, repeat three times.

Push-Up on Knees

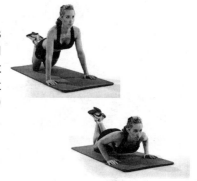

Kneel on a mat on all fours with your knees hip-width apart. Your hands should be slightly wider than shoulder-width apart with your fingers and wrists pointing forward. Feather your breathing as you lower your chest toward the floor through a count of 10 seconds. Hold for 2 seconds at the MTP. Push your body back to starting position through a count of 10 seconds, keeping your elbows slightly bent at the top of the move. Without resting, repeat three times.

Bird Dog

Kneel on all fours with your knees hip-width apart. Keep your head up and abs tight throughout the exercise. Feather your breathing as you simultaneously lift and extend your left arm and your right leg through a count of 10 seconds. Hold and squeeze for 2 seconds at the MTP (when your arm and thigh are parallel to the floor). Return to starting position through a count of 10 seconds. Without resting, repeat once more and then switch sides and complete 2 more reps for a total of 4.

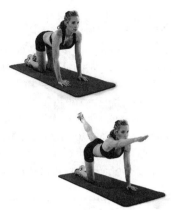

Superman

Lie facedown with your body completely extended, arms parallel to one another, and legs straight. Feather your breathing as you simultaneously lift your arms and your legs through a count of 10 seconds. Hold and squeeze for 2 seconds at the MTP. Return to starting position through a count of 10 seconds. Without resting, repeat three times. (Note: The range of motion is shorter on this exercise so be sure to adjust accordingly.)

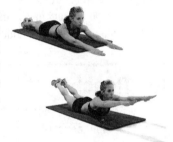

V Push-Up

Plant feet hip-distance apart. Bend forward at the hips to place hands on the floor about 3 feet in front of your toes. Keep abs drawn in, head tucked as if you're holding an orange between your chin and chest (you should look like an upside-down "V" from the side). With hands slightly in front of your shoulders, feather your breathing as you bend your elbows and lower chest and shoulders toward the floor through a count of 10 seconds. Hold for 2 seconds at the MTP. Push back to starting position through a count of 10 seconds. Without resting, repeat three times.

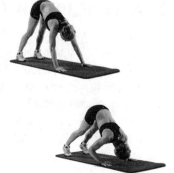

Chair Dip

Sit on the edge of a sturdy chair with your hands behind you, fingers forward and grasping the edge of the chair. Flex your feet so that your weight is on your heels and slide yourself away from the chair. Feather your breathing as you lower yourself through a count of 10 seconds. Hold for 2 seconds at the MTP. Push yourself back up to starting position through a count of 10 seconds. Without resting, repeat three times. (Note: The MTP will depend on how flexible your shoulders are—about 1 inch above your most flexible point.)

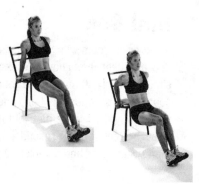

Double Crunch

Lie on a mat with your knees bent and hands behind your head. Raise your feet about 2 inches off the ground. Feather your breathing as you simultaneously crunch and raise your knees through a count of 10 seconds. Hold and squeeze for 2 seconds at the MTP. Return to starting position through a count of 10 seconds. Keep your feet elevated as you transition into the next rep. Without resting, repeat three times.

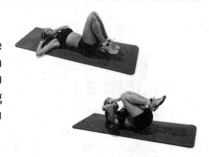

Toe Reach

Lie on your back. Cross your legs, flex your feet, and extend your legs into the air. With your arms extended and chin up, feather your breathing as you crunch up, reaching toward your toes through a count of 10 seconds. Hold and squeeze for 2 seconds at the MTP. Lower yourself to starting position, keeping your shoulder blades from touching the ground, through a count of 10 seconds. Without resting, repeat three times.

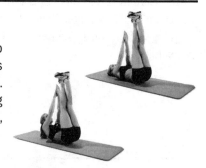

Seated Russian Twist

Sit on the floor with your knees bent, feet together. Keep your chin up and abs tight as you lean back slightly and lift your feet about 2 inches off the floor, engaging your abs. Extend your arms away from your chest with your palms pressed together and turn to one side to begin exercise. Feather your breathing as you slowly rotate your torso as far as possible to the other side through a count of 10 seconds. Hold and squeeze for 2 seconds at the MTP. Rotate back to the other side through a count of 10 seconds. Without resting, repeat three times.

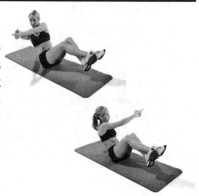

BODY AT HOME™ FOR MEN

PART 2

FOREWORD FOR HIM

By David Barton, fitness expert and owner of
David Barton Gyms (davidbartongym.com)

I ran into a guy on the street the other day. His name is Jack and he was a client of mine when I was a trainer.

Jack was overweight then and still is. I asked how he had been and he recounted a number of enviable business conquests, as well as the recent addition of a wife and two daughters. Then I asked about his weight, still an obvious impediment to various important activities (like tying his shoes). He apparently had just gotten back from a famous retreat where, with the help of a prestigious staff and a ton of broccoli, 20 pounds of unwanted love handle had been temporarily eradicated.

Unfortunately, as anyone who diets without exercising will tell you, those 20 pounds were destined to return with a jiggly vengeance. I then asked Jack what I have asked so many people who are on the fence about exercising: "What would you give to be in great shape? Strong, lean, no gut, lots of energy. If tomorrow morning you could bounce out of bed and feel as good as I do every morning?"

He said "I'd give every cent I have."

But I already knew that.

Whether you drive a Ferrari or a Chevy, your body is the greatest machine you'll ever own. If you don't take care of it, true happiness is almost impossible.

Now the good news: Your body can change. In fact, any image of your body you can dream up is within reach. The science is simple. Taking the first step is usually the hardest part, but if you're reading this book you are halfway there. Look at Jorge Cruise's "before" picture (page 177). He looked just like Jack. The only difference between the two of them is that Jorge made a decision one day to pick up a pair of dumbbells. And so have millions of other guys.

Now go to it. *Jorge's program works.* It's simple, foolproof, and you will see results in a couple of weeks.

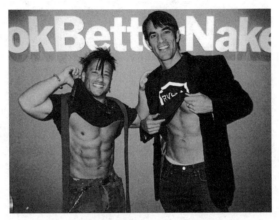

Jorge and David Barton at his New York gym

1 Drop 10 Pounds in Two Weeks at Home

"Your waistline is your lifeline."

—JACK LaLANNE, GODFATHER OF FITNESS

With Body at Home™ you'll lose 10 pounds after just six workouts, and you'll lose them from the most important place: your gut. Nothing in a man's life is as important as getting rid of his gut. *Nothing*. Not money, relationships, kids, sex, the perfect house, or the fastest car. Nothing. Why? If you have a gut, then you have *belly fat*. And belly fat is the most dangerous kind of fat a man can have because it is directly connected to two of the biggest killers of men at any age: cardiovascular disease and type-2 diabetes. None of the great things life has to offer will mean anything if you aren't there to enjoy them, and you could lose them all. This book is for you, and it's going to ensure you lose your gut in two weeks at home—that means *no excuses!*

If you've been carrying around a gut that you can't stand, I know exactly where you're coming from. I used to have 36 pounds of belly fat. But I can personally tell you that once that gut is gone from using my new Body at

Home™ for Men program, you will feel outstanding. You will be able to take off your shirt with confidence. No more feeling embarrassed or dealing with beer-belly jokes from your buddies. And perhaps the best kind of confidence will come from within, knowing that you will not be at risk for heart disease, type-2 diabetes, and other serious health issues. That will be huge burden off your shoulders. It will ensure you live a long, quality life in which you feel good and look good and, I hope, experience years of great sex (keep reading and you'll understand what I'm talking about).

So let's get started right now.

WHY YOUR GUT'S GOTTA GO

Here's what you need to know right now. What I am about to share with you will motivate you for the next two weeks and, I hope, for the rest of your life: Not all fat is the same. Research has confirmed that *belly fat* is the most dangerous fat of all for men (and women) to have on their bodies. Research proves that having a beer belly can harm more than your confidence and self-esteem. It can kill you! That's right, it can kill you. It's not just weight that matters, it's the location of it. As my good friend Dr. Mehmet Oz says, "It's all about your waist." Think: location, location, location.

When you have belly fat, you have what is known as *visceral fat.* Visceral fat is sneaky stuff—it's the fat that dwells deep inside our guts, surrounding our organs and pushing our bellies out and causing the belly to protrude from the inside out. This means even if you're a skinny guy and you've got a belly, you too should listen up. Visceral fat lies inside the *omentum,* a fatty, apron-like organ that hangs down from the bottom of the stomach and is one of the main sites for depositing fat. Visceral fat also gets stored around vital organs, such as the liver and kidneys, which are located in this central cavity of the body. When you have this type of fat, you are at a high risk of premature death. Scary to think about, I know, but it's true—I can't tell you enough how risky this stuff is. Studies have shown that there is a direct link between visceral fat and dangerous diseases such as heart disease, diabetes, cancer, dementia, and Alzheimer's disease . . . the list keeps growing. Breakthrough research points to two reasons why visceral fat leads to these deadly diseases.

Until recently, most researchers thought that this fat was inactive and its sole function was to store energy. However, we now know that when visceral fat accumulates it begins to operate like an endocrine organ such as the pancreas. It actually comes "alive" inside you like some kind of monster lurking deep within your abdomen—think the creature in the movie *Alien*—spewing out toxins, fatty acids, and even hormones and cytokines such as leptin, adiponectin, interleukin-6, and tumor necrosis. Unless you're an endocrinologist, you've probably never heard of these things. But when these substances are released from visceral fat, they cause inflammation throughout your body. This inflammation can lead to cellular irritation, which causes disruption in the function of your arteries and can cause heart disease, stroke, hypertension, high cholesterol, high blood pressure, and heart attack. Talk about a few uninvited guests you don't want crashing your body—these all appear on (or are related to) the list of leading causes of death for men. Heart disease is the number-one cause—nearly 30 percent of deaths in men each year are related to heart disease.

A theory that scientists have named *portal vein theory* provides another explanation of why visceral fat leads to disease. The *portal vein* is the vein that carries blood from the abdominal organs to the liver. When there is an abundance of visceral fat stored in the omentum, the blood begins to dump fatty acids and hormones directly into the liver, causing it to produce too much glucose. As a result, the body produces more and more insulin to try to manage the glucose. This chain of events causes the body to become insulin resistant, which leads to type-2 diabetes. If you think you can live a functional life with diabetes, you're right. But it can have a serious impact on your health. In fact, from the time you become diabetic, you cut every year of your life in half. Diabetes is nothing to mess around with.

Now I've got some great news for you, and it's really the reason why I created the Body at Home™ program: Breakthrough research has shown without question that *resistance training* is one of the most effective solutions to burning visceral belly fat. In my *12-Second Sequence™* book, I go into great detail about the various studies (be sure to pick that book up for more info). But bottom line: You need to know that strength training will help you lose your gut— period. The American Heart Association confirms the power of resistance training to burn belly fat.

Why is resistance training so powerful at burning visceral belly fat? It's the most effective way to create *lean muscle tissue,* which is what gives you the ability to burn fat at rest. Resistance training is the core secret to a revved-up *resting metabolism,* which means how many calories you burn even when you are doing nothing—when you are sleeping, standing, or sitting. Strength training also has the amazing power to create what's called the "after-burn effect." When you do any kind of workout, your body has to do a little extra work after you're done to recover to *homeostasis,* or its resting state. This extra work—or *after-burn*—continues to keep your body burning calories. The problem with most types of exercise is they don't produce enough after-burn to make much of a difference. Strength training, in contrast, has been shown to have an after-burn of *over 16 hours.* It's incredibly effective at keeping your body running hot and burning calories for hours and hours after you finish your workout.

WHY THE BODY AT HOME™ PLAN WORKS

If resistance training is so effective, why doesn't everyone just do it? Here's what has been the main obstacle for almost all people: time. Traditional resistance training has a lot of requirements—hours of gym time, spotters, and so on—a lot of effort, and a lot of time that none of

The Cardio Myth

A lot of guys think that cardio is the best exercise for burning fat. And I tell them it's great for a healthy heart. But if you relied on jogging, the elliptical machine, or running to change your body, I bet you ended up stashing your running shoes in the closet because cardio didn't produce the results you wanted. As wonderful as cardio is for your heart, it isn't the most efficient or effective way to burn belly fat. If the average man did an entire hour of moderately paced walking, he would burn about 240 calories. There are approximately 3,500 calories in just 1 pound. You needn't be a math whiz to figure out that you've got to do a lot of walking to burn the caloric equivalent of only 1 pound.

The other problem with doing only cardio is that once you stop exercising, your body essentially stops burning calories. Remember the after-burn effect I just mentioned? Cardio really doesn't compare to strength training when it comes to after-burn. Many studies have shown that strength training creates a significantly longer after-burn—otherwise known as *excess post-oxygen consumption (EPOC)*—than aerobic activity. One study published in the *International Journal of Sport Nutrition and Exercise Metabolism* tracked the after-burn of people who had recently completed a strength-training session. This is the group I mentioned whose after-burn stayed elevated for 16 hours after they finished exercising. In another study, conducted at Colorado State University, researchers compared the two types of exercise and the length of after-burn they created. Their results revealed that strength training generated a much longer-lasting EPOC compared to the aerobic activity.

us have! In years of working with clients online and face-to-face, I've discovered that most people don't have an hour to put in every day, and they really don't have the time to go to a gym.

So for the past three years, finding a solution to this time problem has been my team's full focus. How could time be compressed? Could I find a way to push a muscle past what is known as the *failure point*—the point at which the muscle changes? And could I do this in less time and let people do it from anywhere, even at home? I became obsessed with finding answers.

I am happy to say that I found a solution: a new way to resistance-train that got rid of my belly fat and helped me get some great-looking abs for a 38-year-old man. Yep, for the first time ever, I am really confident taking off my shirt. The answer is my strength-training technique called the 12-Second Sequence™, on which Body at Home™ is based. The day my book *The 12-Second Sequence™* launched on *The Today Show,* it became a *New York Times* best seller. It became the number-one fitness book in the country. What I revealed was that by slowing down a movement to 10 seconds and holding for 2 seconds, you could fatigue a muscle in just four reps. If you've ever spent time working out, you know that four reps is less than half of the number of reps usually required. Keep reading and I'll tell you how it's possible.

Why did I create this men's-only program? I started to get bombarded by e-mails from men who wanted a specialty book just for them. They wrote telling me they literally hated their guts. Their doctors had told them to lose at least 10 pounds or they would be at risk for heart disease and other serious health issues. Some shared with me that their significant others were no longer attracted to them—and had told them to get to the gym. But here was the big request: The men I heard from wanted to be able to *work out at home and not in the gym.* They felt they didn't have time for the gym. I love going to the gym, but I could completely understand their predicament—they want results but can't get to the gym. I knew what I had to do.

In your hands right now is my brand-new, customized home plan for men. *This new plan is done 100 percent at home and requires no expensive equipment.* Everything you will need—from the exercises to the eating plan, to an important method for staying motivated—is here. You will see extraordinary results no matter how much belly fat you have or what your age is. If you are short on time and want to start immediately, jump to Chapter 2 to read my men's-only strategy to ensure your success on this plan. But if you can, I strongly recommend you read on for an essential overview of my strength-training method.

A BREAKTHROUGH COMBINATION

My Story

As a kid and young man I struggled with my weight. I had no confidence and felt hopeless. I was raised in a Mexican American family, and I was always taught that food was love—and my mom loved me a lot, and it showed in my body. I skipped out on sports as a kid and I never really felt as if I belonged. As I got older, I realized that food had become my best friend and I really needed to change my lifestyle, or I was headed toward a long life of poor health and lousy habits.

I found my way to a life invigorated by a new love of health and fitness, and today I run JorgeCruise.com, write a weekly fitness column for *USA WEEKEND Magazine*, and have a super-busy personal life. My wife, Heather, and I are always on the go with our two small boys, Parker and Owen. I am now almost 40 years old and I can tell you this: I have never been in better shape. Because of Body at Home™ I can see my abs and I feel proud to take my shirt off at the beach! Bottom line: This program will prove to you that the only thing that matters is the quality of the workout, not the number of reps. It will be an eye-opening lesson that I hope will help keep you fit and in shape for the rest of your life!

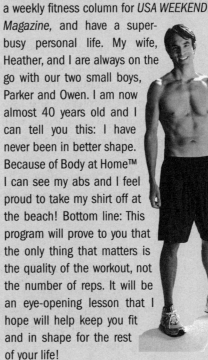

The Body at Home™ program is about simplicity and efficiency. In my opinion, it's the most efficient method to build muscle tissue. Its secret to compressing time is a method I call Controlled Tension™. This unique method forces your muscles to fatigue in just four reps by slowing down each exercise to a 10-second count and a 2-second hold. Remember, fatigue is the critical point your muscles have to get to in order to build new muscle tissue. With Controlled Tension™, you are using the powerful combination of two resistance-training methods that are proven effective at restoring lean muscle tissue. By combining *slow cadence lifting* and *static contraction,* I created a super-powerful and intense method to fatigue your muscles faster than any other technique out there, and I created the ultimate body-sculpting, time-saving method available. Before the 12-Second Sequence™, these two techniques had never been combined. Now, I have built upon this core technique and created the ultimate in fitness customization for men with Body at Home™ for Men. Normally you might need 12 to 14 reps and up to 4 or 5 sets to create fatigue and see results. With this program, all you need is 4 reps and 2 sets. *You will compress a two-hour workout to just a little over half an hour.* With less than a two-hour commitment each week—all done from home—you are going to see phenomenal results (remember to read the success stories throughout the book for proof).

FOR MEN ONLY

This program is designed exclusively for men. Whether you are a student, a business professional, a busy dad, or you're retired, it will help you drop 10 pounds in just two weeks. It incorporates my brand-new life strategy: the Priority Solution™. This strategy is so important that I've given it its own chapter (Chapter 2), and I want to tell you it will be a critical tool for burning your belly fat and ensuring your success with this program. Be sure not to miss that chapter. Its lays out the fundamental groundwork that will help you achieve the best results possible with Body at Home™.

For now, I want to challenge you to make a commitment to yourself to see this program all the way through to the end. Remember, *in only two weeks you will drop 10 pounds!* As you go through the book, you may notice that some of my Body at Home™ Stars lost slightly less than 10 pounds. Depending on your body type and how quickly you add muscle, your scale, like theirs, may tip more slowly. That's why I also recommend measuring your waist to track your success—a lot of my successful clients recorded amazing losses in inches but didn't always register a big loss on the scale. Also remember, there's nothing more dangerous than extra fat in your abdominal area, so making big losses there can be even more important than those made on the scale. By shrinking your waist to a healthy 35 inches or less, you'll reduce your risk for developing life-threatening diseases.

Are you ready to lift some weights, lose your gut, and be on your way to a better life? I know you are. Let's start together and move on to Chapter 2.

13 BODY AT HOME™ STAR   Justin Kroupa

Height: 6'2" | **Age:** 30 | **Lost:** 13 pounds

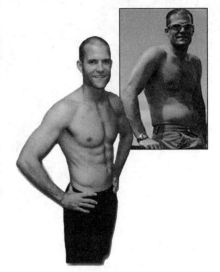

"After battling cancer for a year and a half, my fitness level was not where it was previously. With the Body at Home™ style of lifting, I could feel a difference quickly—within just a few weeks I felt better and looked better. This was confirmed when my friends started commenting on how much leaner I looked and how defined I was becoming— this was the fuel I needed to keep going!

"One thing I really like about the program is how easy it is to get back into the groove if you have a bad weekend or day; it is not hard jump right back in. Another motivating factor is how good you feel and how much time is saved. The diet gives you plenty of energy for the day and the workouts are short and effective, freeing up time normally spent in the gym."

Do This

· Set small goals for yourself so you can see steady progress.

· Sign up for events, such as a race to add a motivational focus.

· Let your friends and family know what you're doing so they can help hold you accountable.

2 A Man's Edge: The Priority Solution™

"I lost 28 pounds with this program and my body is better than ever. I have more energy, more confidence, and I am happier than I have ever been thanks to the Body at Home™!"

—DEVON COLLINS, BODY AT HOME™ STAR, LOST 28 POUNDS

All right—it's time to get the edge. There are two critical elements of this program that will put you on the fast track to losing your gut in two weeks at home: your physical focus and your inner drive. In this chapter you will discover how this program is customized for men with my strategy called the Priority Solution™. The Priority Solution™ is a multifaceted training and life strategy designed to help men create maximum and lasting results. The best part: Just two simple steps will customize the Priority Solution™ to your life. The first will provide the physical structure you're going to follow with the workouts. Think of it as a kind of blueprint for your best body—I call it the "Body Priority." And the second, the "Life Priority," will help you create a powerful inner focus. It's designed to truly get you fired up and motivated.

STEP 1: YOUR BODY PRIORITY

The *Body Priority* is a highly customized training strategy that allows you to boost your resting metabolism while giving special—or "laser"—focus on what all men want to improve: the V-Shape. The V-Shape is without question recognized as *the* symbol of a man's strength and power. What gives a man the V-Shape appearance? A wide, full chest, rounded and broad shoulders, sweeping lats, and a lean waist. Taking all this into account, I knew I had to write a book that would focus on creating the ultimate results with that desired shape in mind. By focusing on these areas, you build and strengthen your power zones while adding critical muscle to your body. Why is this muscle critical? It's what is going to increase your metabolism and help you burn through your gut in just two weeks. And your time commitment will be just three 33.5-minute, at-home workouts per week. So your total investment will be less than two hours a week.

As you already know from Chapter 1, all Body at Home™ workouts are strength-training based, which means they will efficiently restore precious fat-burning muscle mass. My 12-Second Sequence™ program uses a circuit-training format, which produces some amazing results but isn't designed to give special focus to the body parts guys most want to improve. If you followed that program, you may notice that there are three workouts a week with the Body at Home™ plan instead of two. This critical third day is added to create the maximum results in your V-Shape. Plus, it's going to guarantee you lose your gut in two weeks, while revealing your best body ever only six weeks later.

Bottom line: When you want to lose your gut and build a powerful V-Shape, you need something much more focused—a training structure in which your overall effort is not divided into various muscle groups during a session. That's why this men's-only program focuses on one muscle group for three or four exercises before moving on to the next body part. You also will be given a little rest time in between sets to help maximize your recovery.

This is how the training cycle will look: Each workout will pair a primary "large" muscle group with a secondary "smaller" muscle group, and abs will end each workout. You can work your abs more frequently than other muscle groups because they recover more quickly. On day one, you will focus on your chest, shoulders, and abs. Focusing on these body parts at the start of the week and doing the workouts in the exact order in which they appear in this book will be critical. Do your best to get this workout in on Mondays because you then will have six days of rest before hitting these important body parts again. Remember, during the workout is when you break your muscles down; only when you rest do you create strong, new, fat-burning muscle. Really allowing your body that time to recharge itself is critical. So, chest, shoulders, abs . . . and you're done with day one.

After the day one workout you might be thinking, "I don't need to exercise more body parts.

Genetically Speaking—Your Abs

I hear guys say, "I want my abs to look just like that," and then point to a guy with perfectly symmetrical six-pack abs. They often get discouraged when, despite their strict dieting, cardio, and training, their abs don't look exactly the way they were hoping. What I want you to know is this: The shape and appearance of your abs all comes down to one thing—genetics. Abs are like fingerprints; no two people will have the same set. Some guys can be completely ripped, yet you may see only a four pack. Others may not even be in the same condition yet appear to have an eight pack. The blueprint and design of how your abs look all comes down to genetics, which is something you cannot change or control. The goal is to reach the top level of your genetic potential. Being fully dialed into the factors that you can control, such as training, diet, and consistency, will allow you to do this. This program will give you the tools to lose your gut in two weeks, and then get ready to see your abs—however they may take shape. Depending on your genetics, you might develop abs that have deep grooves, or you might get a great six pack yet your abs appear "flat" like Brad Pitt's in the movie *Fight Club*. Or your abs could be symmetrical "stacks" or be offset. Just know that if you complete the eight-week program, you're going to reveal some great abs for *your* body.

I've hit the key body parts to help me lose my gut and get a V-Shape, right?" Unfortunately, that's not how it works! Half of the secret to losing your gut is building muscle tissue, but the other and equally critical half of the secret lies in maximizing your resting metabolism. In order to do this, you've got to add lean muscle tissue *all over* your body. Your body is covered in muscle, and to create maximum results, you've got to get all those muscles working in your favor, burning calories and fat all day long. Ignoring the other body parts will prevent you from accomplishing the best results. So on day two you will hit your back and biceps, which I suggest doing on a Wednesday. Then during your final workout of the week, which ideally will be on a Friday, you will work your legs and triceps.

By following this three-day structure, you will be revving your resting metabolism to its maximum and building a powerful-looking V-Shape most effectively.

STEP 2: YOUR LIFE PRIORITY

The second part of the Priority Solution™ is what I call the "Men's Life Priority." It's the next vital secret to ensuring you lose 10 pounds in two weeks at home. The key is to really harness your inner drive—to find the fuel that ignites the fire. I know that may sound silly, but the truth is, if you don't know what that driving force is, you won't succeed—you won't know what to draw from when you need some extra strength to get through that last, crucial set of your workout. The only way you will truly transform your body in 14 days is if you are *consistent*. That means sticking to your three workouts, customized to create the body you want, or else compromising the results you'll see. I know for many men committing to exercise for two weeks, even from home, can be extremely challenging, especially if your inner drive is not

BODY AT HOME™ MY LIFE PRIORITY

SUCCESS CONTRACT

Photocopy and place on refrigerator, pantry, and bedside.

My Name: _____

My Goal: To drop 10 pounds by _____
(Remember, try to start on a Monday; your goal should be 14 days from your start date.)

My Ultimate Goal: To get my best body ever by _____
(8 weeks from your start date)

My Method: Three 33.5-minute workouts per week for two weeks—less than two hours a week

My Top Priority and Reason: Beyond looking better and being healthier . . . Think of what's driving you at the core: Ask yourself, *"What's my ultimate motivation for losing 10 pounds?"*

_____

_____

_____

_____

_____

_____
Signature

fired up. So get ready to discover my secret for creating a powerful inner fire that will help you accomplish initial success and perhaps, even more important, help propel you toward a lifetime of fulfilling results. Sound good? Let me tell you how it works.

In ten-plus years of working with a male clientele, I have discovered that one of the best methods to empower a man is to create a customized "key" to unlock the door to his critical *inner drive*. Even if the hottest sports car in the world is in your driveway, you aren't going *anywhere* without the right key. So I want to make sure you have the right key to get you out of the driveway. I know motivation is a personal matter—you may be motivated by sex, success, or money—but when it comes down to it, there are shared goals or obstacles that men face at different stages in their lives. It's difficult to generalize, but chances are if you are in your twenties, your priorities are going to be very different from the priorities of someone in his forties or fifties.

The first step is for you to come up with your own Life Priority *without* my support. Fill out the chart on page 183 to the best of your ability. Don't spend more than 10 minutes doing this. Just think about what your goals are and what's motivating you to pursue them. Write your responses in pencil in case you want to change something later.

Now that you have filled out your current Life Priority, let's make it stronger. The stronger the items on that list are for you, the stronger your inner drive will become. Depending on your age, jump down to the section that best applies to you. There are common lifestyle challenges that all guys face, and age is the most common denominator for these challenges so that's how you'll see them addressed here. I encourage you to read all the sections, but if you want to save time, skip to your age, and let's get started stoking the fire of your inner drive.

20 to 35 Years Old: Prime Time

It's a fact of life, when you're in your twenties and early thirties, you are in the prime of your life. You are at your most resilient—you abuse your body to an extreme degree and bounce right back. And the reason for this all comes down to evolution. You see, until modern times men usually lived only till about their mid-thirties—that's it! We were designed to reproduce in the early years, which is why your body will take whatever you throw at it and still come back virtually unfazed. However, a wise man chooses to take this time of his life and use it to his advantage. At this stage of life, your hormones that keep you young, resilient, and lean are at their highest levels. Why not take advantage of that? Now is the time to build a strong foundation, not only in your body but also in your self-confidence and career.

That's where Body at Home™ comes in. This program will create for you a level of fitness and health that will translate into a strong sense of self-worth, which will dramatically impact your relationships on every level. Whether you are dating, have a serious relationship, or are married, getting rid of your gut will boost your confidence very quickly. And this higher level of confidence will positively impact your personal life. This result has been documented in various university studies.

A study done at the University of Minnesota evaluated the effect of body image on sexual behavior. Researchers discovered that people who were more satisfied with their physical bodies were more likely to be more confident in intimate relationships; they enjoyed sex more and felt more comfortable when they were naked than those who weren't happy with their physical appearance. I don't mean to suggest it's all about sex, but I know that's certainly near the top of your mind at this point in your life! Ultimately, however, it's about changing how comfortable you feel about yourself in any setting, whether you're out at a bar, at the beach, or in the bedroom. It can be the difference between you walking across the room to talk to the girl of your dreams or staying in the corner chatting with your buddies. It can mean taking your shirt off to play beach volleyball or feeling ashamed to take it off because you don't want to show your gut. It's all about creating a level of confidence that you carry with you all the time; it's about opening doors and never feeling that you can't do something because of how you feel about your body.

Now's the time to take control. As Donald Trump says, "Confidence can get you where you want to go, and getting there is a daily process. It's so much easier when you feel good about yourself, your abilities and talents."

Getting fit with Body at Home™ is going to help empower you in your professional life as well. If you are just starting out in the workforce, here is something critical for you to know: It's not exactly fair, but real-life studies have shown that people who are physically fit and "attractive" earn more money than those who are not. Now, "attractive" can mean different things to different people, but at face value it can come down what someone judges you on when he or she first meets you—how you wear your clothes, your personal hygiene, and your level of fitness. Ultimately, it's all about how you present yourself. If you respect yourself and your appearance conveys this, then others are likely to respect you.

There are university studies that confirm this, but chances are they are not going to be highlighted in your employee handbook. In one study, researchers asked students at a university to judge the appearance of 94 members of the faculty. Researchers then compared those ratings with others given by students in courses taught by those professors. They used the second set of "scores" to help determine the professors' salary increases. The results revealed an obvious connection between appearance and rating. The more physically fit and attractive a professor was, the higher was his or her student rating—and salary. You see, when you are more fit and take care of yourself, you are more self-assured and you carry yourself with a confidence that people pick up on and feel drawn to. This could be due to the endorphins your body releases when you exercise regularly or to the extra energy you feel when you are fit—you are more dynamic and more outgoing. You carry your head high, you initiate and lead conversations, and you make your presence and contribution known. These are invaluable qualities in the workplace—and they make you attractive to other people.

I'm going to bet that getting that edge in life, creating that thriving confidence, is something that would motivate and drive you. So here is what I invite you to do: Simply add that to your Life Priority chart on page 183. Jot down the areas in which you want to build confidence—hopefully, some from both the personal and the professional perspectives—and get started with your first workout. You are on your way!

(14) PRIMETIME SUPERSTAR   Chance Miles

Height: 6'5" | **Age:** 25 | **Lost:** 14 pounds

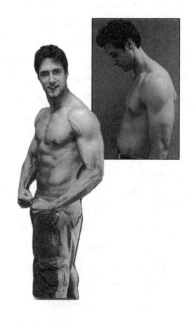

"When I was younger, I would play my Nintendo all the time and eat candy all day. Consequently, I was fat and didn't have the best self-esteem. I joined some sports teams to try to lose weight, but I still ate the same way, and I was never cut or ripped. Once I got to college, I played college sports but still spent hours in the gym trying to keep the weight off.

"Now, that I am in the real world, I have found that I just don't have the kind of time I once did to dedicate to the gym. Body at Home™ has been my answer to staying fit, lean, and ripped without being in the gym hours a day. I have more time to do the things I want! I will definitely incorporate this program into my life to stay active and healthy! Now I can go to the beach, take my shirt off, and have the confidence to talk to the ladies and strut my stuff!"

Do This

· Schedule your workouts to be at the same time each day so there is no question about when you will work out.

· Always take your protein with you and have snacks in your car all the time. This will give you no excuses to fail or cheat!

· Find some motivating pictures and refer to them all the time to stay motivated and on track.

36 to 50 Years Old: Staying Young

Let's face it—this is the point in your life when you start to realize things aren't the same as they were when you were in your twenties. Your body is beginning to change; if you abuse it now, you will definitely pay the price. Remember the days when you needed only a couple of hours of sleep a night and even then you still felt as if you could pick up a car? Well, if you're in this age range, you already know that sleep means more to you now than it did before. Your priorities have certainly shifted—staying young and preventing disease are higher on your list than looking good with your shirt off at the beach. Of course you still want look good with your shirt off, but other things have moved up in priority.

One if the biggest obstacles to staying young is stress. In fact, stress has a direct effect on how we age. It is what my friend Dr. Oz calls a "major ager." Even just looking at the word *stress* makes me a bit anxious, and it probably does you too. But unfortunately, we are stuck with stress, so we must figure out the best way to manage it. Part of managing stress is learning to accept it and on some level appreciate it for the drive it adds to our lives. Think about it. Would we ever get anything done if it weren't for stress?

Almost every man at this stage of life feels as if he needs to be Superman. Men in these years have to balance growing career responsibilities, relationships, friendships, maybe kids, and probably borrowing large sums of money to buy a house. This load of responsibility and level of pressure can start to break you down if you don't know how to manage them. And even worse, if you don't handle stress in the right way, it can prevent you from achieving your goals. What's going to be your number-one weapon against crippling stress? Exercise. Your three workouts each week are going to help you fight stress and stay young. Each workout is designed to build muscle tissue, burn fat, and give you some serious stamina to keep you going strong.

Exercise increases the body's concentration of the neurotransmitter *norepinephrine* in the regions of the brain involved in stress response, which means that exercise directly improves your ability to respond to stress. Exercise also produces the euphoria, or "high," that results from the release of *endorphins,* opiate-like compounds that are released into your body when you work out. Endorphins can make you feel exhilarated and energized but also can make you feel calm and relaxed. Nothing helps me deal with stress better than a good, intense workout. It's on the days when stress is at its highest that I have the best workouts. But don't take my word for it; try it for yourself.

As I mentioned before, besides making you feel overwhelmed, stress also ages you. But in addition to stress, you're also dealing with that whole getting older thing. Guess what? Your workouts are going to help you combat that as well. That's right. There is solid scientific proof that shows a direct connection between rate of aging and exercise. A study of 2,402 twins found that the ones who were fit were biologically *10 years younger* than the ones who were not. So what exactly is it about exercise that keeps us from aging? Well, it all comes down *telomeres,* which are little parts of your DNA that protect the end of your chromosomes from being destroyed. The longer your telomeres are, the less you age. Research has proven that men who exercise three times a week have longer telomeres and thus age more slowly. One of the ways exercise helps keep telomeres in top shape is by reducing the oxidation processes that damage and age the body.

So here is what I will ask you to do if managing stress and staying young sound like something that would help motivate you to a level of accomplishment at which you can stay consistent and live a life of fulfillment, not one of fatigue and disappointment. Add "stay young" and "manage stress" to your list on the Life Priority chart on page 183. Write down that your Body at Home™ workouts will help promote the release of stress-reducing, energizing endorphins and help you manage everything a tough day throws at you. Plus, exercise will help protect your telomeres from wear and tear—and they will preserve your vital chromosomes. You're going to feel a difference even after your first workout. So what are you waiting for? Get started!

10 STAYING YOUNG SUPERSTAR Jimm Johnson

Height: 6'0" | **Age:** 40 | **Lost:** 10 pounds

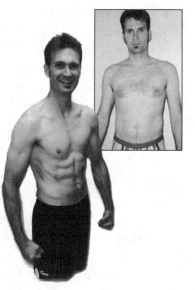

"The Body at Home™ workouts were easy to follow, and I had no problem making time in my hectic schedule to complete them. I'm still amazed how such a little time commitment has given me such great results! Plus, I actually look forward to my workouts, and my stress levels have dropped tremendously.

"I lost my expanding midsection, my arms and chest feel much more muscular, some of my shirts are a bit tighter, and all my pants are loose again. Overall, I feel much healthier, happier, and more attractive! I can now flash my tight, visible abs or flex my bigger, more muscular biceps with popping veins and feel great about it!"

Do This

· Keep track of your progress every week, and don't be discouraged by minor changes—celebrate them! Whether it's a fraction of an inch or a pound, it all adds up by the end of the eight weeks to create a new you.

· Find pictures that represent the body you'd like to have, and use them to visualize what you're becoming. Use multiple pictures if necessary (one for arms, another for legs, and so on).

· Be honest with yourself—with your expectations, your emotions, your behavior, everything! 'Fess up if you cheat, and record and celebrate your successes.

Fifties-Plus: Longevity

At this point in their lives, most men choose to give up on being healthy and fit, if they didn't do so years ago. They choose to believe that it's all over, and that if they aren't in shape now, they will never be. Well, I'm here to tell you that you can make a different choice—and that choice can change your life. The things you choose to make your priorities will affect how you age. Some of the most fit people I know are in this stage of their life. My good friend Jack LaLanne, who is in his nineties, is in better shape than most 20-year-olds! It all comes down to your life priorities. At this point, your priorities should be undoubtedly focused on living a long and healthy life, free of disease.

If your health isn't what you want it to be now, it's time to be proactive about rediscovering a life of health and fitness—a life that doesn't stop you from participating in any activity you wish or experiencing your life to the fullest. If you are already fit and you've picked up this book to stay fit or maybe drop a few pounds, then congratulations on continuing to make your health a priority! Losing your gut or maintaining a healthy weight will help you feel energized and help keep your body strong and resilient against the effects of age. If you are like a lot of men in their fifties and up, years of neglect might have caught up with you—but you have the power to take back control of your life right now. Studies have even shown that exercise can take years off your age. One study done at the University of Wisconsin revealed that previously sedentary people in their fifties who participated in an exercise program increased their fitness level by 23 percent. Plus, they reduced the occurrence of functional decline often attributed to age. That means that by simply getting in your three workouts each week, not only can you maintain a good quality of life, but you can improve it as you get older.

Now, I want to talk about another subject that may not be at the top of your list: E.D. For most guys in their fifties, these two letters can evoke a unique kind of fear. I'm talking about the ever-dreaded *erectile dysfunction,* also known as *impotence.* Anyone who currently has E.D. or has ever had the unfortunate experience can tell you it can take the wind right out of your sails. It not only decreases a man's quality of life but strikes at the very core of his confidence. According to the *Journal of the American Medical Association,* E.D. may affect as many as 30 million men in the United States. This means even if you aren't currently experiencing this problem, you are still at risk.

What causes E.D.? Researchers used to believe it was all a mental condition, and in some rare cases that is true. But what research now tells us is that several factors contribute to erectile dysfunction. Bottom line: How you live you life could put you at risk of getting a kink in your hose. You see, diabetes, heart disease, and high blood pressure all restrict your blood flow and circulation. As a result, certain areas of the body "lose pressure" and that equals no erection. But I have good news for you. You can do something about it, and I'm not talking about taking little blue pills. Men who are overweight and have that visceral belly fat we talked about in Chapter 1 are carrying around the very causes of E.D. Remember that visceral belly fat can lead to heart disease, diabetes, high blood pressure, and high cholesterol, which are not only serious health risks but are the very causes of E.D. (which for some men is a fate worse than death).

There are four simple steps you can take to avoid this problem: (1) Eat a healthy diet. (2) Reduce stress. (3) Quit smoking. (4) Do your Body at Home™ workouts. A study conducted by Harvard professionals and published in the *Annals of Internal Medicine* determined that men who exercise three to five hours a week have 30 percent less risk of having E.D. And here's one more reason to exercise: Working out increases your sex drive. That's right. Just by working out, you kill two birds with one stone. Following this plan will provide the healthy lifestyle you need to live a longer, better life, and it will even help ensure you continue to have great sex during the later years of your life.

In addition to helping alleviate issues with E.D., you can of course improve your quality of life in other ways. Regular exercise can increase heart and lung capacity and lower blood pressure, increase strength, reduce body fat, and reduce susceptibility to depression and disease. Pick up your weights now—it will change your life.

My challenge to you right now is to realize that by committing to the Body at Home™ program for the next two weeks, *you can take control of your health* and even reverse damage done by previous neglect. Once you lose your gut, you'll feel energized and ready to rock and roll! Check out my fifties success man, Ron Courtois. He is 55 and he looks phenomenal! Not only that, he experienced some significant health benefits. It's time for you to take control too.

(14) LONGEVITY SUPERSTAR Ron Courtois

Height: 5'4" | **Age:** 55 | **Lost:** 14 pounds

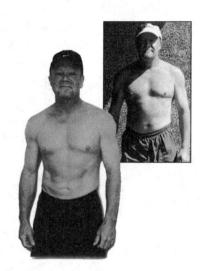

"I've always been athletic, but in 1999 I suffered a serious back injury that eventually resulted in surgery. I was in a body cast for nearly six months and put on a lot of weight. Afterward, I was never able to lose the belly fat I acquired or get back my prior strength and stamina. Add to this a family history of heart disease and it wasn't long before my doctors were concerned about my declining health.

"After two weeks on this plan, I began to see results. I also felt an immediate increase in my energy levels and sex drive. My cholesterol dropped over 150 points on this program—amazing! My doctor was so impressed he asked for information on the program. I have my baseline testosterone checked every few months and my testosterone levels increased 10 percent from my Body at Home™ workouts. I haven't felt this good or been this fit since my thirties."

Do This

· Do your cardio in the morning.

· Plan your meals in advance, as this helps you stay on plan.

· Be flexible on the exercises. If one does not seem to work the muscle group as well as another, pick one for the same body part that you prefer.

Remember that to get on the fast track to losing your gut and getting a V-Shape, you must maximize two critical elements: your *physical focus* and your *inner drive*. The Priority Solution™ will help you identify these elements and allow the Body at Home™ program to work for you. So take a deep breath and commit to the program right now. You will drop 10 pounds in two weeks at home and continue through to the eight-week point where you will reveal your best body ever. With Body at Home™ and the Priority Solution™ you will learn how to keep the weight off and discover the healthiest and best you. You are going to be amazed!

In the next chapter, we'll talk about one of my favorite subjects—eating. You'll read about eating strategies that will accelerate your success.

3 Muscle-Building Foods

"Body at Home™ for Men taught me how to work out, how to eat, and how to most efficiently use my time and energy to create the body that I always wanted."

—JASON KOWALSKIE, BODY AT HOME™ SUCCESS, LOST 8 POUNDS

I've got news for you: If you don't give your body the right foods, nutrients, and muscle-building materials, you're never going to lose 10 pounds from your gut and get the body you want; it's as simple as that. In this chapter, I'm going to give you a quick rundown on how you're going to eat on this plan. Following these guidelines will put you on the fast track to six-pack abs. *Any guy at any age can drop 10 pounds and build muscle with this program.* And best of all—you're never going to walk away from a meal hungry.

The two core elements of this eating plan that will give you the ultimate edge are timing and ingredients. Let me tell you how it works.

CORE ELEMENT 1: TIMING

Timing here has nothing to do with how fast or slow you eat. What's critical is *when* you eat. With this plan, it's crucial that you eat *every three hours.* Eating every three hours will give your body a built-in advantage to burn fat and keep your metabolism running strong. Start your day by drinking 16 ounces of water right after you wake up. Studies have shown this instant shot of hydration speeds your metabolism up 24 percent for the next hour and a half. Plus, it'll quench your body's thirst after a long night of sleep. Next, eat breakfast within an hour of waking. Follow breakfast with a whey protein shake about three hours later, and then lunch three hours after that (I'm sure you're picking up the pattern here). Drink another whey protein shake three hours after lunch; then have dinner three hours later, which for most of us will be around 6 or 7 p.m. Finally, drink one more protein shake before bed.

One of the best things about this plan is that you will not need to keep track of calories. Your focus will be on the ingredients and the quality of the foods you eat. You'll be amazed at how eating protein-packed, nutrient-rich foods will give you the maximum amount of energy and help you feel better than ever before. I promise you, you'll never want to go back to your old diet!

What exactly does eating every three hours do for you? It has a very powerful effect on how your body functions. Eating every three hours helps reduce levels of cortisol, a hormone that contributes to abdominal fat; it helps keep your metabolism running strong throughout the day; and it helps you feel full longer, which reduces the risk of you sabotaging all your success with unnecessary snacking. Bottom line: You're going to feel energized and keep your metabolism revved, and you're never going to feel hungry. That leaves no excuses for failure! Plain and simple: Eat every three hours. If you want to know more about eating every three hours and the research behind it, check out my book *The 3-Hour Diet*.

CORE ELEMENT 2: MUSCLE FOODS

Have you ever built something? It could have been something as small as a model car or as big as house, but I bet one thing was clear no matter the size of your project: To achieve the best end result, you had to start with the right materials. That's how I want you to think about your body. To pack on muscle and lose your gut, it's critical that you provide your body with the right materials—in this case, foods. If you fill up on chips, ice cream, pizza, and so forth, chances are that's what your body's going to resemble—a big, sloppy pile of junk food. If not immediately, junk foods eventually will catch up with you! Besides, you can't see the destruction caused by those foods on your insides, but in the long run, they will turn your body into a broken-down old shack. So how do make sure you give your body the right foods to lose your gut and get your best V-Shape? You follow my Body at Home™ eating plan—a balanced, fiber-dense, and nutrient-rich plan that requires no deprivation and will help your body maximize fat burning and muscle building.

A high-quality diet includes three important macronutrients: protein, carbohydrate, and fat.

Each of these plays an important role in your body by assisting with vital functions such as energy production and tissue development. With this plan, you are going to aim for a 40/40/20 ratio of these nutrients each day: 40 percent protein, 40 percent carbohydrate, and 20 percent fat. You won't have to break out a calculator to keep track of these percentages, but you will want to try to stay as close to this ratio as possible. I'll share a couple of easy ways to do so a little later. But first, let me give you a quick overview of these macronutrients and why they're so important to helping you shed fat and build muscle mass.

Protein

If you like meat, you love protein—and on this plan, you're going to get plenty of it. Proteins consist of chains of *amino acids,* which are organic compounds that are essential to growth and repair of several of your body's tissues. We produce some amino acids naturally in our bodies, but there are other kinds, called *essential amino acids,* that we need to get from foods. If you don't have enough protein in your diet, you risk losing muscle because your body will use it to repair other tissues when it doesn't have an adequate supply of protein. Remember, you are here to *gain* muscle, not lose it, so be sure to give your body the protein it needs to build muscle mass.

To get the right amount of protein in your diet, it's essential to pack your plate with the best type. For example, you can't grab just any steak and grill it and say you've got your protein for the day. Instead, you've got to go for lean, high-quality sources of protein that will fill you up without fattening you up. On this plan, I recommend lean beef and pork cuts, like tenderloin; skinless turkey and chicken (white meat only); cold-water fish like salmon, tuna, and trout; eggs; and low-fat dairy, such as cottage cheese, 2 percent milk, and yogurt. At each meal, you're going to consume about 5 ounces of protein. A 5-ounce serving of most meats will be about the size of a deck and a half of cards, or slightly larger than the palm of your hand.

Besides being an important food in your daily meals, protein is also going to be the ideal snack on this plan. You can find some good sources of protein for your snacks, such as cottage cheese. But my number-one recommendation is a good-quality whey protein shake. You'll find different types of protein shakes on store shelves—soy, casein, and egg—but whey is superior because it has the highest biological value, or bioavailability, of all protein sources. A protein's *bioavailability* determines how quickly and how much of the protein is put to use by your body. Whey trumps egg, milk, and even meat protein, so it can be absorbed more easily and converted more quickly to repair and build tissue than any other protein. *Whey truly is the optimum source of protein for stimulating muscle growth*.

But that's not the end of whey's benefits. It's been shown to have a long list of other advantages. Studies have linked whey to reducing the risk of cardiovascular and other diseases and to helping lower high blood pressure and cholesterol. Plus, it has high levels of *cysteine,* an amino acid that has been associated with lower risk of prostate cancer and is a precursor to a powerful antioxidant. Packed with immunoglobulin, alpha-lactalbumin, and beta-lactalbumin, whey is also effective at fortifying your immune system. In a direct comparison with casein, another type of milk protein, whey even proved to be better at making people feel fuller longer. A study done in England had participants drink a whey shake or a casein shake 90 minutes prior to heading to a buffet. The whey-drinkers ate significantly less than those who consumed the casein shake. Why? Whey was shown to produce greater stimulation of fullness-signaling hormones—people who ingested whey simply felt fuller and more satisfied.

Bottom line: Whey is the number-one snack choice on this plan. Look for a shake that has 100 to 150 calories and gives you at least 20 grams of protein per serving. I created a brand called Jorge's Packs™, which you can check out at jorgespacks.com. Whey shakes taste great, which will help ensure you drink three every day. If you want to mix it up a bit with your snacks as you go through the program, see page 342 of the Resources for Him section for some options.

Carbohydrate

Over the past decade or so, carbs have gotten a bad rap. Sure, there are carbs that can really do some damage to your diet (think a whole bag of chips while you're watching a football game), but ultimately carbs are an essential and important macronutrient just like protein. In fact, they are an invaluable source of energy and, especially when you're exercising, can give you that extra push to get you through a workout. The thing with carbohydrates is you have to know what type to eat and when to eat them. If you eat starchy, simple carbs—white bread, potato chips, pasta—your blood sugar spikes, sometimes by quite a bit, which can lead to an energy "crash." Plus, when your blood sugar fluctuates like that, your appetite does too. My advice: Do your best to skip the simple carbs and aim for whole grains.

Whole grains are complex carbohydrates that actually deliver a slow and steady supply of sugar to your bloodstream, which minimizes false hunger and helps your appetite stabilize. Some good sources of whole grains are whole-wheat pasta, whole-wheat bread and tortillas, brown rice, oatmeal, barley, millet, and quinoa (pronounced "keen-wa"). Plus, plenty of fruits and vegetables are considered complex carbs. Eating complex carbs will also bring some valuable vitamins and minerals into your diet and be an excellent source of fiber. Fiber not only helps you feel full but acts like a broom by sweeping out your insides and eliminating waste that, if left in place, could lead to a higher risk of colon cancer.

On the Body at Home™ eating plan, you're going to aim to eat more complex carbs than simple carbs, but you're not cutting anything out entirely. Simple, starchy carbs are things like bread, rice, potatoes, and corn. Complex, nonstarchy carbs are vegetables like spinach, broccoli, green beans, bell peppers, onions, and garlic. Sweet potatoes and beets aren't on this list because of their high sugar content. Turn to the Ideal Foods List on page 341 in the Resources for Him section for an extended list of starchy and nonstarchy carbs.

My final point on carbs is the most important one: *You have to stop eating starchy carbs after lunch*. You'll get plenty of them with breakfast and lunch, but after that, they're cut out of your diet for the rest of the day. With breakfast and lunch you'll have one serving of a starchy carb, which is the equivalent of about one piece of bread. When you get to dinner, instead of filling up on carbs, you're going pile up the vegetables for a double serving. Here's why: Since you're going to sleep soon, you don't need the energy that's going to be produced from carbs. When that energy isn't used by your body, that unused energy gets stored as fat. So with dinner, instead of having only one serving or about 1 cup of cooked broccoli, you're going to have 2 cups. Depending on the vegetable, you could have up to 4 cups. As I said, you're not going to be hungry on this plan! As for fruit, try to keep it to earlier in the day as well. It tends to have more sugar and can therefore be higher in calories. With breakfast or lunch, eat 1 cup of diced fruit or one piece of fruit, such as an apple. Fruits and vegetables provide essential vitamins and nutrients, so be sure to include plenty of them in your daily diet.

Fat

Many fats deserve the bad reputation they've developed, but some are actually essential to a healthy diet. I'm not talking about the fat that rounded out the edges of the hearty steak you had for dinner. I'm talking about "good" fats. Like proteins, fats are made of a chain of acids, but instead of a chain of aminos, fats consist of fatty acids. Some of them can be generated by the body, but others, the *essential fatty acids,* come from food sources. Fat has a role to play in your body, and it's not just to make your shirts fit tightly. Fat keeps your body warm when it's cold, it helps you digest and absorb vitamins and minerals, it helps maintain cell and organ function, and, most important, it acts as an emergency source of energy if you're ever lacking for food—having some fat on your body could keep you alive in an unfortunate situation.

What's most critical with fats is you've got to know what type to eat, or else you could be in trouble. Several different kinds of fat are found in food: saturated fat, unsaturated fat, and trans (or hydrogenated) fat. *Saturated fat* is easy to spot because it usually is solid at room temperature. You'll find it mostly in foods from animal sources, such as butter, whole milk, chicken skin, lard, beef, and cheese. Research has linked saturated fat to clogged arteries and high levels of cholesterol.

Hydrogenated fat also is solid at room temperature. Often referred to as *trans fat,* this is the kind of fat that manufacturers use to keep foods on supermarket shelves from going bad. The problem is that *trans fat is bad for you*. The Institute of Medicine warns that there is no safe recommended daily amount of trans fat. Hydrogenated fat is created by *hydrogenation,* a process that adds hydrogen molecules to liquid fats such as vegetable oils to make them solid. Trans fat has been shown to increase levels of LDL, or "bad," cholesterol while simultaneously lowering levels of "good" cholesterol, also known as HDL. A study published in the *New En-*

gland Journal of Medicine revealed that trans fat increased the risk of coronary heart disease more than any other macronutrient. Stay away from trans fat, which is found in margarine, shortening, and most store-bought cookies, cakes, and baked goods.

Are you wondering, "What kinds of fat *can* I eat?" The "good" fat to have in your diet is *unsaturated fat*. This kind of fat actually has health benefits, such as helping clear your arteries, reducing the risk of cardiovascular disease and some types of cancer, and lowering cholesterol levels. Unsaturated fat is found in olive, soybean, peanut, sunflower, and canola oils and in avocados. Of all the different types of unsaturated fat available, though, I recommend omega-3 fats most of all.

Omega-3s have unique health and weight-loss benefits. When it comes to keeping your appetite under control, they help you feel full on less food, and they act as an appetite suppressant. Omega-3s also have the rare ability to unlock stored body fat so it can be used as fuel. Plus, they have been shown to aid in the body's ability to maintain muscle tissue and to improve the strength of cell membranes, which allows more oxygen to circulate throughout your body. When your muscles have more oxygen, they're better able to convert body fat into energy. Omega-3s even help signal your body to burn fat by increasing the amount of the hormone glucagon in your body. The best part about omega-3 fats is that your body uses them in so many different ways that there isn't much left over to be stored in your body. This means you get all the benefits and the full flavor of fat without the negative impact on your health.

Look for omega-3 fats in fatty, cold-water fish like trout and salmon, avocados, olive oil, nuts, and soybeans. My personal favorite source of omega-3s is flax oil or fish oil. I've tried a few different brands, but my favorite by far is Barlean's® Organic Omega Swirl Oil Supplement—with a fruit-smoothie look and taste. You can find more info about Barlean's® in the Approved Products List on page 347. You should have one serving of "good" fat with every meal. This is about one slice of avocado or 1 teaspoon of oil, such as flax or olive. If you like nuts, such as almonds, grab a small handful and you're good to go.

Water

Not getting enough water during the day can leave you feeling tired and drained and make your muscles feel weak. Staying hydrated is essential for everyday function, but it's especially crucial when you're exercising. Your body is more than half water, so your cells need replenishing to operate in top form. Since you lose water throughout the day, you've got to consistently put it back in. The average man sweats between 1 and 1.5 liters of liquid a day—and that doesn't include the amount lost when you go to the bathroom. If you fail to keep your body properly hydrated, you risk developing kidney stones and becoming constipated. On top of that, thirst often leads to overeating; your brain sometimes misreads the signal for a big glass of water as the need for a bite to eat.

Maximize Results with the Right Supplements

Guys are lucky because we don't have to deal with constantly fluctuating hormones and something as physically transformative as menopause when we get older. But that doesn't mean our bodies don't change as we age. To help your body function at its best through the ages, I recommend rounding out your diet with some powerful supplements that will help you do such things as build muscle faster and fight the destructive effects of *free radicals,* which are chemical compounds that beat up on your tissues and can cause serious damage over time.

I know how overwhelming it can be to visit a vitamin and supplement store when you don't even know where to start. Before you know it, you could be walking out with boxes full of strangely named supplements such as horny goat weed and milk thistle. Ideally, we should all aim to get most of our nutrients and minerals from food sources, but to ensure your body is truly stocked to perform at its best, I recommend incorporating some quality supplements into your daily routine.

I've broken down the recommendations by ages, but you should start from the top. That means your list grows as you get older. When you're between the ages of 20 and 35, you want to take advantage of your body when it can truly achieve peak form, so your supplements are focused on maximizing muscle growth (adding muscle to your body now will help you stay stronger as you get older). Once you hit 35, things start to change. As your testosterone and growth hormone levels start to decrease, your energy can drop, and it can be tougher to lose fat because your body tends to store more of it. Plus, you've now entered the realm where the term "anti-aging" sounds appealing to you. That's why the supplements that you should add at this point will help you recover faster from workouts and keep your body young and thriving. If you're 50 or over, restoring and maintaining your vitality is the name of the game. If you want to live a long life with good health and to show off your ripped body, you've got to ensure your muscles stay strong and limit your risk of disease, so look into things like saw palmetto. You'll also see additional supplements sprinkled throughout the tips in Chapters 5 and 6. See products for recommended dosages, and always remember to discuss new supplements with a doctor or nutritionist before you use them, to ensure you're taking the right dosage for your personal health.

When you're 20 to 35, take these:

Multivitamin: The first essential move when it comes to supplements is to buy a quality, well-rounded multivitamin. Look for one that is low in iron or has no iron—too much iron can lead to health problems for men. Look for a well-known brand or buy a store brand if the company is reputable. Also, you can check out my brand of supplements, Jorge's Packs™, available at jorgespacks.com. Be sure your multivitamin provides a good supply of vitamin C, which helps protect your immune system and combats free radicals that you produce when working out, and a good supply of vitamin D, which aids in the absorption of calcium and can help increase muscle strength.

Branched-Chain Amino Acids: Research has shown that taking branched-chain amino acids: or BCAAs, after strength training can promote muscle growth. BCAAs consist of three essential amino acids, leucine, isoleucine, and valine, which are all important to the repair and recovery of muscle tissue. Plus, they'll provide you with extra energy and strength to help push you through your workouts. Look for them in powder or liquid form.

L-glutamine: L-glutamine is a real powerhouse when it comes to you and your muscle mass. It aids in recovery from workouts and increases the level of leucine in muscle fibers, which promotes growth and preserves the muscle you already have. It bolsters your immune system to help you stay strong and avoid sickness, and it has been shown to increase growth hormone levels, making it the perfect supplement to take before you go to bed. I recommend taking L-glutamine morning and night, so you may want to try mixing it into your protein shakes for a quick and efficient muscle-boosting snack.

Creatine: Another powerful supplement, creatine is a naturally occurring acid in your body that is essential to quick muscle recovery and growth. It helps your muscles stay strong and resilient during a workout, and it lets you really push yourself by producing energy and pulling extra water into your muscle tissue. It's been linked to numerous health benefits, such as protection from heart disease. Consider taking creatine before and after your workouts.

Nitric Oxide: Otherwise known as NO, this gaseous molecule helps relax your blood vessels, which opens them up to more oxygen. When oxygen is flowing, your muscles are happy and energized and pumped for your workouts. Look for NO in pill or powder form.

L-carnitine: This nutrient helps your body bring fats into your cells to be converted to energy for your muscles to use. It's been shown to improve fat loss when you're exercising, generally helping to keep your energy high and metabolism revved. Plus, it promotes a healthy heart by helping lower blood pressure and levels of "bad" cholesterol.

When you're 35 to 50, take the previously listed supplements, plus these:

Green Tea Extract: Green tea contains *epigallocatechin gallate,* an antioxidant that has been shown to increase your resting metabolic rate and promote fat oxidation. Sure, you can drink green tea, but taking an extract may be more effective. Besides aiding in fat burn, green tea helps protect your cells from free radicals, including those that are generated from sun damage.

Alpha-lipoic Acid: This antioxidant is manufactured in your body and plays an important role in cell protection and toxin removal, making it effective at helping maintain liver health. It also helps promote creatine uptake and has been shown to enhance removal of glucose from the bloodstream, which helps keep your blood sugar stable. Taking it with creatine after a workout can maximize your muscle recovery.

DHEA: Dehydroepiandrosterone, or DHEA, is a precursor to androsterone, the hormone your body uses to form testosterone. Your levels of DHEA begin to drop after age 30, which leads to lower production of testosterone. If you are lacking in DHEA, you may feel tired, depressed, and uninterested in sex. Also, because your testosterone drops as a result of declining DHEA, your body will not maximize muscle tissue growth and recovery. Get your hormone levels checked before using a DHEA supplement, but I recommend it—it could give you the extra boost you've been looking for.

Pregnenolone: Another hormone produced in your body, pregnenolone helps your body make sex hormones such as DHEA and testosterone, so it works well with a DHEA supplement. Pregnenolone can help combat physical and mental decline and has been shown to improve sleep. In one study, it was proven effective at keeping U.S. Army pilots sharp through times of intense stress by helping them fight fatigue. When you have your hormone levels checked, make sure this one's on the list.

Zinc: More than just good for building up your immune system when fighting a cold, zinc is one of the most important trace minerals men can take. It plays an important role in sexual function, prostate health, hormone balances, skin health, protein digestion, and more. Found in every cell of the body, zinc is essential, and if you're deficient, you could experience things like hair loss, fatigue, and fertility problems. Look for zinc in foods such as oysters, red meat, eggs, and pumpkin seeds. Aim to get about 30 milligrams a day of zinc.

When you're 50-plus, take the previously listed supplements, plus these:

Selenium: High levels of this trace mineral have been associated with reduced risk of prostate cancer. In one study, taking 200 micrograms of selenium a day reduced the risk of developing prostate cancer by 63 percent. You can also get selenium from brazil nuts, tuna, and beef. Not just for prostate health, selenium also helps keep your immune system strong and your thyroid in check.

Korean Red Panax Ginseng: Nearly one in five men over 50 reports experiencing erectile dysfunction. You may have heard of people using the herb ginseng, which has long been used by Asian cultures for medicinal purposes, for stimulating their brains. It turns out that ginseng can stimulate other areas as well. A study done in Korea gave patients 900 milligrams of Korean red ginseng three times daily and discovered surprising results: 60 percent of the men in the study reported improved erections.

Coenzyme Q10: CoQ10 is found in mitochondria, which manufacture energy for your cells. It has been shown to help protect the mitochondria from free radical damage by reducing inflammation, and it has been used to treat heart failure. An adequate supply of CoQ10 is important for general health; it can improve general immune function and keep your tissues and organs strong. You'll get some from dark-green leafy vegetables, beef, and some fish, but supplements can be essential as you get older. Aim for about 200 milligrams a day.

I recommend drinking a lot of water throughout the day. Aim to drink at least 8 eight-ounce glasses each day. It's easier than you think to drink this amount of water; it's just a matter of creating the habit. As I mentioned earlier, begin your day with a 16-ounce glass of cold water to get your metabolism charged first thing. Then carry a good, sturdy water bottle with you throughout the day and refill it as needed. I recently discovered reusable bottles by SIGG that are easy to transport and eco-friendly, and because they're made of metal, they don't put you at risk of consuming plastic that's leached from the bottle. Plus, they're nearly unbreakable. Pick up a reusable bottle of your choice and just start drinking—staying hydrated is that simple. You can also mix it up a bit with some flavor, like a squeeze of lemon or lime.

READY FOR ACTION

Now that you've got a good understanding of all the essential elements of the eating plan, you're probably thinking, "That's all great, but what am I really going to *eat?*" Here's a quick preview of a sample day (for recipes, see the Resources for Him section):

SAMPLE DAY

Breakfast 6:30 a.m.	Snack 9:30 a.m.	Lunch 12:30 p.m.	Snack 3:30 p.m.	Dinner 6:30 p.m.	Before-Bed Snack 9:30 p.m.
Breakfast Burrito	Whey protein shake	BBQ Chicken Pita Sandwiches	Whey protein shake	Body at Home™ Burger and Salad	Whey protein shake

That's basically how your day will look on this plan. You're going to be giving your body all the high-quality, nutrient-rich materials it needs to build your muscle mass and burn fat.

To make sure you stick to the plan, I've built in an optional "cheat" day that will allow you to give in to any cravings you've had throughout the week. I know how hard it can be to give up something, so I've made this a realistic plan that works for your life. You get to pick one day a week when you can eat *whatever you want*—pizza, fries, whatever you've been craving all week. I believe that if you try to deprive yourself of things you want, you create weakness that leads to bingeing—I'm talking about stuffing down a bag of potato chips in the middle of the night kind of stuff—and I know guys do it because I was once there myself!

You may be thinking that the last thing you want to do is ruin all of the hard work you've done in just one day. And the choice of whether to use the cheat day or not is completely up to you. But, oddly enough, studies have shown that if you double the amount of calories you normally eat in one day, you actually increase your metabolism by 9 percent for the following

24 hours. The key is to focus on one day of the week when all rules are off. This way you won't lose sight of your goal of losing 10 pounds from your gut. A lot of my clients picked Sunday as their cheat day because it was the perfect day of the week to relax and kick back and drink some beer or have a barbecue.

Use this day to keep yourself on track throughout the rest of the week; in fact, use it as motivation to get through the week if you need to. As soon as you start eating on this plan, though, I think you'll be surprised at how great you feel! You will be giving your body the ingredients it needs to function at its absolute best. You will feel so good that your cheat day may make you feel so lousy that you won't want to continue using it. It will be obvious to you how much what you put in your body controls the amount of energy you have, the kind of sleep you get, how strong you feel in your workouts, and even how good sex is.

Keep in mind that cheat day is optional. If you feel that having a day off will be too much of a distraction, by all means stick to the plan seven days a week. If you need to make a hard and fast commitment for the entire eight weeks, then don't incorporate the cheat day. It's there if you need it but is certainly not required. This eating plan is made to work for your life, so customize it to create results for yourself.

EVERYTHING YOU'LL NEED

If you turn to the Resources for Him section, you'll find some simple and great-tasting recipes that follow the plan. They are delicious; try them out (see page 322). You'll also find a food list (page 341) that will give you a better idea of the best foods to eat to build muscle efficiently. Keep in mind that you can eat out on this plan. When you do, choose dishes that have high-quality, lean protein, double up on the vegetables, and cut out the fries. Making the plan work is simple no matter where you are. Check out the list of fast and frozen foods (page 344) to see what to order at places like KFC and Arby's. I don't recommend eating at such restaurants every day, but if you're on the go, you can still be smart about the foods you choose.

On the next page, you'll see a sample Eating Planner log. Keeping a log of your meals, snacks, and water will be an important way to keep yourself on track. In the Resources for Him section there is a blank Eating Planner log for you to copy and fill out every day (see page 315). You may think it sounds silly, but trust me, it's just as important as logging the weights you use in your workouts. Make notes about what recipes you like and even some modifications, like trying chicken with one of the dishes instead of beef. Using this log will also help you stick to the 40/40/20 ratio by giving you a quick view of what you're eating every day.

Now, it's time to eat!

EATING PLANNER (SAMPLE)

This plan will ensure leaner muscle and a higher metabolism.

Breakfast>time 7:45 am

	Description
● PROTEIN (5oz)	Scrambled Eggs
● CARBS (½ cup or 1 slice of bread)	Tortilla
● FRUIT (1 cup)	Sliced Oranges
● FAT (1 teaspoon)	Flax oil

Snack>time 10:45 am

	Description
● WHEY PROTEIN SHAKE (1 scoop)	Jorge's Packs choc. shake

Jorge recommends Jorge's Packs™ for your protein drinks. **>** See list of other recommended snacks at the back of the book.

Lunch>time 1:45 pm

	Description
● PROTEIN (5oz)	Meatballs
● CARBS (½ cup or 1 slice of bread)	Whole - Grain Bun
● VEGGIES** (2 cups)	Mixed Greens
● FAT (1 teaspoon)	Vinaigrette

Snack>time 4:45 pm

	Description
● WHEY PROTEIN SHAKE (1 scoop)	Jorge's Packs vanilla shake

Dinner>time 7:45 pm

	Description
● PROTEIN (5oz)	Grilled Steak
● VEGGIES* (2–4 cups)	Steamed Broccoli
● FAT (1 teaspoon)	Butter

Snack>time 10:45 pm

	Description
● WHEY PROTEIN SHAKE (1 scoop)	Jorge's Packs choc. shake

*Veggies = nonstarchy vegetables.

Water (eight 8-oz cups) ● ● ● ● ● ● ● ●

Multivitamin ●

Height: 6'1" | **Age:** 46 | **Lost:** 6 pounds

"Before this plan, I was not getting the results that I wanted from my workouts. No matter how much I would do in the gym, I could not get the six-pack abs and nice chest that I was working so hard for. Body at Home™ showed me how to get the results I had been working for all those years. I can see my six pack now—and it took only eight weeks to see the difference!

"My confidence level has increased, and I feel good and I look good! My friends are asking me, 'What program are you on because you are looking good?!' Now that in itself is worth gold to me!"

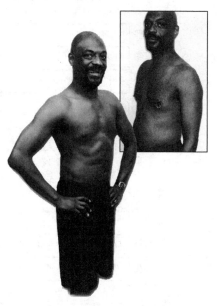

Do This

· Remove all processed foods from the house (white pastas, rice, breads, sugars, etc).

· Keep a healthy snack around at all times. That way, when your body says, "It's been three hours and I want to eat something," you'll have a good option.

· If you have a setback, don't give up. Your body actually remembers where you left off, and it does not take long at all to resume from that point.

4 Getting Started

"I have been thrilled with Jorge's program—the results have been amazing. I am getting lean and toned, and my muscle definition is more pronounced."

—STEVE SHULTZ, BODY AT HOME™ STAR, LOST 11 POUNDS

Body at Home™ for Men has two phases: the Quick-Start Phase and the Power Phase. The phases are designed to build up the challenge to your muscles. I recommend following the plan exactly as it's laid out for you—at least the first time around. If you want to see maximum results, it's critical for you to follow the plan as it was designed.

You will need only a few basic tools to get started with the workouts: a Swiss ball, a set of dumbbells, a mat, a medicine ball, and a simple barbell free weight set. In some of my other workouts, you may have noticed things like bands and cables, which are great, but when it comes down to building as much muscle as possible, free weights are the way to go. Barbells and dumbbells challenge your muscles to another degree by incorporating balancing and stability elements that help engage every fiber of your muscle tissue.

You can get all of the equipment you need at BodyatHome.com, or you can pick it up at your local sporting goods store or in stores such as Target or Wal-Mart. The products I like and the ones I have in my own home gym are made by GoFit™. You can find out more about them on page 347.

QUICK-START PHASE

This two-week phase is specifically designed so you can start losing fat—especially abdominal fat—right away. Remember, you do not need to go to the gym to do this program. Every single one of your workouts can be done from home. Eliminating the "I just couldn't get to the gym" excuse is going to help you stick to this plan.

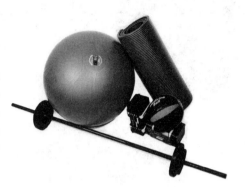

POWER PHASE

Once you're done with the Quick-Start Phase, I hope you're hooked! After just two weeks I know you'll already be impressed with the improvement in your body and the amount of energy you have. My challenge to you is to continue for six more weeks and really see your V-Shape build up and your abs develop even more.

In week three, you'll begin the Power Phase. In this portion of the program you will be building stacks of lean muscle and really adding definition. As the weeks progress, you will find that the program becomes slightly more challenging each week. This is to keep your body changing and adapting so that you avoid plateaus and continue to build that lean muscle. If you kept doing the same exercises, your body would adjust and hit a sort of comfort zone. Guess what? Nobody ever created change when they were comfortable. *You are here to lose 10 pounds from your gut.* That's why the workouts will continue to challenge you throughout the program.

Even though we're going to take it up a notch in the Power Phase, you can continue to do the workouts at home. If you want to mix it up, try doing your workout at the gym or outside, or get a buddy to try the workout with you and use his house for a change of environment. Most important, no matter where or when you do your workouts, devote your full attention for the entire 33.5 minutes. I know how easy it is to get distracted, but you've got to shut everything out for this time. Turn off your Blackberry, close down your computer, and really focus on getting everything you can out of each workout. If you do this, you'll be rewarded with amazing results.

TIME TO WORK OUT

I know you have a busy schedule, but the most important thing you can do to reach your goal is to stay consistent. From training my clients and trying to stick to my own workouts, I can tell you that one of the keys to staying consistent is a solid no-excuses schedule. What I recommend and what works for me is a *Monday, Wednesday, and Friday training schedule*. It gives you a day of rest between each workout day and the entire weekend to recover. Plus, starting the week with such a strong and powerful workout will really get you pumped. Believe me—Monday, Wednesday, and Friday workouts are the way to go. If you absolutely can't work out on these days, be sure to allow at least one day between workouts for essential rest, repair, and recovery.

I have provided some logs for you to use to track your progress through the program. On page 208 there's a filled-out example of the Workout Log that you will use to record each workout, including details such as how much weight you used, the intensity you achieved, and other important information. In the Resources for Him section, on pages 315–319, you'll find blank versions of the Workout Log for all three workout days. Make eight copies of each one to use throughout the program.

On page 209, you'll see a handwritten example of the 8-Week Workout Chart, a simple tracking calendar that lets you cross off each day of the plan. This chart may seem a bit basic, but each workout you log means you are closer to losing your gut and reaching your goal—you will feel good. For a blank version, turn to page 316. Downloadable versions of the logs and chart are available at BodyatHome.com.

Before you start your first workout, I have a few quick essential tips for you. This information will be vital to creating the absolute optimum results on this program. Four simple things can make all the difference in how quickly and effectively you lose your gut and build your V-shape: form, counting, breathing, and intensity.

No Equipment? No Problem

Even if you don't have dumbbells, barbells, or a stability ball, you can get a workout in right now. In the Resources section, on page 338, you'll find my "no excuses workout"—a Weight-Free Routine that you can begin right now. All you need is your body's own resistance, a chair, and a towel. This routine provides a full-body workout in a little over 30 minutes. I use it when I'm traveling and when I can't get away from work long enough to work out. You can do it right in your office. One important point to remember: This routine is not to replace the regular workouts; it's meant to get you started right away. As soon as you can, get the equipment you need and jump to Chapter 5. You need the weighted workouts to create the challenge needed to build your muscle mass.

DAY 1

DATE __Monday__

Start Time __7:00__ Finish Time __7:34__

TOTAL TIME __34 minutes__

Select weights so that by the end of the 4th rep of each exercise you feel an intensity level of 8.

Muscle Group	Exercise	Weight Used	Intensity Level	set 1	set 2
CHEST	Push-up	N/A	9	✓	✓
CHEST	Flat Barbell Pres	35 lbs	8	✓	✓
CHEST	Incline Dumbell Press	25 lbs	9	✓	✓
CHEST	Incline Dumbell Fly	15 lbs	9	✓	✓

At this point you should be about 6 minutes into your workout.

SHOULDERS	Barbell Mil. Press on Ball	20 lbs	8	✓	✓
SHOULDERS	Standing Lateral Raise	5 lbs	10	✓	✓
SHOULDERS	Bent-over Rear Delt Raise	5 lbs	9	✓	✓

At this point you should be about 14 minutes into your workout, including 2 minutes of transition time.

ABS	Medicine Ball Pullover	8 lbs	10	✓	✓
ABS	Reverse Crunch	N/A	8	✓	✓
ABS	Barbell Twist	Bar	9	✓	✓

At this point in your workout you should be at 20 minutes. Congratulations! YOU DID IT!

BONUS CARDIO 20-MINUTE MORNING POWER WALK ●

LARGE

SMALL

ABS

8-WEEK WORKOUT CHART

Start Date **7/2**   Finish Date **8/26**

Monday	Tuesday	Wednesday	Thursday	Friday	Saturday	Sunday	
DAY 1 WORKOUT 7/2	**DAY 2** DAY OFF	**DAY 3** WORKOUT 7/4	**DAY 4** DAY OFF	**DAY 5** WORKOUT 7/6	**DAY 6** DAY OFF	**DAY 7** DAY OFF	WEEK 1
DAY 8 WORKOUT 7/9	**DAY 9** DAY OFF	**DAY 10** WORKOUT 7/11	**DAY 11** DAY OFF	**DAY 12** WORKOUT 7/13	**DAY 13** DAY OFF	**DAY 14** DAY OFF	WEEK 2
DAY 15 WORKOUT 7/16	**DAY 16** DAY OFF	**DAY 17** WORKOUT 7/18	**DAY 18** DAY OFF	**DAY 19** WORKOUT 7/20	**DAY 20** DAY OFF	**DAY 21** DAY OFF	WEEK 3
DAY 22 WORKOUT 7/23	**DAY 23** DAY OFF	**DAY 24** WORKOUT 7/25	**DAY 25** DAY OFF	**DAY 26** WORKOUT 7/27	**DAY 27** DAY OFF	**DAY 28** DAY OFF	WEEK 4
DAY 29 WORKOUT 7/30	**DAY 30** DAY OFF	**DAY 31** WORKOUT 8/1	**DAY 32** DAY OFF	**DAY 33** WORKOUT 8/3	**DAY 34** DAY OFF	**DAY 35** DAY OFF	WEEK 5
DAY 36 WORKOUT 8/6	**DAY 37** DAY OFF	**DAY 38** WORKOUT 8/8	**DAY 39** DAY OFF	**DAY 40** WORKOUT 8/10	**DAY 41** DAY OFF	**DAY 42** DAY OFF	WEEK 6
DAY 43 WORKOUT 8/13	**DAY 44** DAY OFF	**DAY 45** WORKOUT 8/15	**DAY 46** DAY OFF	**DAY 47** WORKOUT 8/17	**DAY 48** DAY OFF	**DAY 49** DAY OFF	WEEK 7
DAY 50 WORKOUT 8/20	**DAY 51** DAY OFF	**DAY 52** WORKOUT 8/22	**DAY 53** DAY OFF	**DAY 54** WORKOUT 8/24	**DAY 55** DAY OFF	**DAY 56** SUCCESS	WEEK 8

*Please photocopy and place on your refrigerator. As you complete your workouts, cross off the days so you can see your success!

Just for Men

Even if you followed my 12-Second Sequence™ program, which requires gym time, the Body at Home™ program will still create amazing results for you. It is designed specifically for guys to create powerful fat-burning muscle mass. Using the Body Priority, you will give special priority to the muscle groups that require more strength and intensity. You'll begin the first training day of the week at your strongest, which is why you'll work chest and shoulders. On the second day, you're going to focus on back and biceps; on the third, legs and triceps. I know abs are number one, so we'll train them during every workout. They recover more quickly than your other muscle groups, so they can be worked each time.

Some of the Body at Home™ movements might seem familiar. Essentially, your muscles can follow only certain *paths of motion*. This means that a squat will always follow the same path, as will a curl, a press, and so forth. What makes the Body at Home™ program different from my other program is the Body Priority. The sequence in which you do the workouts will make all the difference in the results. It's like the way letters come together to form a word. Take the letters L-I-V-E, and you've got a positive, hopeful word. Reverse the letters, and you've got E-V-I-L, a source of darkness and destruction. Bottom line: Because of the order in which you do these workouts, you will pack on muscle in all the right places and create the V-Shape you want, no matter what workouts you've done before.

The Importance of Form

Since the Body at Home™ movements are based on a *slow-lifting technique,* you are already a step ahead when it comes to achieving proper form. Most people (especially guys!) rush through their exercises, which can result in poor form—otherwise known as the fast track to lousy results or (even worse) injury. Don't cheat yourself out of getting the best results by throwing your back to lift a weight or engaging your biceps when you're trying to work your triceps. If you have improper form, you won't fully fatigue the right muscle group and you won't see the results you want. Don't waste your time with bad form—it won't get you where you want to go.

In Chapter 5, you will see a brief description for each move accompanied by two main photographs. To make sure you have correct form on each exercise, read through the descriptions before you begin your workout, and pay attention to the notes! The descriptions are brief, but they provide critical information such as how to grip the weights and where to position your feet. Although they will help you with each specific exercise, there are some other steps you can take to ensure you get the most out of each workout.

First, I recommend doing a "dry run" before each workout. Read through the exercises and do each move once (without weights) to get your body familiar with the MTP of each move. You'll get the movement down pretty quickly, but don't get frustrated if it feels a little strange at first. Remember, you can always use your 30-second break between moves to review something if you have to.

Visit BodyatHome.com for videos you can watch to help with proper form.

Counting

Counting is going to be critical to your success, and it's incredibly important that you do not cheat! As I mentioned before, you are going to begin each move with a 10-second motion, hold for 2 seconds at the MTP, and then return to the starting position through another count of 10 seconds. Stick to a slow and deliberate count—don't rush or cut the crucial 2-second hold short. Remember, timing is the revolutionary core of Body at Home™; doing it right is what's going to transform your body. Each workout is just 33.5 minutes, so every second that you make the most of puts you one step closer to losing your gut.

Breathing Right

I'm sure you've seen guys whose faces turn bright red face when they work out and who literally look as if they're going to explode. The problem is those guys aren't breathing properly while they're lifting. This not only puts a dangerous amount of stress on their hearts but does a disservice to their muscles. Your muscles use oxygen as fuel, and when you don't give them enough, they become weak and fatigue faster. Oxygen combines with glycogen and fat to produce energy and keep you going strong. To make sure you keep your muscles fueled during your workouts, I recommend a technique called *feathered breathing*. It is a breathing pattern that prevents you from holding your breath throughout your four reps by creating a continuous, steady stream of oxygen. Simply take a deep breath in before beginning an exercise, and then exhale in small short bursts until you have expelled all of the air out of your lungs. Then repeat. There's a video of me demonstrating feathered breathing at BodyatHome.com. Feathered breathing may feel a bit awkward at first, but stick with it. This breathing pattern will start to feel natural while you are doing your workouts. And I guarantee it will keep you feeling strong and energized throughout each workout.

Intensity

I'm sure you've thought there's no way you're really going to see impressive results in just over 30 minutes. Well, if you don't put in an intense workout, you might not. The exercises and structure to build muscle mass and help you lose your gut are here in this program, but your intensity is going to determine how rapidly you see results. Bottom line: You get out of it what you put into it. The right level is different for everyone. What's important is that you achieve the most challenging workout *for your body*. Here are some tips on creating the right intensity:

- *Pick the right weight.* If you can lift a weight past four reps, then the weight you are working with is not heavy enough. If you can get in only two or three reps, your weight is too heavy. I know, it's not rocket science, but it really is the best way to determine if you're creating the right level of intensity for your body. If you don't create a challenge for your muscles, you will not accelerate the development of new muscle mass.

- *Perform a gut check.* At the end of each workout ask yourself, "Did I really work as hard as I could today?" Be honest! If you don't push yourself, you're never going to change your body. Don't be afraid to really take it to the next level—you'll be rewarded with truly incredible results.

ACCELERATE RESULTS FOR YOUR BODY TYPE

To accelerate your results on this plan, I recommend 20 minutes of pre-breakfast cardio done at an incline. Why should you do it in the morning? Well, research at Kansas State University and at the University of California, Berkeley, confirms that cardio done on an empty stomach is more effective than cardio performed after eating. Studies at these universities found that fasting exercisers burned more than exercisers who ate beforehand. *How often you should do this cardio depends on your particular body type.*

Everyone's genetics are different, and let's face it, some people have it easier than others when it comes to staying in shape. Merely looking at a slice of pizza can make some guys feel as if they just put on 5 pounds. Other guys can literally eat all day long, consuming tons of calories yet still look as if they are starving. And then of course there are guys who are genetically lucky and don't have to put in much effort but still have mountains of muscle and more definition than Webster's dictionary.

But wait—even though you may not have perfect genetics, you still can have an amazing body. You just need to know how to make a few small adjustments to suit your specific body type. There are basically three different body types: endomorphs, mesomorphs, and ectomorphs. Modify your cardio training to reflect the category that you fall into:

Endomorphs: Endomorphs are naturally large people who usually build muscle fairly easily but often carry more fat. Characteristics of endomorphs are large, thick, dense bone structure, wide hips, and round face. Endomorphs usually have a slower metabolism and seem to find it a little more difficult to shed fat. If you are an endomorph, it is going to be critical for you to do morning cardio six or seven days a week. The good news is you will have an advantage when it comes to building fat-burning lean muscle, so you can keep your metabolism at full throttle!

Mesomorphs: Mesomorphs are naturally muscular. They are identified by their wide shoulders, small waists, and long, full-muscle bellies. Building lean muscle and losing body fat isn't very difficult for mesomorphs. If you are a mesomorph, you should generally do you morning cardio two or three days a week, but not more or less than that.

Ectomorphs: Ectomorphs are the skinny guys, Think about Lance Armstrong or Michael Phelps—these are prime examples of ectomorphs. Ectomorphs have extremely fast metabolism. Characteristics of ectomorphs are narrow bones and joints, such as the wrist, very low body fat, and long, thin, sinewy muscles. If you are an ectomorph, you should stay away from cardio altogether. You need to put all of your focus on building muscle mass. If you are very thin yet have some fat around your midsection, the added muscle mass will take care of that area.

Now, let's get to the workout! If you forget anything about breathing, counting, or form, remember to flip back to this chapter for a quick review. The Body at Home™ for Men is going to help you drop 10 pounds from your gut and develop your V-Shape. Following these guidelines will ensure you accomplish this as quickly, effectively, and safely as possible. Now let's get started!

Height: 6'3" | **Age:** 32 | **Lost:** 10 pounds (Plus restored 2 pounds of lean muscle)

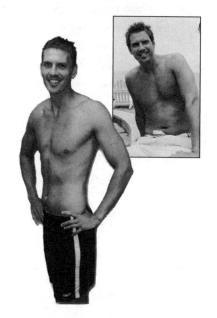

"I am so busy all the time that I never could fit eating right and working out into my busy schedule. After hearing about this program, I was skeptical that it would make managing the workouts and eating easy enough for my lifestyle. Eight weeks later, I realize how easy living a healthy, active lifestyle is. Eating is like clockwork now and the exercises take no time at all! I couldn't believe the results I have seen—I look great and feel great, and now I have found a program that is manageable with my busy schedule. Body at Home™ is great for anyone who thinks they don't have time to exercise!"

Do This

· Try to create a schedule that works for your lifestyle. Don't force yourself to do the workouts in the morning if you're not a morning person. Do them when you know you'll be most motivated.

· Find a friend/spouse to team up with. This helps you stay focused and motivated.

· Definitely have a cheat meal or day on weekends to reward yourself. It gives you something to look forward to.

5 Quick-Start Phase

WEEKS 1 AND 2

20 to 35 PRIME TIME

Stand Tall

Nothing says confidence more than walking into a room with your back straight, shoulders wide, and head up. Add a slight, assured smile and you're likely to win anyone over, whether it's a prospective boss or a potential first date. Having good posture doesn't just make you look better; it can make you feel better too. When you make a physiological change—even something as simple as pulling your shoulders back and lifting your chest—you change your emotional state as well. When you stand or sit up straight, you open up your lungs and allow oxygen to flow better throughout your body. And when the cells and tissues in your body are fully oxygenated, you feel energized and calm, and your organs have the space they need to function at their best. Slouching or slumping limits the flow of oxygen through your body, and the physical "depression" can literally make you feel down, anxious, and tense because your body isn't getting enough of this crucial element. Plus, good posture can make your voice sound stronger and fuller, which can give you a commanding presence on the field, in the office, and anywhere else you'd like to take the lead.

35 to 50 STAY YOUNG

Skin Care

I hate to say it, but wrinkles catch up even to us guys! We're fortunate because our skin tends to be more resilient than women's, but wrinkles still become a dead giveaway of our age. To help protect your skin and keep it healthy, be sure you have a skin-care routine. There was a time when it was hard to find cleansers or moisturizers that were good for men's skin, but now we can get nearly everything a woman can. From eye creams to masks, products catering to men's grooming are available at most department stores. If you want to keep it simple, look for a good face soap and a moisturizer with SPF 30. One brand I trust and use every day is Alba, found at many grocery stores. Dry skin doesn't look good on anyone, and if you've been using bar soap on your face and skipping a daily moisturizer, chances are your skin could use some hydration. Lack of sleep and drinking alcohol or smoking also can lead to dry skin. At the very least, skip the cigarettes and get some sleep. If you do have a few drinks on your free day, remember to get a lot of water that night or the next day—your skin, and your body, will thank you. Taking care of your skin now will keep you looking younger, so don't neglect it!

WEEK 1

As you gear up to start your week, use these tips based on your Life Priority to create extra inner drive and motivation. They are customized to your age category, but I recommend you read every one of them. You'll find valuable information in each tip, no matter what your age.

50-Plus LONGEVITY

Get a Physical

If you have this book in your hands, chances are you want to be strong and fit for life—and prove that even a guy in his fifties or older can get rid of his gut. Body at Home™ is going to give you the workouts and the proper nutrition to get you there, but you've got to hold up your end of the bargain. What do I mean? Well, if you want to ensure longevity, you've got to stay on track with regular doctor's visits and checkups. At this point in your life, you should be getting a physical every year. It should include getting your blood pressure checked and blood work done; a rectal exam; an EKG and heart-health check; a prostate-specific antigen (PSA) test; and inspection of your skin to check for discolored moles and bumps and other signs of skin cancer. The American Cancer Society suggests taking steps to ensure early detection of types of cancer besides prostate. They recommend a test that checks for both polyps and cancer, such as a sigmoidoscopy or a double-contrast barium enema, every five years or a colonoscopy every ten years. Remember too to tell your doctor about your family history; this information can let your doctor know how aggressively to monitor your health.

MONDAY

Push-Up

Lie on a mat with your hands slightly wider than shoulder-width apart and your fingers pointing forward. Press up to starting position, keeping your back straight, abs tight, and head up. Feather your breathing as you lower your chest toward the floor through a count of 10 seconds. Hold for 2 seconds at the MTP. Push your body back to starting position through a count of 10 seconds, keeping your elbows slightly bent. Without resting, repeat three times. Rest for 30 seconds and then repeat the entire sequence.

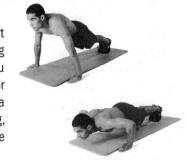

Flat Barbell Press

Hold the barbell and lie on the ball so that it comfortably supports your shoulder blades. Extend your arms in front of you pressing the weight up. Feather your breathing as you lower the weight through a count of 10 seconds. Hold for 2 seconds at the MTP (about 1 inch above your chest). Press the barbell back to starting position through a count of 10 seconds. Without resting, repeat three times. Rest for 30 seconds and then repeat the entire sequence.

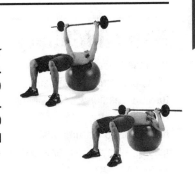

Incline Dumbbell Press

Hold a pair of dumbbells and lie on the ball so that your head and neck are supported. Allow your hips to drop almost to the ground. Press the weights up and together, with a slight bend in the elbows so that the upper chest is targeted. Feather your breathing as you lower the weights through a count of 10 seconds. Hold for 2 seconds at the MTP. Press the dumbbells up to starting position through a count of 10 seconds. Without resting, repeat three times. Rest for 30 seconds and then repeat the entire sequence.

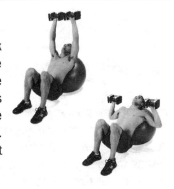

Key

MTP: Maximum tension point.

Feather your breathing: Inhale deeply and exhale in short bursts.

Timing: Each exercise should take 90 seconds and be followed by a 30-second rest. The workout should take a total of 20 minutes.

Incline Dumbbell Fly

Hold a pair of dumbbells and lie on the ball with your head and neck supported. Roll down the ball until your hips drop almost to the ground. Extend the dumbbells over your chest, palms facing each other, elbows slightly bent. Feather your breathing as you lower the weights down and out through a count of 10 seconds. Hold for 2 seconds at the MTP (when your arms are open in a "T" position). Raise the weights to starting position in a "bear hug" type motion through a count of 10 seconds. Without resting, repeat three times. Rest for 30 seconds and then repeat the entire sequence.

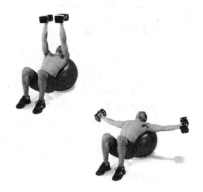

Barbell Military Press on Swiss Ball

Hold the barbell and sit on the ball with your back straight, abs tight, and chin up. Extend the barbell up and directly over your head, palms facing forward. Feather your breathing as you lower the weight through a count of 10 seconds. Hold for 2 seconds at the MTP (chin level). Press the barbell up to starting position through a count of 10 seconds. Without resting, repeat three times. Rest for 30 seconds and then repeat the entire sequence.

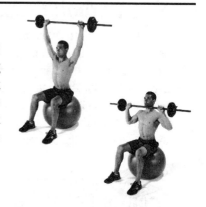

Standing Lateral Raise

Hold a pair of dumbbells and stand with your back straight and abs tight. With your arms against your sides and elbows slightly bent, feather your breathing as you raise the weights up through a count of 10 seconds. Hold and squeeze for 2 seconds at the MTP ("T" position). Lower the weights to starting position through a count of 10 seconds. Without resting, repeat three times. Rest for 30 seconds and then repeat the entire sequence.

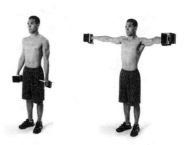

Bent-Over Rear Delt Raise

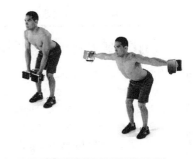

Hold a pair of dumbbells, palms facing each other. Bend at the waist as if you were about to tie your shoes; then lift only your chin and chest, creating a slight arch in your back. Feather your breathing as you raise the weights to your sides through a count of 10 seconds. Hold and squeeze for 2 seconds at the MTP. Lower the weights to starting position through a count of 10 seconds. Without resting, repeat three times. Rest for 30 seconds and then repeat the entire sequence.

Medicine Ball Pull-Over

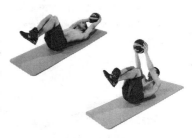

Lie on a mat and bring your knees up to a 90-degree angle. Grasp a medicine ball and extend it over your head, keeping a slight bend in your elbows. Keep your abs tight and feather your breathing as you raise the ball over your head and crunch up through a count of 10 seconds. Hold for 2 seconds at the MTP. Lower the ball to starting position through a count of 10 seconds. Without resting, repeat three times.

Reverse Crunch

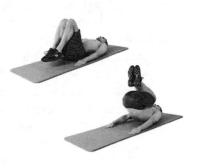

Lie on a mat with your hands by your sides, palms down. Pull your heels up as close to your butt as possible. Raise your heels about 2 inches off the ground. Keep your chin tucked and abs tight. Feather your breathing as you pull your knees toward your chest, using your lower abdominals, through a count of 10 seconds. Hold and squeeze for 2 seconds at the MTP (when your butt is completely off the ground). Lower your body to starting position through a count of 10 seconds. Without resting, repeat three times.

Barbell Twist

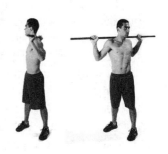

Grip an empty barbell, placing it across the back of your shoulders. Stand with your legs about 3 feet apart. Twist your upper body to one side. With your chin up and abs squeezed tight, feather your breathing as you slowly twist to the other side through a count of 10 seconds. At the MTP of your twist, hold and squeeze for 2 seconds. Return to starting position through a count of 10 seconds. Without resting, repeat three times. (Note: If you can do more than 4 reps, you're not squeezing your abs hard enough throughout the exercise.)

Dumbbell Pull-Over

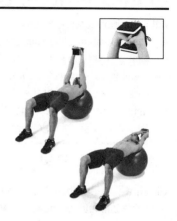

Grasp a dumbbell using the "diamond grip." Lie on the ball with your head and neck supported. Keep your hips up and abs tight throughout the exercise. Extend the weight over your chest with a slight bend in the elbows. Feather your breathing as you lower the weight behind your head through a count of 10 seconds. Hold for 2 seconds at the MTP. Raise the weight to starting position through a count of 10 seconds. Without resting, repeat three times. Rest for 30 seconds and then repeat the entire sequence. (Note: How far you can stretch your arms back will determine your MTP.)

Bent-Over Dumbbell Row (Underhand Grip)

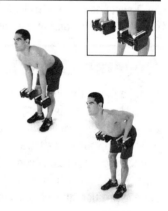

Hold a pair of dumbbells, using the underhand grip, arms extended. Stand with your feet hip-width apart. Bend at the waist as if tying your shoes. Raise your head and chest to create a slight arch in the back. Bend your knees slightly. Feather your breathing as you pull the dumbbells up in a fluid rowing motion through a count of 10 seconds, keeping your elbows close to your body. Hold and squeeze your shoulder blades together for 2 seconds at the MTP. Lower your arms to starting position through a count of 10 seconds. Without resting, repeat three times. Rest for 30 seconds and then repeat the entire sequence.

Bent-Over Barbell Row (Overhand Grip)

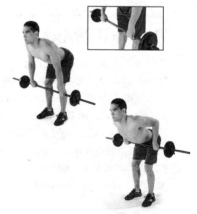

Hold the barbell with your arms extended, using the overhand grip. Stand with your feet hip-width apart. Bend at the waist as if you were about to tie your shoes; then lift only your chin and chest, creating a slight arch in your back. Keeping a bend in your knees, feather your breathing as you pull the weight up toward your hips in a fluid rowing motion through a count of 10 seconds. Hold and squeeze your shoulder blades together for 2 seconds at the MTP. Lower your arms to starting position through a count of 10 seconds. Without resting, repeat three times. Rest for 30 seconds and then repeat the entire sequence.

Hyperextension

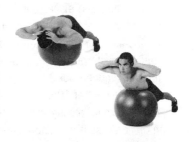

Lie facedown on the ball with your hips supported and your hands behind your head. Bend at the waist and feather your breathing as you lift your upper body through a count of 10 seconds, using your lower back. Hold for 2 seconds at the MTP. Return to starting position through a count of 10 seconds. Without resting, repeat three times. Rest for 30 seconds and then repeat the entire sequence.

Standing Barbell Curl (Wide Grip)

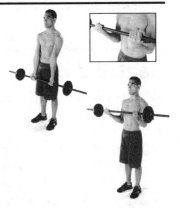

Hold the barbell using the wide grip. Stand with your feet shoulder-width apart and your arms extended by your sides, knees slightly bent. Feather your breathing as you curl the weight up through a count of 10 seconds. Hold and squeeze for 2 seconds at the MTP. Keep your elbows close against your body as you lower the weight to starting position through a count of 10 seconds. Without resting, repeat three times. Rest for 30 seconds and then repeat the entire sequence.

Standing Side Curl

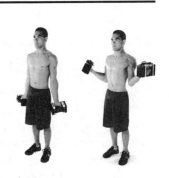

Hold a pair of dumbbells with your palms turned out, elbows to your side. Keep your chest up, feet hip-width apart, knees slightly bent, and abs tight throughout the exercise. Feather your breathing as you curl the weight up through a count of 10 seconds, keeping your elbows close to your body. Hold and squeeze for 2 seconds at the MTP. Lower the weights to starting position through a count of 10 seconds until your arms are completely straight (do not lock your elbows). Without resting, repeat three times. Rest for 30 seconds and then repeat the entire sequence.

Hammer Curl

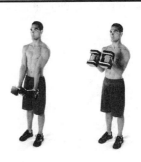

Holding a pair of dumbbells, stand with your feet shoulder-width apart, your arms extended slightly in front of your thighs, palms facing each other, and knees slightly bent. Feather your breathing as you curl the weights up through a count of 10 seconds, keeping your palms facing each other. Hold and squeeze for 2 seconds at the MTP. Lower the weights to starting position through a count of 10 seconds. Without resting, repeat three times. Rest for 30 seconds and then repeat the entire sequence.

Double Crunch

Lie on a mat and place your hands behind your head, elbows up, chin up, and abs tight. Pull your heels toward your butt as far as you can. Using your upper abs, feather your breathing as you crunch up while simultaneously pulling your knees in through a count of 10 seconds. Hold and squeeze for 2 seconds at the MTP. Return to starting position through a count of 10 seconds, never letting your upper back touch the ground. Without resting, repeat three times. (Note: The range of motion on this exercise is very short so be sure to adjust your speed so that you hit the MTP on the count of 10.)

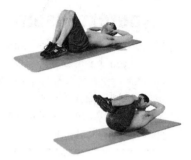

Seated V-Up

Sit on the ground with your arms slightly behind you, elbows bent, and fingertips pointed forward. Start with your knees together, legs extended, and heels off the ground about 2 inches. Support your upper body weight with your palms. Feather your breathing as you pull the knees into your chest for a count of 10 seconds. Hold and squeeze for 2 seconds at the MTP. Return to starting position through a count of 10 seconds, keeping your abs tight. Without resting, repeat three times.

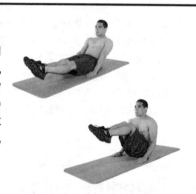

Bicycle Crunch

Lie flat on your back. Place your hands behind your head and raise your heels about 2 inches from the ground, keeping your chin up and abs tight throughout the exercise. Bring your right elbow to your left knee and feather your breathing as you rotate to the other side for a count of 10 seconds. Hold and squeeze for 2 seconds at the MTP (where your left elbow meets your right knee). Return to starting position through a count of 10 seconds. Without resting, repeat three times.

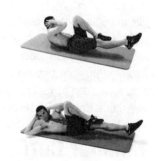

FRIDAY

Dumbbell Squat

Hold a pair of dumbbells with your arms extended against your sides, and stand with your feet shoulder-width apart. Feather your breathing as you slowly squat through a count of 10 seconds, keeping your back straight, abs tight, and chest up. Hold for 2 seconds at the MTP (when your legs are almost at a 90-degree angle). Return to starting position through a count of 10 seconds. Without resting, repeat three times. Rest for 30 seconds and then repeat the entire sequence.

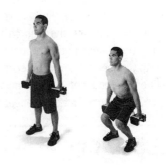

Dumbbell Sumo Squat

Hold a pair of dumbbells, palms facing back, arms extended in front of your body. Stand with your feet about two times wider than shoulder-width apart, toes turned out to the sides, and knees aligned over the toes. Feather your breathing as you squat through a count of 10 seconds. Hold for 2 seconds at the MTP. Push through your heels to return to starting position through a count of 10 seconds. Without resting, repeat three times. Rest for 30 seconds and then repeat the entire sequence.

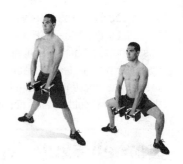

Lunge

Hold a dumbbell in one hand and rest the other on the back of a sturdy chair for balance. Stand in a lunge position. Keep your back straight, chest up, and abs tight. Feather your breathing as you drop your back knee toward the ground through a count of 10 seconds. Hold for 2 seconds at the MTP (a couple of inches above the ground). Return to starting position through a count of 10 seconds. Without resting, repeat one more time on this leg and then perform 2 more reps on the other side for a total of 4. Rest for 30 seconds and then repeat the entire sequence. (Note: To avoid injury, make sure that your front knee stays aligned with your toes and doesn't bend farther than a 90-degree angle.)

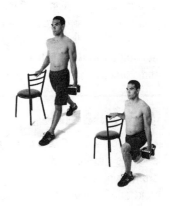

Swiss Ball Hamstring Curl

Lie on your back with your arms at your sides, palms flat on the floor. Place your heels on the ball, knees straight but not completely locked; then lift your butt and hips off the ground. With your abs tight, feather your breathing and bend your knees as you roll the ball toward your butt with your heels. Hold for 2 seconds at the MTP. Return to starting position through a count of 10 seconds. Without resting, repeat three times. Rest for 30 seconds and then repeat the entire sequence.

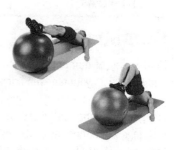

Chair Dip

Sit at the front edge of a sturdy chair or exercise bench, hands close to your sides, fingers forward, and legs extended. Flex your feet so that your weight is on your heels and slide yourself away from the chair. Feather your breathing as you lower yourself through a count of 10 seconds. Hold for 2 seconds at the MTP (when your arms are at a 90-degree angle). Push yourself back up to starting position through a count of 10 seconds. Without resting, repeat three times. Rest for 30 seconds and then repeat the entire sequence. (Note: The MTP will depend on how flexible your shoulders are—about 1 inch above your most flexible point.)

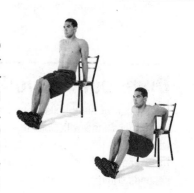

Barbell Skull Crusher

Hold a barbell and lie on the ball so that your head and neck are supported. Elevate your hips slightly and keep your abs tight. Extend the barbell straight up with your palms facing out. Drop your arms back toward your head slightly. Feather your breathing as you bend your elbows and lower the weight through a count of 10 seconds. Hold for 2 seconds at the MTP (a few inches above your forehead). Raise the barbell to starting position through a count of 10 seconds. Without resting, repeat three times. Rest for 30 seconds and then repeat the entire sequence.

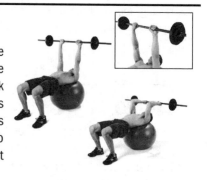

Toe Reach

Lie on your back. Cross your legs, flex your feet, and extend your arms and legs into the air. Keep your chin up and feather your breathing as you crunch up, reaching toward your toes through a count of 10 seconds. Hold and squeeze for 2 seconds at the MTP. Lower yourself to starting position, keeping your shoulder blades from touching the ground, through a count of 10 seconds. Without resting, repeat three times.

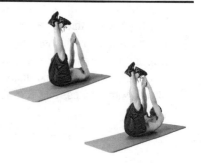

Standing Kickback

Hold a pair of dumbbells, palms facing each other. Bend at the waist as if you were about to tie your shoes; then lift only your chin and chest, creating a slight arch in your back, keeping a slight bend in your knees. Raise your elbows as high as possible while keeping them close to your body. Feather your breathing as you extend the weights back and out (without moving the upper part of the arm) through a count of 10 seconds. Hold and squeeze for 2 seconds at the MTP. Return the weights to starting position through a count of 10 seconds. Without resting, repeat three times. Rest for 30 seconds and then repeat the entire sequence.

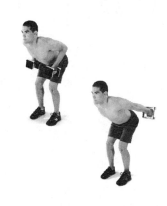

Chair Tuck-Up

Sit on the front edge of a sturdy chair. Reach your hands behind you and grab the sides of the chair. Extend your legs out and allow your upper body to lean back slightly. Feather your breathing as you slowly draw your knees in and up toward your chest through a count of 10 seconds. Hold and squeeze for 2 seconds at the MTP. Return legs to starting position through a count of 10 seconds. Without resting, repeat three times.

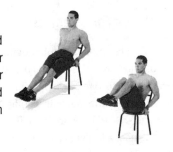

Russian Twist

Sit on the mat with your knees bent, feet together. Keep your chin up and abs tight as you lean back slightly, engaging your abs. Extend your arms away from your chest with your palms pressed together and turn to one side to begin exercise. Feather your breathing as you slowly rotate your torso as far as possible to the other side through a count of 10 seconds. Hold and squeeze for 2 seconds at the MTP. Rotate back to the other side through a count of 10 seconds. Without resting, repeat three times.

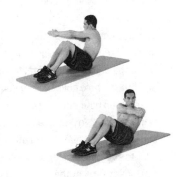

WEEK 2

As you gear up to start your week, use these tips based on your Life Priority to create extra inner drive and motivation. They are customized to your age category, but I recommend you read every one of them. You'll find valuable information in each tip, no matter what your age.

20 to 35 PRIME TIME

Dress for Success

It is important to remember that people make quick judgments about you based on your appearance. One study done in the medical field determined that patients significantly favored doctors wearing white coats. The professional look inspired trust and confidence. Even if you're not a doctor, this study reveals an obvious link between dress and people's perceptions. You could be overlooked for a shot at something just because you don't look the part. To make sure you're taken seriously, be smart about your wardrobe choices. Don't feel the need to run out and buy a whole collection of suits; simply sharpen up your clothing options with some nice-fitting clothes. Invest in a quality suit that you can wear to interviews and other business events. If your office or profession doesn't require business attire, at the very least get to know your iron—nothing looks sloppier than a wrinkled T-shirt or button-down. If you are going to stick to casual, aim for neat casual. *Neat* means clean clothes that have at the very least been folded—not pulled from the bottom pile of laundry on your way out the door!

35 to 50 STAY YOUNG

Skip the Mustache

Facial hair—long sideburns, goatees, and so forth—can age you. In your twenties, facial hair can be fun to mix it up or maybe even make you feel a bit distinguished. But as you get older, it may make you look older than you want—according to some experts, up to 10 years older. To stay looking young, go for a clean shave. It opens up your face and can reveal good facial features, such as a strong jaw line. If you think a clean shave is boring, think about its interesting history: Alexander the Great made his soldiers shave because he thought facial hair only gave their enemies something else to grab during battle. Even if you won't be on the battlefield anytime soon, keep your razor handy. Most women prefer guys to be clean-shaven. Plus, as all that new muscle on your body continues to help you drop fat, you'll probably notice your face become lean and your features sharpen. Getting that extra facial hair out of the way will help you show off your new chiseled look.

50-Plus LONGEVITY

Protect Your Prostate

Saw palmetto may sound kind of like a guy you used to know in high school, but it's actually an herb that comes from the fruit of a dwarf palm tree and has proven effective at treating benign prostatic hyperplasia (BPH). An enlargement of the prostate gland, BPH affects an estimated 50 percent of men over age 50. Your prostate may start growing in your thirties, but you may not see any symptoms of BPH until you reach 50. BPH is not considered a precursor to cancer, but it certainly can become a hindrance in your life by causing symptoms such as the frequent need to urinate, repeated bathroom trips throughout the night, and the feeling that you never quite empty your bladder. If you think you have BPH, talk to your doctor and ask about saw palmetto. In a study published in the *Journal of the American Medical Association,* researchers reported that saw palmetto improved symptoms and increased urologic flow. When compared to a common prescription for BPH, finasteride, saw palmetto showed similar improvements *without* side effects such as decreased interest in sex and problems getting an erection.

Incline Barbell Press

Hold the barbell with your palms facing out and lie on the ball so that your head and neck are supported. Allow your hips to drop almost to the ground. Press the weight up over your nose, keeping a slight bend in the elbows so that the upper chest is targeted. Feather your breathing as you lower the weight through a count of 10 seconds. Hold for 2 seconds at the MTP (when the barbell is only a couple of inches from your chest). Press the bar up to starting position through a count of 10 seconds. Without resting, repeat three times. Rest for 30 seconds and then repeat the entire sequence.

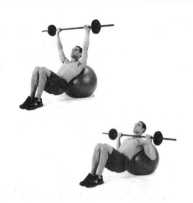

Push-Up

Lie on a mat with your hands slightly wider than shoulder-width apart and your fingers pointing forward. Press up to starting position, keeping your back straight, abs tight, and head up. Feather your breathing as you lower your chest toward the floor through a count of 10 seconds. Hold for 2 seconds at the MTP. Push your body back to starting position through a count of 10 seconds, keeping your elbows slightly bent. Without resting, repeat three times. Rest for 30 seconds and then repeat the entire sequence.

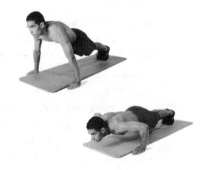

Flat Dumbbell Press

Hold a pair of dumbbells and lie on the ball so that it comfortably supports your shoulder blades. Extend your arms in front of you, pressing the weights together. Feather your breathing as you lower the weights through a count of 10 seconds. Hold for 2 seconds at the MTP (about 1 inch above your chest). Press the dumbbells up and together, then back to starting position through a count of 10 seconds. Without resting, repeat three times. Rest for 30 seconds and then repeat the entire sequence.

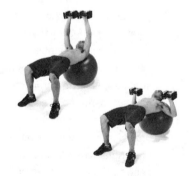

Flat Dumbbell Fly on Swiss Ball

Hold a pair of dumbbells and lie on the ball with your head and neck supported. Extend the dumbbells over your chest, palms facing each other, elbows slightly bent. Feather your breathing as you lower the weights down and out through a count of 10 seconds. Hold for 2 seconds at the MTP (when your arms are open in a "T" position). Raise the weights to starting position in a "bear hug" type motion through a count of 10 seconds. Without resting, repeat three times. Rest for 30 seconds and then repeat the entire sequence.

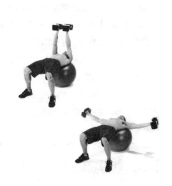

Standing Military Press

Hold a barbell and take a wide step forward with one foot, keeping your back straight, abs tight, knees slightly bent, and chin up. Extend the weight up directly over your head, palms facing forward. Feather your breathing as you lower the barbell through a count of 10 seconds. Hold for 2 seconds at the MTP (chin level). Press the weight up to starting position through a count of 10 seconds. Without resting, repeat three times. Rest for 30 seconds and then repeat the entire sequence.

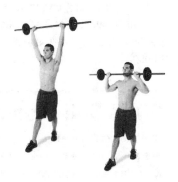

Upright Barbell Row

Hold a barbell with your arms extended in front of you, palms facing your body, thumbs placed along the bar. Place your feet about hip-width apart, keeping your knees slightly bent, back straight, abs tight, and chin up. Feather your breathing as you draw the bar up toward your chin through a count of 10 seconds. Hold for 2 seconds at the MTP (right below your chin). Return to starting position through a count of 10 seconds. Without resting, repeat three times. Rest for 30 seconds and then repeat the entire sequence. (Note: You should not feel a strain in your neck. If you do, relax your neck muscles and focus the exertion on your shoulders.)

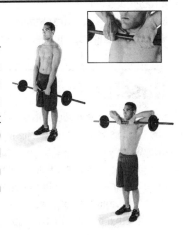

Seated Lateral Raise

Hold a pair of dumbbells and sit on a ball with your feet together, back straight, and abs tight. With your arms against your sides and elbows slightly bent, feather your breathing as you raise the weights through a count of 10 seconds. Hold and squeeze for 2 seconds at the MTP ("T" position). Lower the weights to starting position through a count of 10 seconds. Without resting, repeat three times. Rest for 30 seconds and then repeat the entire sequence.

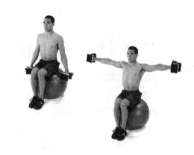

Toe Reach

Lie on your back. Cross your legs, flex your feet, and extend your arms and legs into the air. Keep your chin up and feather your breathing as you crunch up reaching toward your toes through a count of 10 seconds. Hold and squeeze for 2 seconds at the MTP. Lower yourself to starting position, keeping your shoulder blades from touching the ground, through a count of 10 seconds. Without resting, repeat three times.

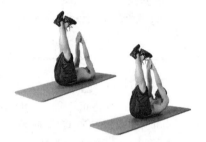

Swiss Ball Crunch

Sit on the ball with your feet on the floor. Walk your feet out until your hips are slightly lower than your knees but your lower back is still firmly supported. Place your hands behind your head to support your neck. Feather your breathing and, using your abs only, slowly crunch up through a count of 10 seconds. Hold and squeeze for 2 seconds at the MTP. Lower yourself to starting position through a count of 10 seconds. Without resting, repeat three times.

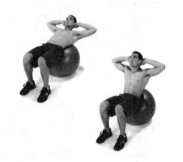

Russian Twist

Sit on the mat with your knees bent, feet together. Keep your chin up and abs tight as you lean back slightly, engaging your abs. Extend your arms away from your chest with your palms pressed together and turn to one side to begin exercise. Feather your breathing as you slowly rotate your torso as far as possible to the other side through a count of 10 seconds. Hold and squeeze for 2 seconds at the MTP. Rotate back to the other side through a count of 10 seconds. Without resting, repeat three times.

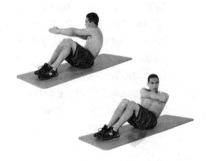

WEDNESDAY

Barbell Pull-Over

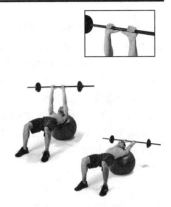

Grasp the barbell with a close grip. Lie on the ball with your head and neck supported. Keep your hips up and abs tight throughout the exercise. Extend the weight over your chest with a slight bend in the elbows. Feather your breathing as you lower the weight behind your head through a count of 10 seconds. Hold for 2 seconds at the MTP. Raise the weight to starting position through a count of 10 seconds. Without resting, repeat three times. Rest for 30 seconds and then repeat the entire sequence. (Note: How far you can stretch your arms back will determine your MTP.)

Bent-Over Dumbbell Row (Standard Grip)

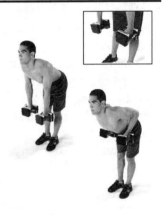

Hold a pair of dumbbells, arms extended, palms facing each other. Stand with your feet hip-width apart. Bend at the waist as if you were about to tie your shoes; then lift only your chin and chest, creating a slight arch in your back. Bend your knees slightly. Feather your breathing as you pull the dumbbells up in a fluid rowing motion through a count of 10 seconds, keeping your elbows close to your body. Hold and squeeze your shoulder blades together for 2 seconds at the MTP. Lower your arms to starting position through a count of 10 seconds. Without resting, repeat three times. Rest for 30 seconds and then repeat the entire sequence. (Note: Keep your elbows close to your body throughout the exercise.)

Bent-Over Barbell Row (Underhand Grip)

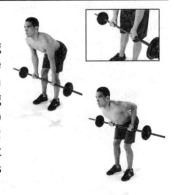

Grasp the barbell using the underhand grip. Bend at the waist as if tying your shoes, keeping your knees slightly bent. Grasp the bar using the underhand grip and raise your head and chest to create a slight arch in the back. Feather your breathing as you pull the bar up in a fluid rowing motion through a count of 10 seconds, keeping your elbows close to your body. Hold and squeeze your shoulder blades together for 2 seconds at the MTP. Lower your arms to starting position through a count of 10 seconds. Without resting, repeat three times. Rest for 30 seconds and then repeat the entire sequence.

Reverse Hyperextension

Lie facedown on the ball. Roll yourself forward until the ball is under your hips and your upper body is slightly angled toward the ground. Place your palms on the floor about shoulder-width apart. With legs together, feather your breathing as you raise your heels toward the ceiling through a count of 10 seconds, using your lower back and hamstrings. Hold and squeeze for 2 seconds at the MTP. With straight legs, lower through a count of 10 seconds to starting position, about 2 inches from the ground. Without resting, repeat three times. Rest for 30 seconds and then repeat the entire sequence.

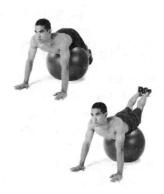

Standing Dumbbell Curl

Hold a pair of dumbbells, arms extended, palms facing out, and your feet shoulder-width apart. Keep your knees slightly bent. Feather your breathing as you curl the dumbbells up through a count of 10 seconds. Hold and squeeze for 2 seconds at the MTP. Keep your elbows tight against your body as you lower the weights to starting position through a count of 10 seconds. Without resting, repeat three times. Rest for 30 seconds and then repeat the entire sequence. (Note: Be sure to not let your elbows move away from your sides throughout the exercise.)

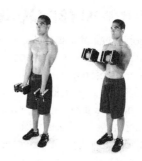

Standing Side Curl

Hold a pair of dumbbells with your palms turned out, elbows to your side. Keep your chest up, feet hip-width apart, knees slightly bent, and abs tight throughout the exercise. Feather your breathing as you curl the weights up through a count of 10 seconds, keeping your elbows close to your body. Hold and squeeze for 2 seconds at the MTP. Lower the weights to starting position through a count of 10 seconds, until your arms are completely straight (do not lock your elbows). Without resting, repeat three times. Rest for 30 seconds and then repeat the entire sequence.

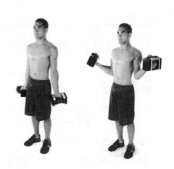

Barbell Reverse Curl

Grip a barbell with both hands, palms facing back. Stand with your feet shoulder-width apart and your arms extended by your sides, knees slightly bent. Feather your breathing as you curl the bar up through a count of 10 seconds to just past a 90-degree angle. Hold and squeeze for 2 seconds at the MTP (when your hands reach chest height). Keep your elbows tight against your body as you lower the weight through a count of 10 seconds. Without resting, repeat three times. Rest for 30 seconds and then repeat the entire sequence. (Note: Keep your elbows tight against your sides throughout the exercise.)

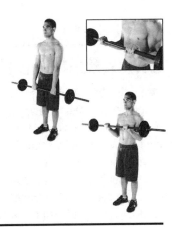

Double Crunch

Lie on a mat and place your hands behind your head, elbows up, chin up, and abs tight. Pull your heels toward your butt as far as you can. Using your upper abs, feather your breathing as you crunch up while simultaneously pulling your knees in through a count of 10 seconds. Hold and squeeze for 2 seconds at the MTP. Return to starting position through a count of 10 seconds, never letting your upper back touch the ground. Without resting, repeat three times. (Note: The range of motion on this exercise is very short so be sure to adjust your speed so that you hit the MTP on the count of 10.)

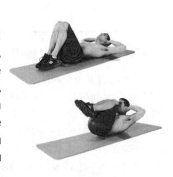

Chair Tuck-Up

Sit on the front edge of a sturdy chair. Reach your hands behind you and grab the sides of the chair. Extend your legs out and allow your upper body to lean back slightly. Feather your breathing as you slowly draw your knees in and up toward your chest through a count of 10 seconds. Hold and squeeze for 2 seconds at the MTP. Return legs to starting position through a count of 10 seconds. Without resting, repeat three times.

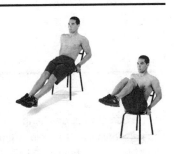

Lying Oblique Twist

Lie on your back with your arms outstretched, palms facing down. Raise your knees up to a 90-degree angle, and drop your knees down to one side. Feather your breathing as you rotate your knees to the other side through a count of 10 seconds. Hold and squeeze for 2 seconds at the MTP (when your knees are a few inches from the ground). Rotate to the other side through a count of 10 seconds. Without resting, repeat three times.

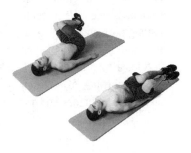

FRIDAY

Swiss Ball Squat

Place the ball against a wall and position yourself with the ball supporting your middle to upper back. Hold a pair of dumbbells with your arms against your sides. Move your feet forward about 1 foot, keeping them about hip-width apart. Feather your breathing as you slowly squat down through a count of 10 seconds. Hold for 2 seconds at the MTP (when your knees are at a 90-degree angle). Return to starting position through a count of 10 seconds. Without resting, repeat three times. Rest for 30 seconds and then repeat the entire sequence.

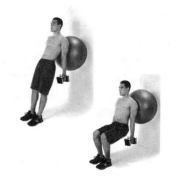

Dumbbell Squat

Hold a pair of dumbbells with your arms extended against your sides, and stand with your feet shoulder-width apart. Feather your breathing as you slowly squat through a count of 10 seconds, keeping your back straight, abs tight, and chest up. Hold for 2 seconds at the MTP (when your legs are almost at a 90-degree angle). Return to starting position through a count of 10 seconds. Without resting, repeat three times. Rest for 30 seconds and then repeat the entire sequence.

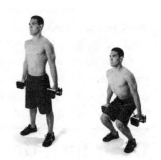

Lunge

Hold a dumbbell in one hand and rest the other on the back of a sturdy chair for balance. Stand in a lunge position. Keep your back straight, chest up, and abs tight. Feather your breathing as you drop your back knee toward the ground through a count of 10 seconds. Hold for 2 seconds at the MTP (a couple of inches above the ground). Return to starting position through a count of 10 seconds. Without resting, repeat one more time on this leg and then perform 2 more reps on the other side for a total of 4. Rest for 30 seconds and then repeat the entire sequence. (Note: To avoid injury, make sure that your front knee stays aligned with your toes and doesn't bend farther than a 90-degree angle.)

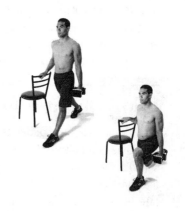

Quadriceps Flex

Stand with feet shoulder-width apart. Grasp the back of a sturdy chair for support at about hip level. Feather your breathing as you bend your knees and allow your body to fall backwards, letting your heels come off the floor, through a count of 10 seconds. Hold and squeeze your quads for 2 seconds at the MTP (when your knees are near the floor). Return to starting position through a count of 10 seconds. Without resting, repeat three times. Rest for 30 seconds and then repeat the entire sequence.

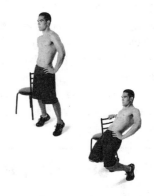

Diamond Push-Up

Lie on a mat with your hands in the "diamond" position. Press up to starting position, keeping your back straight, abs tight, and head up. Feather your breathing as you lower your body through a count of 10 seconds, allowing your elbows to move outward. Hold for 2 seconds at the MTP (about 2 inches above the ground). Push your body back to starting position through a count of 10 seconds. Without resting, repeat three times. Rest for 30 seconds and then repeat the entire sequence.

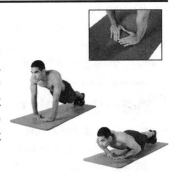

Barbell Skull Crusher

Hold a barbell and lie on the ball so that your head and neck are supported. Elevate your hips slightly and keep your abs tight. Extend the barbell straight up with your palms facing out. Drop your arms back toward your head slightly. Feather your breathing as you bend your elbows and lower the weight through a count of 10 seconds. Hold for 2 seconds at the MTP (a few inches above your forehead). Raise the barbell to starting position through a count of 10 seconds. Without resting, repeat three times. Rest for 30 seconds and then repeat the entire sequence.

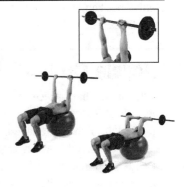

Overhead Barbell Triceps Extension

Grasp the barbell, palms facing out. Sit on a ball with your chest up, back straight, feet together. Extend your arms with your elbows slightly bent, keeping your biceps close to your head. Feather your breathing as you drop the bar back through a count of 10 seconds. Hold for 2 seconds at the MTP (when your elbows are at about a 90-degree angle). Press the bar up to starting position through a count of 10 seconds. Without resting, repeat three times. Rest for 30 seconds and then repeat the entire sequence.

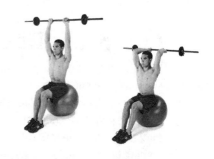

Medicine Ball Pull-Over

Lie on a mat and bring your knees up to a 90-degree angle, crossing your feet. Grasp a medicine ball and extend it over your head, keeping a slight bend in your elbows. Keep your abs tight and feather your breathing as you raise the ball over your head and crunch up through a count of 10 seconds. Hold for 2 seconds at the MTP (when your arms are extending straight up). Lower the ball to starting position through a count of 10 seconds. Without resting, repeat three times.

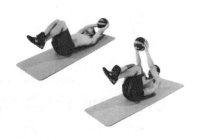

Reverse Crunch

Lie on a mat with your hands by your sides, palms down. Pull your heels up as close to your butt as possible. Raise your heels about 2 inches off the ground. Keep your chin tucked and abs tight. Feather your breathing as you pull your knees toward your chest, using your lower abdominals, through a count of 10 seconds. Hold and squeeze for 2 seconds at the MTP (when your butt is completely off the ground). Lower your body to starting position through a count of 10 seconds. Without resting, repeat three times.

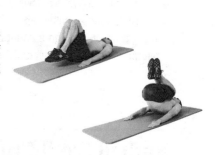

Bicycle Crunch

Lie flat on your back. Place your hands behind your head and raise your heels about 2 inches from the ground, keeping your chin up and abs tight throughout the exercise. Bring your right elbow to your left knee and feather your breathing as you rotate to the other side for a count of 10 seconds. Hold and squeeze for 2 seconds at the MTP (where your left elbow meets your right knee). Return to starting position through a count of 10 seconds. Without resting, repeat three times.

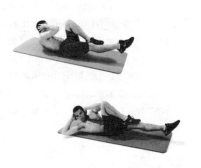

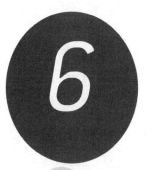

6

Power Phase

WEEKS 3 THROUGH 8

20 to 35 PRIME TIME

Personal Grooming

We have more options than ever before when it comes to hair maintenance. Whether we're talking latest hairstyles or body hair, somebody out there has an opinion on what guys should do. I say go with what makes you comfortable. But if you really want to stand out with your ripped new body, here are a few tips. As your workouts start to build and define your muscles, think about shaving your chest and ab area. This really brings the definition out and can make the cuts in your muscles pop. To look even better with your shirt off, assess the state of the rest of your body hair. Unruly back hair can not only be a turn off for some but will hide all the hard work you've done with your body. Using tweezers can work for some guys, but if you've got more hair than you can handle on your own, head to the salon. Add on a massage while you're there to reward yourself for getting through the pain. It will all be worth it when you strip your shirt off at the beach and feel more confident than ever.

35 to 50 STAY YOUNG

The Power of Sleep

Getting enough sleep is one of the best things you can do to keep looking and feeling young. It may sound simple, but it's true that getting eight hours of sleep a night can really make all the difference in your life. According to *Harvard Health Watch,* sleep improves your learning and memory skills, helps manage your weight by balancing your hormones, keeps you safer when you do things that require alertness, such as driving, improves your mood, and helps maintain heart health. It also boosts your immune system, protecting you from cell damage and sickness. Staying well rested can also improve your sex life. Just being tired can make you feel disinterested in sex, but people with sleep problems also report decreased libido. When you're sleep deprived, your hormones are out of balance and this impacts your physiological response to sex. Bottom line: Skipping sleep can lead to a lousy sex life and a load of other problems. To make sure you get enough shut-eye each night, make sure you're getting your Body at Home™ workouts in—studies have shown that people who exercise get better sleep. But try not to work out too late; otherwise your adrenaline will keep you up for a while. Also, have a cup of chamomile tea before bed. I do this each night and it helps me de-stress and relax so sleep comes easily.

WEEK 3

As you gear up to start your week, use these tips based on your Life Priority to create extra inner drive and motivation. They are customized to your age category, but I recommend you read every one of them. You'll find valuable information in each tip, no matter what your age.

50-Plus LONGEVITY

Refuel Your Joints

Just like your car's brake pads, your cartilage can start to wear down as you put more miles on your body. Your cartilage is made up of two types of molecules—*glucosamine,* which is responsible for the makeup and repair of cartilage, and *chondroitin,* which helps it stay strong. When your cartilage starts to thin, your joints weaken and you risk injury or, worse, you develop osteoarthritis. Symptoms of osteoarthritis are joint aching and soreness, swelling and stiffness. And while there is no known direct cause of osteoarthritis, obesity is considered a major contributing factor—another reason to get rid of that excess fat on your body. In addition to losing weight, you can take glucosamine and chondrointin in supplement form to help relieve symptoms of osteoarthritis and protect your cartilage from breaking down further. Studies have shown that taking these in supplement form helps ease pain associated with osteoarthritis even as much as ibuprofen—with fewer side effects—and may be effective at preventing decline of cartilage.

MONDAY

Flat Dumbbell Press

Hold a pair of dumbbells and lie on the ball so that it comfortably supports your shoulder blades. Extend your arms in front of you, pressing the weights together. Feather your breathing as you lower the weights through a count of 10 seconds. Hold for 2 seconds at the MTP (about 1 inch above your chest). Press the dumbbells up and together, then back to starting position through a count of 10 seconds. Without resting, repeat three times. Rest for 30 seconds and then repeat the entire sequence.

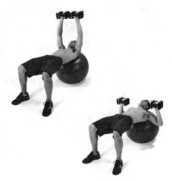

Incline Dumbbell Press

Hold a pair of dumbbells and lie on the ball so that your head and neck are supported. Allow your hips to drop almost to the ground. Press the weights up and together, with a slight bend in the elbows so that the upper chest is targeted. Feather your breathing as you lower the weights through a count of 10 seconds. Hold for 2 seconds at the MTP. Press the dumbbells up to starting position through a count of 10 seconds. Without resting, repeat three times. Rest for 30 seconds and then repeat the entire sequence.

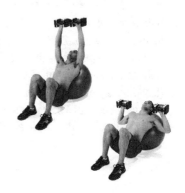

Incline Barbell Press

Hold the barbell with your palms facing out and lie on the ball so that your head and neck are supported. Allow your hips to drop almost to the ground. Press the weight up over your nose, keeping a slight bend in the elbows so that the upper chest is targeted. Feather your breathing as you lower the weight through a count of 10 seconds. Hold for 2 seconds at the MTP (when the barbell is only a couple of inches from your chest). Press the bar up to starting position through a count of 10 seconds. Without resting, repeat three times. Rest for 30 seconds and then repeat the entire sequence.

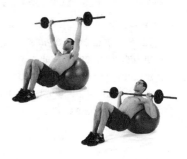

Chair Push-Up

Place two sturdy chairs in front of you and place your hands on the seats, slightly wider than shoulder-width apart, arms extended. Feather your breathing as you lower your chest toward the chairs through a count of 10 seconds, keeping your back straight and abs tight. Hold for 2 seconds at the MTP. Push your body back to starting position through a count of 10 seconds, keeping your elbows slightly bent at the top of the move. Without resting, repeat three times. Rest for 30 seconds and then repeat the entire sequence.

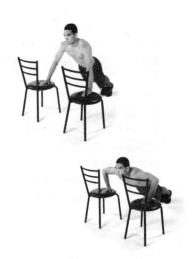

Seated Shoulder Press

Hold a pair of dumbbells and sit on the ball with your back straight, abs tight, and chin up. Extend the dumbbells up and together directly over your head, palms facing forward. Feather your breathing as you lower the weights through a count of 10 seconds. Hold for 2 seconds at the MTP (just above chin level). Press the dumbbells up to starting position through a count of 10 seconds. Without resting, repeat three times. Rest for 30 seconds and then repeat the entire sequence.

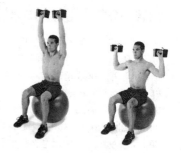

Seated Lateral Raise

Hold a pair of dumbbells and sit on a ball, your back straight and abs tight. With your arms against your sides and elbows slightly bent, feather your breathing as you raise the weights through a count of 10 seconds. Hold and squeeze for 2 seconds at the MTP ("T" position). Lower your arms to starting position through a count of 10 seconds. Without resting, repeat three times. Rest for 30 seconds and then repeat the entire sequence.

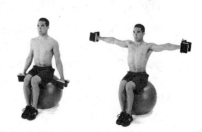

Bent-Over Rear Delt Raise

Hold a pair of dumbbells, palms facing each other. Bend at the waist as if you were about to tie your shoes; then lift only your chin and chest, creating a slight arch in your back. Feather your breathing as you raise the weights to your sides through a count of 10 seconds. Hold and squeeze for 2 seconds at the MTP. Lower the weights to starting position through a count of 10 seconds. Without resting, repeat three times. Rest for 30 seconds and then repeat the entire sequence.

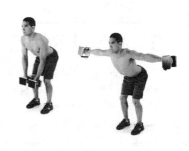

Medicine Ball Pull-Over

Lie on a mat and bring your knees up to a 90-degree angle. Grasp a medicine ball and extend it over your head, keeping a slight bend in your elbows. Keep your abs tight and feather your breathing as you raise the ball over your head and crunch up through a count of 10 seconds. Hold for 2 seconds at the MTP. Lower the ball to starting position through a count of 10 seconds. Without resting, repeat three times.

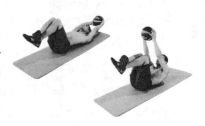

Reverse Crunch

Lie on a mat with your hands by your sides, palms down. Pull your heels up as close to your butt as possible. Raise your heels about 2 inches off the ground. Keep your chin tucked and abs tight. Feather your breathing as you pull your knees toward your chest, using your lower abdominals, through a count of 10 seconds. Hold and squeeze for 2 seconds at the MTP (when your butt is completely off the ground). Lower your body to starting position through a count of 10 seconds. Without resting, repeat three times.

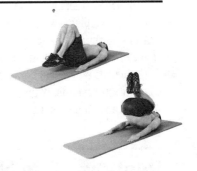

Weighted Russian Twist

Sit on the mat with your knees bent, feet together. While holding a medicine ball lean back slightly, engaging your abs. Extend your arms away from your chest and turn to one side to begin exercise. Keep your chin up and abs tight as you feather your breathing and slowly rotate your torso as far as possible to the other side through a count of 10 seconds. Hold and squeeze for 2 seconds at the MTP. Rotate back to the other side through a count of 10 seconds. Without resting, repeat three times.

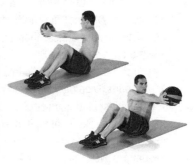

WEDNESDAY

Dumbbell Pull-Over

Grasp a dumbbell using the "diamond grip." Lie on the ball with your head and neck supported. Keep your hips up and abs tight throughout the exercise. Extend the weight over your chest with a slight bend in the elbows. Feather your breathing as you lower the weight behind your head through a count of 10 seconds. Hold for 2 seconds at the MTP. Raise the weight to starting position through a count of 10 seconds. Without resting, repeat three times. Rest for 30 seconds and then repeat the entire sequence. (Note: How far you can stretch your arms back will determine your MTP.)

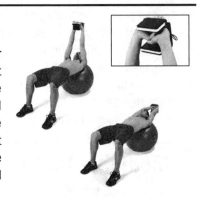

Bent-Over Barbell Row (Overhand Grip)

Hold the barbell with your arms extended, using the overhand grip. Stand with your feet hip-width apart. Bend at the waist as if you were about to tie your shoes; then lift only your chin and chest, creating a slight arch in your back. Keeping a bend in your knees, feather your breathing as you pull the weight up toward your hips in a fluid rowing motion through a count of 10 seconds. Hold and squeeze your shoulder blades together for 2 seconds at the MTP. Lower your arms to starting position through a count of 10 seconds. Without resting, repeat three times. Rest for 30 seconds and then repeat the entire sequence.

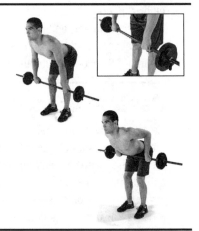

Bent-Over Dumbbell Row (Standard Grip)

Hold a pair of dumbbells, arms extended, palms facing each other. Stand with your feet hip-width apart. Bend at the waist as if you were about to tie your shoes; then lift only your chin and chest, creating a slight arch in your back. Bend your knees slightly. Feather your breathing as you pull the dumbbells up in a fluid rowing motion through a count of 10 seconds, keeping your elbows close to your body. Hold and squeeze your shoulder blades together for 2 seconds at the MTP. Lower your arms to starting position through a count of 10 seconds. Without resting, repeat three times. Rest for 30 seconds and then repeat the entire sequence. (Note: Keep your elbows close to your body throughout the exercise.)

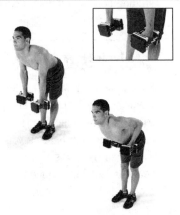

Dumbbell Dead Lift

Stand holding a dumbbell in each hand, palms facing back, feet about hip-width apart. Bend over at the waist as if you were about to tie your shoes; then lift your chin and chest, creating a slight arch in your back. Feather your breathing as you lift your upper body through a count of 10 seconds, driving through your heels and using your lower back and hamstrings. Hold for 2 seconds at the MTP (at the top of the movement). Return to starting position through a count of 10 seconds. Without resting, repeat three times. Rest for 30 seconds and then repeat the entire sequence.

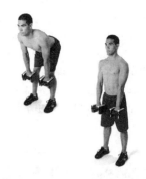

Standing Barbell Curl (Wide Grip)

Hold the barbell using the wide grip. Stand with your feet shoulder-width apart and your arms extended by your sides, knees slightly bent. Feather your breathing as you curl the barbell up through a count of 10 seconds to just past a 90-degree angle. Hold and squeeze for 2 seconds at the MTP. Keep your elbows tight against your body as you lower the weight through a count of 10 seconds. Without resting, repeat three times. Rest for 30 seconds and then repeat the entire sequence. (Note: Keep the elbows tight against your sides throughout the exercise.)

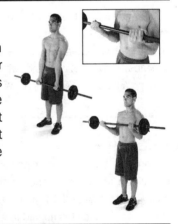

Dumbbell Preacher Curl

Hold a pair of dumbbells and rest over the ball with your knees on the floor and a 6- to 8-inch gap between your arms. Lift your arms to starting position, with your elbows bent at about a 90-degree angle. Feather your breathing as you lower the weights through a count of 10 seconds. Hold for 2 seconds at the MTP. Lift the dumbbells to starting position through a count of 10 seconds. Without resting, repeat three times. Rest for 30 seconds and then repeat the entire sequence.

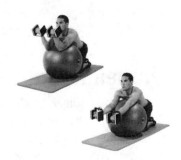

Reverse Barbell Curl

Grip a barbell with both hands, palms facing back. Stand with your feet shoulder-width apart and your arms extended by your sides, knees slightly bent. Feather your breathing as you curl the bar up through a count of 10 seconds to just past a 90-degree angle. Hold and squeeze for 2 seconds at the MTP. Keep your elbows tight against your body as you lower the weight through a count of 10 seconds. Without resting, repeat three times. Rest for 30 seconds and then repeat the entire sequence. (Note: Keep your elbows tight against your sides throughout the exercise.)

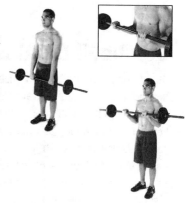

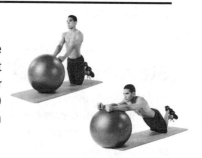

Swiss Ball Ab Roll

Kneel on a mat in front of a ball and cross your ankles behind you. Close both hands into fists and place on the ball, keeping your elbows straight but not locked. Keep your head up, back straight, and abs tight. Feather your breathing as you roll forward on the ball through a count of 10 seconds. Hold for 2 seconds at the MTP. Return to starting position through a count of 10 seconds. Without resting, repeat three times.

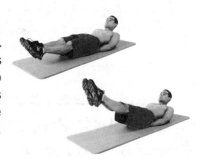

Leg Lift

Lie on your back with your palms down, hands underneath your butt. Crunch up and hold your upper abs tight so that your shoulder blades are just off the ground. Lift your legs about 2 inches off the ground. Keep your abs tight and chin up and feather your breathing as you lift your legs through a count of 10 seconds. Hold and squeeze for 2 seconds at the MTP. Lower your legs to starting position through a count of 10 seconds. Without resting, repeat three times.

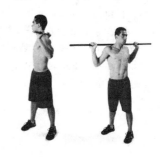

Barbell Twist

Grip an empty barbell, placing it across the back of your shoulders. Stand with your legs about 3 feet apart. Twist your upper body to one side. With your chin up and abs squeezed tight, feather your breathing as you slowly twist to the other side through a count of 10 seconds. At the MTP of your twist, hold and squeeze for 2 seconds. Return to starting position through a count of 10 seconds. Without resting, repeat three times. (Note: If you can do more than 4 reps, you're not squeezing your abs hard enough throughout the exercise.)

FRIDAY

Barbell Squat

Stand with your feet hip-width apart and hold a weighted barbell across your shoulders. Keep your back straight, abs tight, and head up. Feather your breathing as you squat through a count of 10 seconds. Hold for 2 seconds at the MTP. Push through your heels as you stand and return to starting position through a count of 10 seconds. Without resting, repeat three times. Rest for 30 seconds and then repeat the entire sequence.

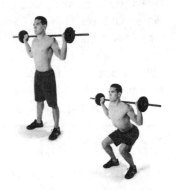

Swiss Ball Squat

Place the ball against a wall and position yourself with the ball supporting your middle to upper back. Hold a pair of dumbbells with your arms against your sides. Move your feet forward about 1 foot, keeping them about hip-width apart. Feather your breathing as you slowly squat down through a count of 10 seconds. Hold for 2 seconds at the MTP (when your knees are at a 90-degree angle). Return to starting position through a count of 10 seconds. Without resting, repeat three times. Rest for 30 seconds and then repeat the entire sequence.

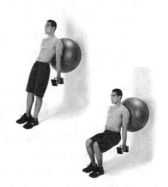

Dumbbell Sumo Squat

Hold a pair of dumbbells, palms facing back, arms extended in front of your body. Stand with your feet about two times wider than shoulder-width apart, toes turned out to the sides, and knees aligned over the toes. Feather your breathing as you squat through a count of 10 seconds. Hold for 2 seconds at the MTP. Push through your heels to return to starting position through a count of 10 seconds. Without resting, repeat three times. Rest for 30 seconds and then repeat the entire sequence.

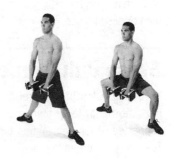

Swiss Ball Hamstring Curl

Lie on your back with your arms at your sides, palms flat on the floor. Place your heels on the ball, knees straight but not completely locked; then lift your butt and hips off the ground. With your abs tight, feather your breathing and bend your knees as you roll the ball toward your butt with your heels. Hold for 2 seconds at the MTP. Return to starting position through a count of 10 seconds. Without resting, repeat three times. Rest for 30 seconds and then repeat the entire sequence.

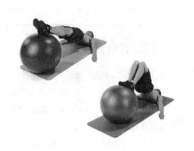

Barbell Skull Crusher

Hold a barbell and lie on the ball so that your head and neck are supported. Elevate your hips slightly and keep your abs tight. Extend the barbell straight up with your palms facing out. Drop your arms back toward your head slightly. Feather your breathing as you bend your elbows and lower the weight through a count of 10 seconds. Hold for 2 seconds at the MTP (a few inches above your forehead). Raise the barbell to starting position through a count of 10 seconds. Without resting, repeat three times. Rest for 30 seconds and then repeat the entire sequence.

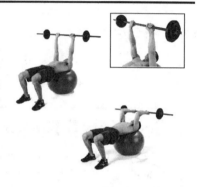

Close-Grip Barbell Press

Hold a barbell with a close grip, and lean back onto a ball so that your head and neck are supported. Elevate your hips slightly and keep your abs tight. Extend your arms in front of you, pressing the weight up. Feather your breathing as you lower the barbell through a count of 10 seconds. Hold for 2 seconds at the MTP (about 1 inch above your chest). Press the bar back to starting position through a count of 10 seconds. Without resting, repeat three times. Rest for 30 seconds and then repeat the entire sequence.

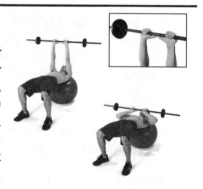

Swiss Ball Crunch

Sit on the ball with your feet on the floor. Walk your feet out until your hips are slightly lower than your knees but your lower back is still firmly supported. Place your hands behind your head to support your neck. Feather your breathing and, using your abs only, slowly crunch up through a count of 10 seconds. Hold and squeeze for 2 seconds at the MTP. Lower yourself to starting position through a count of 10 seconds. Without resting, repeat three times.

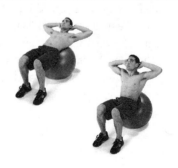

Chair Dip

Sit on the front edge of a sturdy chair, hands close to your sides, fingers forward, and legs extended. Flex your feet so that your weight is on your heels and slide yourself away from the chair. Feather your breathing as you lower yourself through a count of 10 seconds. Hold for 2 seconds (when your arms are at a 90-degree angle) at the MTP. Push yourself back up to starting position through a count of 10 seconds. Without resting, repeat three times. Rest for 30 seconds and then repeat the entire sequence. (Note: The MTP will depend on how flexible your shoulders are. Your MTP will be about 1 inch above your most flexible point. If this exercise is too difficult, move your feet closer to your body for more stability.)

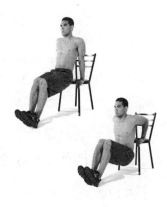

Chair Tuck-Up

Sit on the front edge of a sturdy chair. Reach your hands behind you and grab the sides of the chair. Extend your legs out and allow your upper body to lean back slightly. Feather your breathing as you slowly draw your knees in and up toward your chest through a count of 10 seconds. Hold and squeeze for 2 seconds at the MTP. Return legs to starting position through a count of 10 seconds. Without resting, repeat three times.

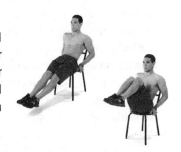

Bicycle Crunch

Lie flat on your back. Place your hands behind your head and raise your heels about 2 inches from the ground, keeping your chin up and abs tight throughout the exercise. Bring your right elbow to your left knee and feather your breathing as you rotate to the other side for a count of 10 seconds. Hold and squeeze for 2 seconds at the MTP (where your left elbow meets your right knee). Return to starting position through a count of 10 seconds. Without resting, repeat three times.

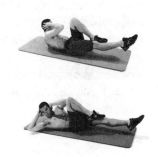

WEEK 4

As you gear up to start your week, use these tips based on your Life Priority to create extra inner drive and motivation. They are customized to your age category, but I recommend you read every one of them. You'll find valuable information in each tip, no matter what your age.

20 to 35 PRIME TIME

Time for a Tan

Despite rising cases of skin cancer, tan skin still strikes many as synonymous with healthy. We associate tan bodies with active, healthy lifestyles and sunny locales. When you're tan, your body looks better, your teeth look whiter, and studies have even linked UV exposure to an endorphin rush. To get a tan and minimize the dangerous effects of too much sun, consider alternatives or be smart about the amount of time you spend in the sun. Try to limit your outdoor activities between 10 a.m. and 2 p.m. If you are outside during these peak hours, slap on some sunscreen of at least SPF 30. And try using SunGuard detergent when you do your laundry. It's a powder that creates an "invisible shield," giving your clothes an SPF of 30. To go an entirely sun-free route, explore spray tanning options, such as Mystic Tan. These offer a safe alternative to sun exposure and can give you a healthy, bronzed look that typically lasts four to seven days.

35 to 50 STAY YOUNG

Yoga Keeps You Young

Our muscles and tendons naturally lose flexibility as we age, and guys are especially susceptible to tightness because chances are we've skipped out on things like stretching and yoga. The problem with tight muscles is they can lead to injuries, and they leave areas such as your lower back especially susceptible to strains. If you can't touch your toes when you bend over, your hamstrings are too tight—and tight hamstrings are one of the main culprits in back and hip pain. If you want to keep your body feeling young and active, try a yoga class. Besides increasing flexibility and reducing muscle soreness, yoga has a built-in stress reliever: deep breathing. Most yoga instructors will have you perform deep breathing exercises, which are proven effective at reducing tension and anxiety—so effective that the U.S. Army has started using yoga as treatment for soldiers who return from war with post-traumatic stress disorder. I recommend exploring different types of yoga. Some are done at a slow pace and really focus on breathing and held poses. Others, like bikram, my personal favorite, are done in a hot room, which creates a vigorous, intense experience—and makes you sweat like crazy! Don't be surprised if it takes you a while to loosen up. Try a few classes and you'll be happy to discover that reaching down to tie your shoes is a little bit easier.

50-Plus LONGEVITY

More MSM

Methylsulfonylmethane (MSM) is a form of sulfur that occurs naturally in foods such as tomatoes, chard, milk, and some fish. You may not know it, but sulfur is more than just matchstick-material. It's an essential element found in many of your body's tissues and organs, and it plays a crucial role in cell structure by helping maintain tissue integrity in everything from your skin to your liver cells. Like just about everything, though, the amount of MSM in your body declines as you age and this can lead to less than optimum cell and connective tissue function. Studies have shown that MSM supplements help ease pain and joint soreness associated with arthritis. Even if you don't have arthritis, MSM has a long list of other benefits: helps the proteins methionine and cysteine detoxify your body; keeps your hair, nails, and skin strong; reduces muscle cramps; and may help your body maintain insulin balance.

MONDAY

Incline Dumbbell Press

Hold a pair of dumbbells and lie on the ball so that your head and neck are supported. Allow your hips to drop almost to the ground. Press the weights up and together with a slight bend in the elbows so that the upper chest is targeted. Feather your breathing as you lower the weights through a count of 10 seconds. Hold for 2 seconds at the MTP. Press the dumbbells up to starting position through a count of 10 seconds. Without resting, repeat three times. Rest for 30 seconds and then repeat the entire sequence.

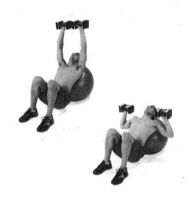

Flat Barbell Press

Hold the barbell and lie on the ball so that it comfortably supports your shoulder blades. Extend your arms in front of you, pressing the weight up. Feather your breathing as you lower the weight through a count of 10 seconds. Hold for 2 seconds at the MTP (about 1 inch above your chest). Press the barbell back to starting position through a count of 10 seconds. Without resting, repeat three times. Rest for 30 seconds and then repeat the entire sequence.

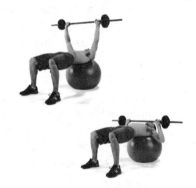

Flat Dumbbell Press

Hold a pair of dumbbells and lie on the ball so that it comfortably supports your shoulder blades. Extend your arms in front of you, pressing the weights together. Feather your breathing as you lower the weights through a count of 10 seconds. Hold for 2 seconds at the MTP (about 1 inch above your chest). Press the dumbbells up and together then back to starting position through a count of 10 seconds. Without resting, repeat three times. Rest for 30 seconds and then repeat the entire sequence.

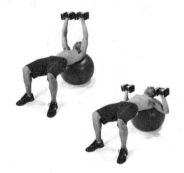

Chair Push-Up

Place two sturdy chairs in front of you and place your hands on the seats, slightly wider than shoulder-width apart, arms extended. Feather your breathing as you lower your chest toward the chairs through a count of 10 seconds, keeping your back straight and abs tight. Hold for 2 seconds at the MTP. Push your body back to starting position through a count of 10 seconds, keeping your elbows slightly bent at the top of the move. Without resting, repeat three times. Rest for 30 seconds and then repeat the entire sequence.

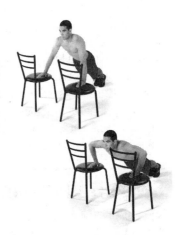

Barbell Military Press on Swiss Ball

Hold the barbell and sit on the ball with your back straight, abs tight, and chin up. Extend the barbell up and directly over your head, palms facing forward. Feather your breathing as you lower the weight through a count of 10 seconds. Hold for 2 seconds at the MTP (chin level). Press the barbell up to starting position through a count of 10 seconds. Without resting, repeat three times. Rest for 30 seconds and then repeat the entire sequence.

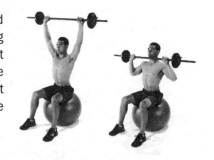

Chicken Wing

Hold a pair of dumbbells and stand with feet hip-width apart and knees slightly bent. Bend your elbows, holding the dumbbells in front of you at a 45-degree angle. Keep your forearms tight and feather your breathing as you raise your elbows up and out through a count of 10 seconds. Hold and squeeze for 2 seconds at the MTP. Return to starting position through a count of 10 seconds. Without resting, repeat three times. Rest for 30 seconds and then repeat the entire sequence. (Note: Be sure to relax your neck and avoid shrugging the shoulders.)

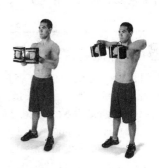

Upright Row

Hold a pair of dumbbells and stand with your feet together, knees slightly bent, and arms extended in front of you with a slight bend in your elbows, palms facing your body. Feather your breathing as you draw the weights up toward your chin through a count of 10 seconds. Hold for 2 seconds at the MTP (right below your chin). Return to starting position through a count of 10 seconds. Without resting, repeat three times. Rest for 30 seconds and then repeat the entire sequence. (Note: You should not feel a strain in your neck. If you do, relax your neck muscles and focus the exertion on your shoulders.)

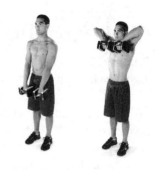

Swiss Ball Crunch with Elevated Feet

Sit on the ball about 2 feet away from a wall, arms behind your head. Walk your feet out and place them against the wall. Feather your breathing as you crunch up through a count of 10 seconds, using only your abs. Hold and squeeze for 2 seconds at the MTP. Return to starting position through a count of 10 seconds. Without resting, repeat three times. (Note: The range of motion is significantly shorter on this exercise so be sure to adjust your pace.)

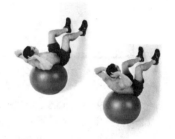

Chair Tuck-Up

Sit on the front edge of a sturdy chair. Reach your hands behind you and grab the sides of the chair. Extend your legs out and allow your upper body to lean back slightly. Feather your breathing as you slowly draw your knees in and up toward your chest through a count of 10 seconds. Hold and squeeze for 2 seconds at the MTP. Return legs to starting position through a count of 10 seconds. Without resting, repeat three times.

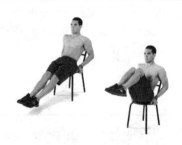

Bicycle Crunch

Lie flat on your back. Place your hands behind your head and raise your heels about 2 inches from the ground, keeping your chin up and abs tight throughout the exercise. Bring your right elbow to your left knee and feather your breathing as you rotate to the other side for a count of 10 seconds. Hold and squeeze for 2 seconds at the MTP (where your left elbow meets your right knee). Return to starting position through a count of 10 seconds. Without resting, repeat three times.

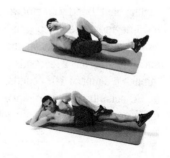

Barbell Pull-Over

Grasp the barbell with a close grip. Lie on the ball with your head and neck supported. Keep your hips up and abs tight throughout the exercise. Extend the weight over your chest with a slight bend in the elbows. Feather your breathing as you lower the weight behind your head through a count of 10 seconds. Hold for 2 seconds at the MTP. Raise the weight to starting position through a count of 10 seconds. Without resting, repeat three times. Rest for 30 seconds and then repeat the entire sequence. (Note: How far you can stretch your arms back will determine your MTP.)

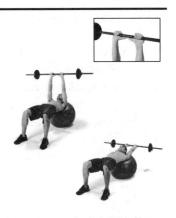

Bent-Over Row (Underhand Grip)

Hold a pair of dumbbells, arms extended, using the underhand grip. Bend at the waist as if tying your shoes. Raise your head and chest to create a slight arch in the back. Bend your knees slightly. Feather your breathing as you pull the dumbbells up in a fluid rowing motion through a count of 10 seconds, keeping your elbows close to your body. Hold and squeeze your shoulder blades together for 2 seconds at the MTP. Lower your arms to starting position through a count of 10 seconds. Without resting, repeat three times. Rest for 30 seconds and then repeat the entire sequence.

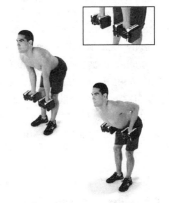

Bent-Over Barbell Row (Overhand Grip)

Hold the barbell with your arms extended, using the overhand grip. Stand with your feet hip-width apart. Bend at the waist as if you were about to tie your shoes; then lift only your chin and chest, creating a slight arch in your back. Keeping a bend in your knees, feather your breathing as you pull the weight up toward your hips in a fluid rowing motion through a count of 10 seconds. Hold and squeeze your shoulder blades together for 2 seconds at the MTP. Lower your arms to starting position through a count of 10 seconds. Without resting, repeat three times. Rest for 30 seconds and then repeat the entire sequence.

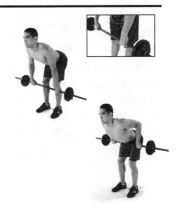

Barbell Dead Lift

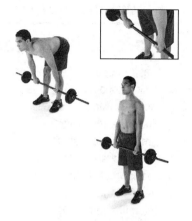

Grip the barbell with one palm facing forward, one palm facing back, and your feet about 6 to 8 inches apart. Bend over at the waist as if you were about to tie your shoes, knees slightly bent. Lift your chin and chest, creating a slight arch in your back. Feather your breathing as you lift your upper body through a count of 10 seconds, driving through your heels and using your lower back and hamstrings. Hold for 2 seconds at the MTP (at the top of the movement). Return to starting position through a count of 10 seconds. Without resting, repeat three times. Rest for 30 seconds and then repeat the entire sequence.

Standing Dumbbell Curl

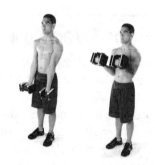

Hold a pair of dumbbells, palms facing out. Stand with your feet shoulder-width apart and your arms extended by your sides, knees slightly bent. Feather your breathing as you curl the dumbbells up through a count of 10 seconds. Hold and squeeze for 2 seconds at the MTP. Keep your elbows tight against your body as you lower the weights for 10 seconds to starting position. Without resting, repeat three times. Rest for 30 seconds and then repeat the entire sequence. (Note: Keep your elbows tight against your sides throughout the exercise.)

Incline Curl

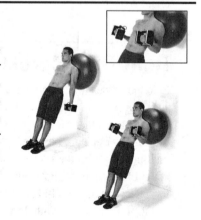

Hold a pair of dumbbells and stand with a ball against a sturdy wall, the ball between your shoulder blades. Bend your knees slightly. Keep your abs tight and chest up. Feather your breathing as you curl the weights up through a count of 10 seconds. Hold and squeeze for 2 seconds at the MTP. Lower the weights to starting position through a count of 10 seconds, until your arms are completely straight (do not lock your elbows). Without resting, repeat three times. Rest for 30 seconds and then repeat the entire sequence. (Note: As you perform the exercise, be sure to not let your elbows move away from the sides of your body.)

Reverse Barbell Curl

Grip a barbell with both hands, palms facing back. Stand with your feet shoulder-width apart and your arms extended by your sides, knees slightly bent. Feather your breathing as you curl the bar up through a count of 10 seconds to just past a 90-degree angle. Hold and squeeze for 2 seconds at the MTP. Keep your elbows tight against your body as you lower the weight through a count of 10 seconds. Without resting, repeat three times. Rest for 30 seconds and then repeat the entire sequence. (Note: Keep your elbows tight against your sides throughout the exercise.)

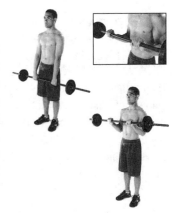

Chair Tuck-Up

Sit on the front edge of a sturdy chair. Reach your hands behind you and grab the sides of the chair. Extend your legs out and allow your upper body to lean back slightly. Feather your breathing as you slowly draw your knees in and up toward your chest through a count of 10 seconds. Hold and squeeze for 2 seconds at the MTP. Return legs to starting position through a count of 10 seconds. Without resting, repeat three times.

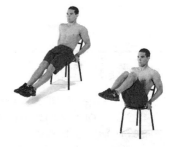

Toe Reach

Lie on your back. Cross your legs, flex your feet, and extend your legs into the air. Hold a medicine ball and extend your arms toward your toes. Keep your chin up and feather your breathing as you crunch up, reaching toward your toes through a count of 10 seconds. Hold and squeeze for 2 seconds at the MTP. Lower yourself to starting position, keeping your shoulder blades from touching the ground, through a count of 10 seconds. Without resting, repeat three times.

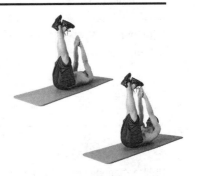

Bicycle Crunch

Lie flat on your back. Place your hands behind your head and raise your heels about 2 inches from the ground, keeping your chin up and abs tight throughout the exercise. Bring your right elbow to your left knee and feather your breathing as you rotate to the other side for a count of 10 seconds. Hold and squeeze for 2 seconds at the MTP (where your left elbow meets your right knee). Return to starting position through a count of 10 seconds. Without resting, repeat three times.

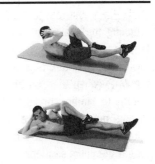

FRIDAY

Dumbbell Squat

Hold a pair of dumbbells, with your arms against your sides, and stand with your feet shoulder-width apart. Feather your breathing as you slowly squat through a count of 10 seconds, keeping your back straight, abs tight, and chest up. Hold for 2 seconds at the MTP. Return to starting position through a count of 10 seconds. Without resting, repeat three times. Rest for 30 seconds and then repeat the entire sequence.

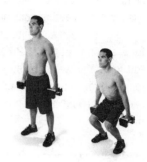

Barbell Sumo Squat

Rest the barbell across your back and stand with your feet about two times wider than shoulder-width apart, toes turned out to the sides, and knees aligned over the toes. Feather your breathing as you squat through a count of 10 seconds. Hold for 2 seconds at the MTP. Push through your heels to return to starting position through a count of 10 seconds. Without resting, repeat three times. Rest for 30 seconds and then repeat the entire sequence.

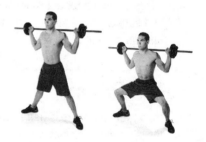

Split Squat

Hold a dumbbell in one hand and stand about 3 feet in front of a sturdy chair. Place your rear foot on the chair with the top of your shoe lightly touching the chair. With your back straight, chest up, and abs tight, feather your breathing as you bend your front knee, lowering yourself toward the ground through a count of 10 seconds. Hold for 2 seconds at the MTP (when there is about a 90-degree bend in the front knee). Return to starting position through a count of 10 seconds. Without resting, repeat once more and then switch sides (including dumbbell) and perform 2 more reps for a total of 4. Rest for 30 seconds and then repeat the entire sequence.

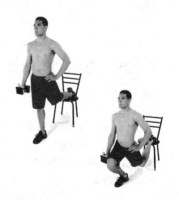

Quadriceps Flex

Stand with feet shoulder-width apart. Grasp the back of a sturdy chair for support at about hip level. Feather your breathing as you bend your knees and allow your body to fall backwards, letting your heels come off the floor, through a count of 10 seconds. Hold and squeeze your quads for 2 seconds at the MTP (when your knees are near the floor). Return to starting position through a count of 10 seconds. Without resting, repeat three times. Rest for 30 seconds and then repeat the entire sequence.

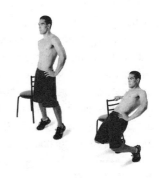

Overhead Barbell Triceps Extension

Grasp the barbell, palms facing out. Sit on a ball with your chest up, back straight, feet together. Extend your arms with your elbows slightly bent, keeping your biceps close to your head. Feather your breathing as you drop the bar back through a count of 10 seconds. Hold for 2 seconds at the MTP (when your elbows are at about a 90-degree angle). Press the bar up to starting position through a count of 10 seconds. Without resting, repeat three times. Rest for 30 seconds and then repeat the entire sequence.

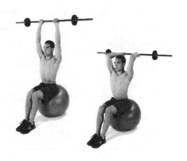

Barbell Skull Crusher

Hold a barbell and lie on the ball so that your head and neck are supported. Elevate your hips slightly and keep your abs tight. Extend the barbell straight up with your palms facing out. Drop your arms back toward your head slightly. Feather your breathing as you bend your elbows and lower the weight through a count of 10 seconds. Hold for 2 seconds at the MTP (a few inches above your forehead). Raise the barbell to starting position through a count of 10 seconds. Without resting, repeat three times. Rest for 30 seconds and then repeat the entire sequence.

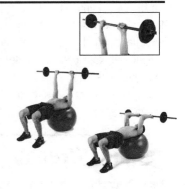

Standing Kickback

Hold a pair of dumbbells, palms facing each other. Bend at the waist as if you were about to tie your shoes; then lift only your chin and chest, creating a slight arch in your back, keeping a slight in bend your knees. Raise your elbows as high as possible, keeping them close to your body. Feather your breathing as you extend the weight back and out (without moving the upper part of the arm) through a count of 10 seconds. Hold and squeeze for 2 seconds at the MTP. Return the weights to starting position through a count of 10 seconds. Without resting, repeat three times. Rest for 30 seconds and then repeat the entire sequence.

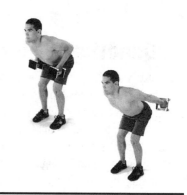

Double Crunch

Lie on a mat and place your hands behind your head, elbows up, chin up, and abs tight. Pull your heels toward your butt as far as you can. Using your upper abs, feather your breathing as you crunch up while simultaneously pulling your knees in through a count of 10 seconds. Hold and squeeze for 2 seconds at the MTP. Return to starting position through a count of 10 seconds, never letting your upper back touch the ground. Without resting, repeat three times. (Note: The range of motion on this exercise is very short so be sure to adjust your speed so that you hit the MTP on the count of 10.)

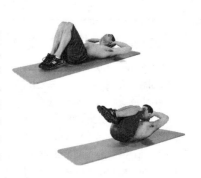

Seated V-Up

Sit on the ground with your arms slightly behind you, elbows bent, and fingertips pointed forward. Start with your knees together, legs extended, and heels off the ground about 2 inches. Support your upper body weight with your palms. Feather your breathing as you pull your knees into your chest for a count of 10 seconds. Hold and squeeze for 2 seconds at the MTP. Return to starting position through a count of 10 seconds, keeping your abs tight. Without resting, repeat three times.

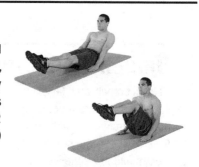

Oblique Crunch

Lie on your side on a mat with your knees bent and angled toward one side. Place hands behind your head. Look up at the ceiling, tighten your abs, and feather your breathing as you crunch up through a count of 10 seconds. Hold and squeeze for 2 seconds at the MTP. Maintain tension in your obliques as you lower yourself to starting position through a count of 10 seconds. Without resting, repeat once more on this side and then switch sides and complete 2 more reps for a total of 4.

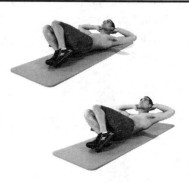

WEEK 5

As you gear up to start your week, use these tips based on your Life Priority to create extra inner drive and motivation. They are customized to your age category, but I recommend you read every one of them. You'll find valuable information in each tip, no matter what your age.

20 to 35 PRIME TIME

Time to Ditch Your Friends?

Having good friends can help you de-stress and stay healthy. But what if it turns out your friends may be what's keeping you from getting healthy? One study published in the *New England Journal of Medicine* revealed that obesity can spread through social networks. In fact, your chance of being obese increases 59 percent if you have an obese friend—and jumps to a whopping 171 percent if it's a close friend. This doesn't mean you have to cut overweight friends out of your life. I'd like to think of it more as a wake-up call: Pay attention to the choices you make. If your buddy opts to chow down potato skins and beer for dinner, what are you most likely to do? Eat the same thing! When you make the commitment to the Body at Home™ workouts and eating plan, tell all your friends about it. Try turning the tide by becoming the one who sets the example. If you are looking to surround yourself with people with the same goals, visit BodyatHome.com. If they aren't up for the challenge as you are, they will be when you take your shirt off in a few weeks!

35 to 50 STAY YOUNG

Healthy Sex

Just what every guy has always wanted to hear: Sex is good for you. Studies have shown that sex—with a partner or through masturbation—has a long list of health benefits. When you get turned on or have an orgasm, your body releases more of the "feel-good" hormone oxytocin. Oxytocin has been shown to have a calming effect by balancing out stress hormones. It also can help counteract impotence. Plus, sex helps your body naturally combat pain because it releases endorphins, which can mirror the effects of opiates by creating a sense of relaxation and euphoria. A study published in the *Journal of the American Medical Association* investigated the relationship between ejaculation frequency and risk for prostate cancer. The researchers found that a high rate of ejaculation was associated with a lower risk for prostate cancer. While the exact reasons are unknown, scientists speculate that having an orgasm helps "cleanse" the prostate of toxins that could build up into tumors. So don't just do it, do it often—all in the name of your health!

50-Plus LONGEVITY

Baby Aspirin: Not Just for Babies

You may remember all the hype associated with aspirin as a preventive against heart attack . . . and then of course the backlash. Aspirin helps thin the blood, which reduces the risk of blood clots that can lead to heart attacks, but too-thin blood can produce nosebleeds and bleeding in your brain. So how do you get the benefits without the risk? Try baby aspirin. In their fantastic book *YOU: Staying Young,* Dr. Mehmet C. Oz and Dr. Michael F. Roizen recommend 162 milligrams a day of baby aspirin. A study done at the University of Kentucky indicated that the lower dosage (compared to adult aspirin) posed less risk of gastrointestinal bleeding yet had protective benefits. Studies also have linked a daily aspirin with reduced risk of certain cancers, such those occurring in the colon and prostate. The theory behind this is aspirin helps limit inflammation, which can lead to cancer-causing enzymes that eventually produce tumors. While the jury's still out on the true benefits of aspirin and cancer prevention, the link to heart health is definite. Take two baby aspirin a day with food. Of course, check first with your doctor to make sure it's right for you.

MONDAY

Flat Dumbbell Press

Hold a pair of dumbbells and lie on the ball so that it comfortably supports your shoulder blades. Extend your arms in front of you, pressing the weights together. Feather your breathing as you lower the weights through a count of 10 seconds. Hold for 2 seconds at the MTP (about 1 inch above your chest). Press the dumbbells up and together, then back to starting position through a count of 10 seconds. Without resting, repeat three times. Rest for 30 seconds and then repeat the entire sequence.

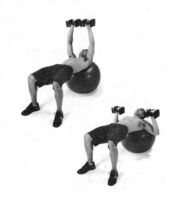

Incline Barbell Press

Hold the barbell with your palms facing out and lie on the ball so that your head and neck are supported. Allow your hips to drop almost to the ground. Press the weight up over your nose, keeping a slight bend in the elbows so that the upper chest is targeted. Feather your breathing as you lower the weight through a count of 10 seconds. Hold for 2 seconds at the MTP (when the barbell is only a couple of inches from your chest). Press the bar up to starting position through a count of 10 seconds. Without resting, repeat three times. Rest for 30 seconds and then repeat the entire sequence.

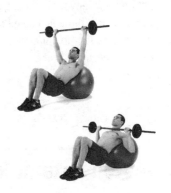

Incline Unilateral Dumbbell Press

Grasp a dumbbell in one hand and lie on the ball so that your head and neck are supported. Allow your hips to drop almost to the ground. Press the weight up with one hand, keeping your free hand on your hip. Feather your breathing as you slowly lower the weight toward your chest through a count of 10 seconds. Hold and squeeze for 2 seconds at the MTP (about 2 inches above your chest). Return to starting position through a count of 10 seconds. Without resting, repeat once more on this side and then switch sides and complete 2 more reps for a total of 4. Rest for 30 seconds and then repeat the entire sequence.

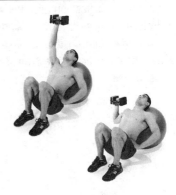

Flat Dumbbell Fly

Hold a pair of dumbbells and lie on the ball with your head and neck supported. Extend the dumbbells over your chest, palms facing each other, elbows slightly bent. Feather your breathing as you lower the weights down and out through a count of 10 seconds. Hold for 2 seconds at the MTP. Raise the weights to starting position in a "bear hug" type motion through a count of 10 seconds. Without resting, repeat three times. Rest for 30 seconds and then repeat the entire sequence.

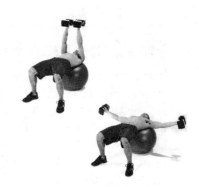

V Push-Up

Stand with your feet shoulder-width apart, bend forward, and walk your hands out to create an upside-down "V" with your body. Keep your abs tight and feather your breathing as you lower your head and upper body toward the mat through a count of 10 seconds. Hold for 2 seconds at the MTP. Press back up through a count of 10 seconds. Without resting, repeat three times. Rest for 30 seconds and then repeat the entire sequence.

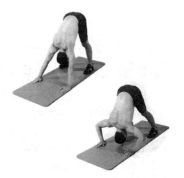

Seated Lateral Raise

Hold a pair of dumbbells and sit on a ball, your back straight and abs tight. With your arms against your sides and elbows slightly bent, feather your breathing as you raise the weights through a count of 10 seconds. Hold and squeeze for 2 seconds at the MTP ("T" position). Lower your arms to starting position through a count of 10 seconds. Without resting, repeat three times. Rest for 30 seconds and then repeat the entire sequence.

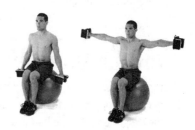

Upright Barbell Row

Grasp the barbell using the grip shown, palms facing your body. Stand upright with your back straight and abs tight. Feather your breathing as you raise the bar to your chin through a count of 10 seconds. Hold and squeeze for 2 seconds at the MTP. Lower the weight to starting position through a count of 10 seconds. Without resting, repeat three times. Rest for 30 seconds and then repeat the entire sequence.

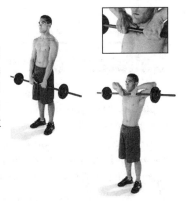

Jackknife

Stand about 3 feet in front of the ball and place your palms on the ground, hands shoulder-width apart. Put one foot on the ball about mid-shin level. Once you are stabilized, place the other foot on the ball, keeping your head forward, spine straight, and abs tight. Slowly pull your knees up to your chin through a count of 10 seconds, as you concentrate on maintaining stability by squeezing your abs tight. Hold and squeeze for 2 seconds at the MTP. Return to starting position through a count of 10 seconds. Without resting, repeat three times.

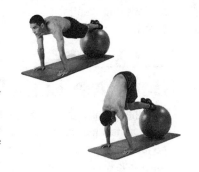

Swiss Ball Ab Roll

Kneel on a mat in front of a ball and cross your ankles behind you. Close both hands into fists and place on the ball, keeping your elbows straight but not locked. Keep your head up, back straight, and abs tight. Feather your breathing as you roll forward on the ball through a count of 10 seconds. Hold for 2 seconds at the MTP. Return to starting position through a count of 10 seconds. Without resting, repeat three times.

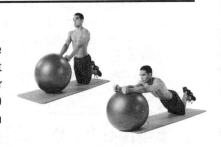

Weighted Russian Twist

Sit on the mat with your knees bent, feet together. While holding a medicine ball, lean back slightly, engaging your abs. Extend your arms away from your chest and turn to one side to begin exercise. Keep your chin up and abs tight as you feather your breathing and slowly rotate your torso as far as possible to the other side through a count of 10 seconds. Hold and squeeze for 2 seconds at the MTP. Rotate back to the other side through a count of 10 seconds. Without resting, repeat three times.

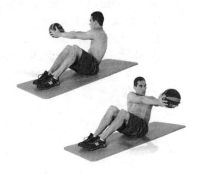

WEDNESDAY

Unilateral Dumbbell Pull-Over

Grasp a dumbbell and lie on the ball with your head and neck supported. Keep your hips up and abs tight throughout the exercise. With one arm, extend the weight over your chest, keeping a slight bend in the elbows; place other arm on your hip. Feather your breathing as you lower the weight behind your head through a count of 10 seconds. Hold for 2 seconds at the MTP. Raise the weight to starting position through a count of 10 seconds. Without resting, repeat once more on this side and then switch sides and complete 2 more reps for a total of 4. Rest for 30 seconds and then repeat the entire sequence. (Note: How far you can stretch your arms back will determine your MTP.)

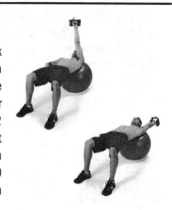

Bent-Over Barbell Row (Overhand Grip)

Hold the barbell with your arms extended, using the overhand grip. Stand with your feet hip-width apart. Bend at the waist as if you were about to tie your shoes; then lift only your chin and chest, creating a slight arch in your back. Keeping a bend in your knees, feather your breathing as you pull the weight up toward your hips in a fluid rowing motion through a count of 10 seconds. Hold and squeeze your shoulder blades together for 2 seconds at the MTP. Lower your arms to starting position through a count of 10 seconds. Without resting, repeat three times. Rest for 30 seconds and then repeat the entire sequence.

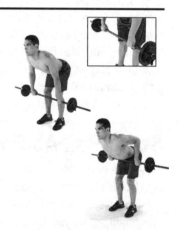

Bent-Over Dumbbell Row (Underhand Grip)

Hold a pair of dumbbells, using the underhand grip, arms extended. Stand with your feet hip-width apart. Bend at the waist as if tying your shoes. Raise your head and chest to create a slight arch in the back. Bend your knees slightly. Feather your breathing as you pull the dumbbells up in a fluid rowing motion through a count of 10 seconds, keeping your elbows close to your body. Hold and squeeze your shoulder blades together for 2 seconds at the MTP. Lower your arms to starting position through a count of 10 seconds. Without resting, repeat three times. Rest for 30 seconds and then repeat the entire sequence.

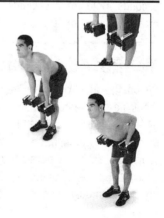

Hyperextension

Lie facedown on the ball with your hips supported and your hands behind your head. Bend at the waist. Feather your breathing as you lift your upper body through a count of 10 seconds, using your lower back. Hold for 2 seconds at the MTP. Return to starting position through a count of 10 seconds. Without resting, repeat three times. Rest for 30 seconds and then repeat the entire sequence.

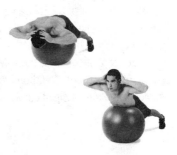

Standing Side Curl

Hold a pair of dumbbells with your palms turned out, elbows to your side. Keep your chest up, feet hip-width apart, knees slightly bent, and abs tight throughout the exercise. Feather your breathing as you curl the weights up through a count of 10 seconds. Hold and squeeze for 2 seconds at the MTP. Lower the weights to starting position through a count of 10 seconds until your arms are completely straight (do not lock your elbows). Without resting, repeat three times. Rest for 30 seconds and then repeat the entire sequence.

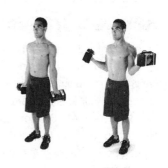

Barbell Preacher Curl

Hold the barbell and rest over the ball with your knees on the floor and a 6- to 8-inch gap between your arms. Lift your arms to starting position with your elbows bent at about a 90-degree angle. Feather your breathing as you lower the weight through a count of 10 seconds. Hold for 2 seconds at the MTP. Lift the barbell to starting position through a count of 10 seconds. Without resting, repeat three times. Rest for 30 seconds and then repeat the entire sequence.

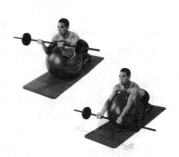

Hammer Curl

Holding a pair of dumbbells, stand with your feet shoulder-width apart, your arms extended slightly in front of your thighs, palms facing each other, and knees slightly bent. Feather your breathing as you curl the weights up through a count of 10 seconds, keeping your palms facing each other. Hold and squeeze for 2 seconds at the MTP. Lower the weights to starting position through a count of 10 seconds. Without resting, repeat three times. Rest for 30 seconds and then repeat the entire sequence.

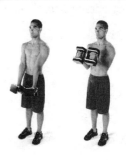

Swiss Ball Crunch with Elevated Feet

Sit on the ball about 2 feet away from a wall, arms crossed. Walk your feet out and place them against the wall. Feather your breathing as you crunch up through a count of 10 seconds, using only your abs. Hold and squeeze for 2 seconds at the MTP. Return to starting position through a count of 10 seconds. Without resting, repeat three times. (Note: The range of motion is significantly shorter on this exercise so be sure to adjust your pace.)

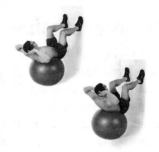

Reverse Crunch

Lie on a mat with your hands by your sides, palms down. Pull your heels up as close to your butt as possible. Raise your heels about 2 inches off the ground. Keep your chin tucked and abs tight. Feather your breathing as you pull your knees toward your chest, using your lower abdominals, through a count of 10 seconds. Hold and squeeze for 2 seconds at the MTP (when your butt is completely off the ground). Lower your body to starting position through a count of 10 seconds. Without resting, repeat three times.

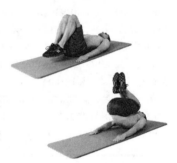

Oblique Crunch

Lie on your side on a mat with your knees bent and angled toward one side. Place hands behind your head. Look up at the ceiling, tighten your abs, and feather your breathing as you crunch up through a count of 10 seconds. Hold and squeeze for 2 seconds at the MTP. Maintain tension in your obliques as you lower yourself to starting position through a count of 10 seconds. Without resting, repeat once more on this side and then switch sides and complete 2 more reps for a total of 4.

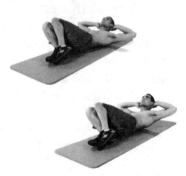

FRIDAY

Swiss Ball Squat

Place the ball against a wall and position yourself with the ball supporting your middle to upper back. Hold a pair of dumbbells with your arms against your sides. Move your feet forward about 1 foot, keeping them about hip-width apart. Feather your breathing as you slowly squat down through a count of 10 seconds. Hold for 2 seconds at the MTP (when your knees are at a 90-degree angle). Return to starting position through a count of 10 seconds. Without resting, repeat three times. Rest for 30 seconds and then repeat the entire sequence.

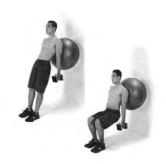

Barbell Squat

Stand with your feet hip-width apart and hold a weighted barbell across your shoulders. Keep your back straight, abs tight, and head up. Feather your breathing as you squat through a count of 10 seconds. Hold for 2 seconds at the MTP. Push through your heels as you stand and return to starting position through a count of 10 seconds. Without resting, repeat three times. Rest for 30 seconds and then repeat the entire sequence.

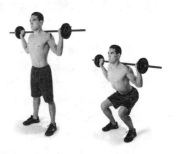

Dumbbell Sumo Squat

Hold a pair of dumbbells, palms facing back, arms extended in front of your body. Stand with your feet about two times wider than shoulder-width apart, toes turned out to the sides, and knees aligned over the toes. Feather your breathing as you squat through a count of 10 seconds. Hold for 2 seconds at the MTP. Push through your heels to return to starting position through a count of 10 seconds. Without resting, repeat three times. Rest for 30 seconds and then repeat the entire sequence.

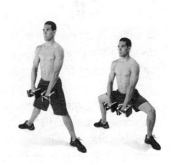

Swiss Ball Hamstring Curl

Lie on your back with your arms at your sides, palms flat on the floor. Place your heels on the ball, knees straight but not completely locked; then lift your butt and hips off the ground. With your abs tight, feather your breathing and bend your knees as you roll the ball toward your butt with your heels. Hold for 2 seconds at the MTP. Return to starting position through a count of 10 seconds. Without resting, repeat three times. Rest for 30 seconds and then repeat the entire sequence.

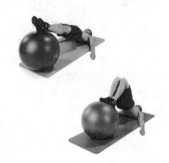

Barbell Skull Crusher

Hold a barbell and lie on the ball so that your head and neck are supported. Elevate your hips slightly and keep your abs tight. Extend the barbell straight up with your palms facing out. Drop your arms back toward your head slightly. Feather your breathing as you bend your elbows and lower the weight through a count of 10 seconds. Hold for 2 seconds at the MTP (a few inches above your forehead). Raise the barbell to starting position through a count of 10 seconds. Without resting, repeat three times. Rest for 30 seconds and then repeat the entire sequence.

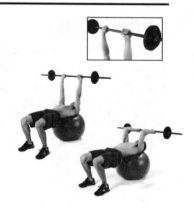

Chair Dip

Sit on the front edge of a sturdy chair, hands close to your sides, fingers forward, and legs extended. Feather your breathing as you lower yourself through a count of 10 seconds. Hold for 2 seconds at the MTP. Push yourself back up to starting position through a count of 10 seconds. Without resting, repeat three times. Rest for 30 seconds and then repeat the entire sequence. (Note: The MTP will depend on how flexible your shoulders are. Your MTP will be about 1 inch above your most flexible point. If this exercise is too difficult, move your feet closer to your body for more stability.)

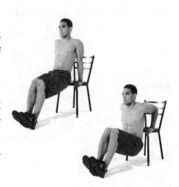

Overhead Barbell Triceps Extension

Grasp the barbell, palms facing out. Sit on a ball with your chest up, back straight, feet together. Extend your arms with your elbows slightly bent, keeping your biceps close to your head. Feather your breathing as you drop the bar back through a count of 10 seconds. Hold for 2 seconds at the MTP (when your elbows are at about a 90-degree angle). Press the bar up to starting position through a count of 10 seconds. Without resting, repeat three times. Rest for 30 seconds and then repeat the entire sequence.

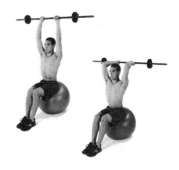

Swiss Ball Ab Roll

Kneel on a mat in front of a ball and cross your ankles behind you. Close both hands into fists and place on the ball, keeping your elbows straight but not locked. Keep your head up, back straight, and abs tight. Feather your breathing as you roll forward on the ball through a count of 10 seconds. Hold for 2 seconds at the MTP. Return to starting position through a count of 10 seconds. Without resting, repeat three times.

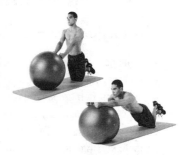

Leg Lift

Lie on your back with your palms down, hands underneath your butt. Crunch up and hold your upper abs tight so that your shoulder blades are off the ground. Lift your legs about 2 inches off the ground. Keep your abs tight and chin up and feather your breathing as you lift your legs through a count of 10 seconds. Hold and squeeze for 2 seconds at the MTP. Lower your legs to starting position through a count of 10 seconds. Without resting, repeat three times.

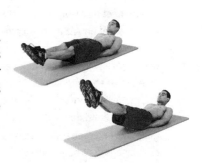

Bicycle Crunch

Lie flat on your back. Place your hands behind your head and raise your heels about 2 inches from the ground, keeping your chin up and abs tight throughout the exercise. Bring your right elbow to your left knee and feather your breathing as you rotate to the other side for a count of 10 seconds. Hold and squeeze for 2 seconds at the MTP (where your left elbow meets your right knee). Return to starting position through a count of 10 seconds. Without resting, repeat three times.

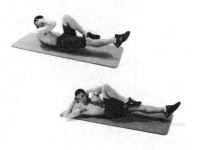

WEEK 6

As you gear up to start your week, use these tips based on your Life Priority to create extra inner drive and motivation. They are customized to your age category, but I recommend you read every one of them. You'll find valuable information in each tip, no matter what your age.

20 to 35 PRIME TIME

Making a Good First Impression

Whether you're meeting someone for the first time at the office or a bar, first impressions are lasting ones. Remember, dress to impress and keep your head up and shoulders back. But what do you do from there? First off, have a good handshake. A handshake is a universal greeting that can set the tone for a relationship. Avoid a grip of the bone-crunching variety—whether you're meeting a guy or a girl. The receiver will wonder what you're trying to prove. And never offer a "dead fish" handshake that will say "I'm weak" or convey a lack of respect for the receiver. When I meet someone new, I make sure to stand tall, make eye contact, smile, and offer a firm but courteous handshake. Be enthusiastic. But keep your cool and repeat the person's name after he or she says it, to help yourself remember it. This way, whatever your outcome, the person will know you mean business.

35 to 50 STAY YOUNG

Know Your Levels

After you hit age 30, your testosterone levels start to drop by 1.5 percent each year. Low testosterone levels can lead to decreased bone density and muscle mass; they can cause decreased energy levels, make you feel depressed, lead to insulin resistance, and lower your sex drive. Worst of all, they also have been linked to high risk of cardiovascular disease. Other hormone levels—such as growth hormone, DHEA, and insulin—change as we age, as do our triglyceride and cholesterol levels. This shifting body chemistry can create health issues ranging from minor to serious and make it difficult for you to achieve the body you want. For example, when your body doesn't have enough bioavailable testosterone, it could be tougher for you to achieve your desired muscle mass. That's why it's important for you to check in on your body now to see where you stand. Why wait until you are older, when it will take longer and be more difficult to put your body on the right course? I had my hormones tested and complete blood work done at age 37, and that's helped me create a supplement plan that allows me to live life in optimum health. Ask for a test that will evaluate your endocrine functions, in addition to traditional testing that will show your metabolic panel.

50-Plus LONGEVITY

Sharpen Your Memory

From forgetting phone numbers, birthdays, and people's names to losing our keys, memory can play a tricky game of hide-and-seek on us sometimes. Good thing there are things you can do now to keep your mind sharp and functioning at its best. First tip: Take your B vitamins. Nearly one out of five people is deficient in vitamin B12, which plays a critical role in forming red blood cells. When you don't have enough B12, your body may not get enough oxygen because it's short on red blood cells—the delivery trucks that carry oxygen into your bloodstream. If this shortage affects your brain, you could experience nerve damage that triggers depression, dementia, and Alzheimer's disease. Aim to get 800 to 1,000 micrograms of B12 a day. Another tip for keeping your memory sharp: Exercise. Three Body at Home™ workouts a week will help your body produce new brain cells that help in the areas of learning and memory. Research done at the Salk Institute in California found that exercise increased the survival and birth of brain cells in the hippocampus, the part of the brain associated with long-term memory and spatial awareness. So put this book down and get to those weights—before you forget!

MONDAY

Incline Dumbbell Press

Hold a pair of dumbbells and lie on the ball so that your head and neck are supported. Allow your hips to drop almost to the ground. Press the weights up and together, with a slight bend in the elbows so that the upper chest is targeted. Feather your breathing as you lower the weights through a count of 10 seconds. Hold for 2 seconds at the MTP. Press the dumbbells up to starting position through a count of 10 seconds. Without resting, repeat three times. Rest for 30 seconds and then repeat the entire sequence.

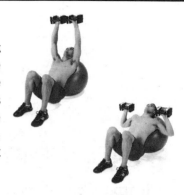

Flat Barbell Press

Hold the barbell and lie on the ball so that it comfortably supports your shoulder blades. Extend your arms in front of you, pressing the weight up. Feather your breathing as you lower the weight through a count of 10 seconds. Hold for 2 seconds at MTP (about 1 inch above your chest). Press the barbell back to starting position through a count of 10 seconds. Without resting, repeat three times. Rest for 30 seconds and then repeat the entire sequence.

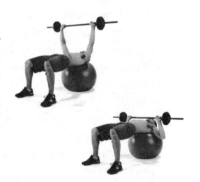

Unilateral Flat Dumbbell Press

Grasp a dumbbell in one hand and lie on the ball so that your head and neck are supported, keeping your hips and abs tight. Press the weight up with one hand, keeping your free hand on your hip. Feather your breathing as you slowly lower the weight toward your chest through a count of 10 seconds. Hold and squeeze for 2 seconds at the MTP (about 2 inches above your chest). Return to starting position through a count of 10 seconds. Without resting, repeat once more on this side and then switch hands and complete 2 more reps for a total of 4. Rest for 30 seconds and then repeat the entire sequence.

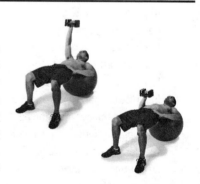

Push-Up

Lie on a mat with your hands slightly wider than shoulder-width apart and your fingers pointing forward. Press up to starting position, keeping your back straight, abs tight, and head up. Feather your breathing as you lower your chest toward the floor through a count of 10 seconds. Hold for 2 seconds at the MTP. Push your body back to starting position through a count of 10 seconds, keeping your elbows slightly bent. Without resting, repeat three times. Rest for 30 seconds and then repeat the entire sequence.

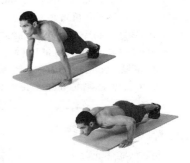

Seated Shoulder Press (Neutral Position)

Hold a pair of dumbbells in the neutral position and sit on the ball with your back straight, abs tight, and chin up. Extend the weights up and together directly over your head, palms facing each other. Feather your breathing as you lower the weights through a count of 10 seconds. Hold for 2 seconds at the MTP (chin level). Press the dumbbells up to starting position through a count of 10 seconds. Without resting, repeat three times. Rest for 30 seconds and then repeat the entire sequence.

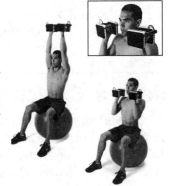

Standing Lateral Raise

Hold a pair of dumbbells and stand with your feet slightly apart, back straight, and abs tight. With your arms against your sides and elbows slightly bent, feather your breathing as you raise the weights up through a count of 10 seconds. Hold and squeeze for 2 seconds at the MTP ("T" position). Lower the weights to starting position through a count of 10 seconds. Without resting, repeat three times. Rest for 30 seconds and then repeat the entire sequence.

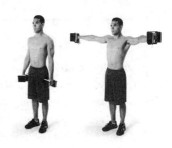

Bent-Over Rear Delt Raise

Hold a pair of dumbbells, palms facing each other. Bend at the waist as if you were about to tie your shoes; then lift only your chin and chest, creating a slight arch in your back. Feather your breathing as you raise the weights to your sides through a count of 10 seconds. Hold and squeeze for 2 seconds at the MTP. Lower the weights to starting position through a count of 10 seconds. Without resting, repeat three times. Rest for 30 seconds and then repeat the entire sequence.

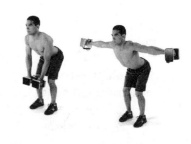

Toe Reach

Lie on your back on a mat. Cross your legs, flex your feet, and extend your legs into the air. With your arms extended and chin up, feather your breathing as you crunch up, reaching toward your toes through a count of 10 seconds. Hold and squeeze for 2 seconds at the MTP. Lower yourself to starting position, keeping your shoulder blades from touching the ground, through a count of 10 seconds. Without resting, repeat three times.

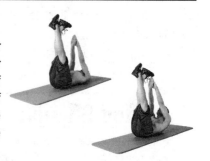

Reverse Crunch

Lie on a mat with your hands by your sides, palms down. Pull your heels up as close to your butt as possible. Raise your heels about 2 inches off the ground. Keep your chin tucked and abs tight. Feather your breathing as you pull your knees toward your chest, using your lower abdominals, through a count of 10 seconds. Hold and squeeze for 2 seconds at the MTP (when your butt is completely off the ground). Lower your body to starting position through a count of 10 seconds. Without resting, repeat three times.

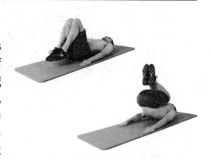

Barbell Twist

Grip an empty barbell, placing it across the back of your shoulders. Stand with your legs about 3 feet apart. Twist your upper body to one side. With your chin up and abs squeezed tight, feather your breathing as you slowly twist to the other side through a count of 10 seconds. At the MTP of your twist, hold and squeeze for 2 seconds. Return to starting position through a count of 10 seconds. Without resting, repeat three times. (Note: If you can do more than 4 reps, you're not squeezing your abs hard enough throughout the exercise.)

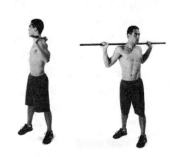

Barbell Pull-Over

Grasp the barbell with a close grip. Lie on the ball with your head and neck supported. Keep your hips up and abs tight throughout the exercise. Extend the weight over your chest with a slight bend in the elbows. Feather your breathing as you lower the weight behind your head through a count of 10 seconds. Hold for 2 seconds at the MTP. Raise the weight to starting position through a count of 10 seconds. Without resting, repeat three times. Rest for 30 seconds and then repeat the entire sequence. (Note: How far you can stretch your arms back will determine your MTP.)

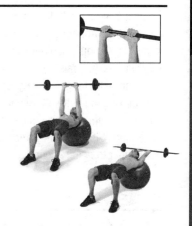

Bent-Over Dumbbell Row (Standard Grip)

Hold a pair of dumbbells, arms extended, palms facing each other. Stand with your feet hip-width apart. Bend at the waist as if you were about to tie your shoes; then lift only your chin and chest, creating a slight arch in your back. Bend your knees slightly. Feather your breathing as you pull the dumbbells up in a fluid rowing motion through a count of 10 seconds. Hold and squeeze your shoulder blades together for 2 seconds at the MTP. Lower your arms to starting position through a count of 10 seconds. Without resting, repeat three times. Rest for 30 seconds and then repeat the entire sequence. (Note: Keep your elbows close to your body throughout the exercise.)

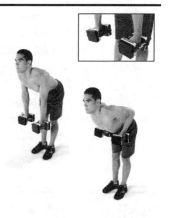

Bent-Over Barbell Row (Underhand Grip)

Grasp the barbell using the underhand grip. Bend at the waist as if tying your shoes, keeping your knees slightly bent. Raise your head and chest to create a slight arch in the back. Feather your breathing as you pull the bar up in a fluid rowing motion through a count of 10 seconds, keeping your elbows close to your body. Hold and squeeze your shoulder blades together for 2 seconds at the MTP. Lower your arms to starting position through a count of 10 seconds. Without resting, repeat three times. Rest for 30 seconds and then repeat the entire sequence.

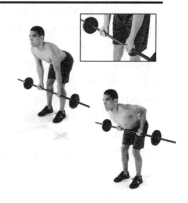

Reverse Hyperextension

Lie facedown on the ball. Roll yourself forward until the ball is under your hips and your upper body is angled toward the ground. Place your palms on the floor about shoulder-width apart. With legs together, feather your breathing as you raise your heels toward the ceiling using your lower back and hamstrings. Raise your legs through a count of 10 seconds. Hold and squeeze for 2 seconds at the MTP. With straight legs, lower through a count of 10 seconds to starting position, about 2 inches from the ground. Without resting, repeat three times. Rest for 30 seconds and then repeat the entire sequence.

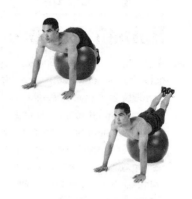

Standing Barbell Curl (Wide Grip)

Grasp a barbell using a wide grip, palms facing up. Stand with your feet shoulder-width apart and your arms extended by your sides, knees slightly bent. Feather your breathing as you curl the barbell up through a count of 10 seconds to just past a 90-degree angle. Hold and squeeze for 2 seconds at the MTP. Keep your elbows close to your body as you lower the weight through a count of 10 seconds. Without resting, repeat three times. Rest for 30 seconds and then repeat the entire sequence. (Note: Keep the elbows tight against your sides throughout the exercise.)

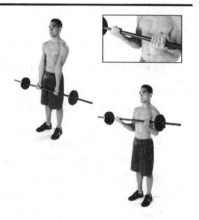

Incline Curl

Hold a pair of dumbbells and stand with a ball against a sturdy wall, the ball between your shoulder blades. Bend your knees slightly. Keep your abs tight and chest up. Feather your breathing as you curl the weights up through a count of 10 seconds. Hold and squeeze for 2 seconds at the MTP. Lower the weights to starting position through a count of 10 seconds, until your arms are completely straight (do not lock your elbows). Without resting, repeat three times. Rest for 30 seconds and then repeat the entire sequence. (Note: As you perform the exercise, be sure to not let your elbows move away from the sides of your body.)

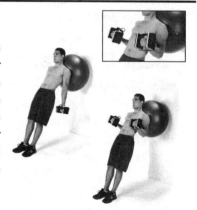

Reverse Barbell Curl

Grip a barbell with both hands, palms facing back. Stand with your feet shoulder-width apart and your arms extended by your sides, knees slightly bent. Feather your breathing as you curl the bar up through a count of 10 seconds to just past a 90-degree angle. Hold and squeeze for 2 seconds at the MTP. Keep your elbows tight against your body as you lower the weight through a count of 10 seconds. Without resting, repeat three times. Rest for 30 seconds and then repeat the entire sequence. (Note: Keep your elbows tight against your sides throughout the exercise.)

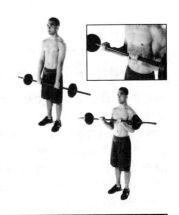

Double Crunch

Lie on a mat and place your hands behind your head, elbows up, chin up, and abs tight. Pull your heels toward your butt as far as you can. Using your upper abs, feather your breathing as you crunch up while simultaneously pulling your knees in through a count of 10 seconds. Hold and squeeze for 2 seconds at the MTP. Return to starting position through a count of 10 seconds, never letting your upper back touch the ground. Without resting, repeat three times. (Note: The range of motion on this exercise is very short so be sure to adjust your speed so that you hit the MTP on the count of 10.)

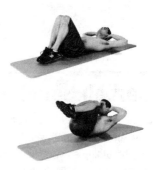

Leg Lift

Lie on your back with your palms down, hands underneath your butt. Crunch up and hold your upper abs tight so that your shoulder blades are off the ground. Lift your legs about 2 inches off the ground. Keep your abs tight and chin up and feather your breathing as you lift your legs through a count of 10 seconds. Hold and squeeze for 2 seconds at the MTP. Lower your legs to starting position through a count of 10 seconds. Without resting, repeat three times.

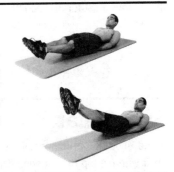

Bicycle Crunch

Lie flat on your back. Place your hands behind your head and raise your heels about 2 inches from the ground, keeping your chin up and abs tight throughout the exercise. Bring your right elbow to your left knee and feather your breathing as you rotate to the other side for a count of 10 seconds. Hold and squeeze for 2 seconds at the MTP (where your left elbow meets your right knee). Return to starting position through a count of 10 seconds. Without resting, repeat three times.

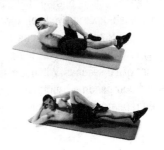

FRIDAY

Barbell Sumo Squat

Rest the barbell across your back and stand with your feet about two times wider than shoulder-width apart, toes turned out to the sides, and knees aligned over the toes. Feather your breathing as you squat through a count of 10 seconds. Hold for 2 seconds at the MTP. Push through your heels to return to starting position through a count of 10 seconds. Without resting, repeat three times. Rest for 30 seconds and then repeat the entire sequence.

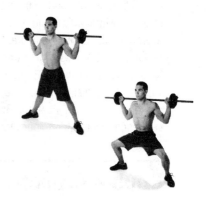

Barbell Squat

Stand with your feet hip-width apart and hold a weighted barbell across your shoulders. Keep your back straight, abs tight, and head up. Feather your breathing as you squat through a count of 10 seconds. Hold for 2 seconds at the MTP. Push through your heels as you stand and return to starting position through a count of 10 seconds. Without resting, repeat three times. Rest for 30 seconds and then repeat the entire sequence.

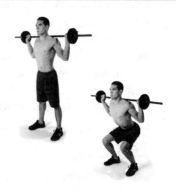

Split Squat

Stand about 3 feet in front of a sturdy chair. Place your rear foot on the chair with the top of your shoe lightly touching the chair. With your back straight, chest up, and abs tight, feather your breathing as you bend your front knee, lowering yourself toward the ground through a count of 10 seconds. Hold for 2 seconds at the MTP (when there is about a 90-degree bend in the front knee). Return to starting position through a count of 10 seconds. Without resting, repeat once more and then switch sides and perform 2 more reps for a total of 4. Rest for 30 seconds and then repeat the entire sequence.

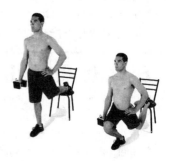

Quadriceps Flex

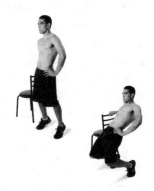

Stand with feet shoulder-width apart. Grasp the back of a sturdy chair for support at about hip level. Feather your breathing as you bend your knees and allow your body to fall backward, letting your heels come off the floor, through a count of 10 seconds. Hold and squeeze your quads for 2 seconds at the MTP (when your knees are near the floor). Return to starting position through a count of 10 seconds. Without resting, repeat three times. Rest for 30 seconds and then repeat the entire sequence.

Barbell Skull Crusher

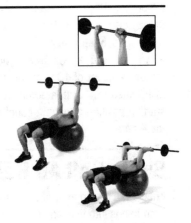

Hold a barbell and lie on the ball so that your head and neck are supported. Elevate your hips slightly and keep your abs tight. Extend the barbell straight up with your palms facing out. Drop your arms back toward your head slightly. Feather your breathing as you bend your elbows and lower the weight through a count of 10 seconds. Hold for 2 seconds at the MTP (a few inches above your forehead). Raise the barbell to starting position through a count of 10 seconds. Without resting, repeat three times. Rest for 30 seconds and then repeat the entire sequence.

Incline Diamond Push-Up

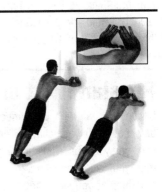

Place your hands in a push-up position against a wall; then shift your hands into the center to form a "diamond." Be sure that your upper body is elevated above your feet. Keep your head up, back straight, and abs tight. Feather your breathing as you lower yourself through a count of 10 seconds. Hold for 2 seconds at the MTP. Return to starting position through a count of 10 seconds. Without resting, repeat three times. Rest for 30 seconds and then repeat the entire sequence.

Standing Kickback

Hold a pair of dumbbells, palms facing each other. Bend at the waist as if you were about to tie your shoes; then lift only your chin and chest, creating a slight arch in your back, keeping a slight bend in your knees. Raise your elbows as high as possible, keeping them close to your body. Feather your breathing as you extend the weights back and out (without moving the upper part of the arm) through a count of 10 seconds. Hold and squeeze for 2 seconds at the MTP. Return the weights to starting position through a count of 10 seconds. Without resting, repeat three times. Rest for 30 seconds and then repeat the entire sequence.

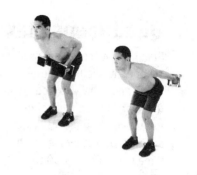

Reverse Crunch

Lie on a mat with your hands by your sides, palms down. Pull your heels up as close to your butt as possible. Raise your heels about 2 inches off the ground. Keep your chin tucked and abs tight. Feather your breathing as you pull your knees toward your chest, using your lower abdominals, through a count of 10 seconds. Hold and squeeze for 2 seconds at the MTP (when your butt is completely off the ground). Lower your body to starting position through a count of 10 seconds. Without resting, repeat three times.

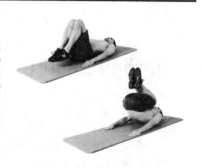

Swiss Ball Ab Roll

Kneel on a mat in front of a ball and cross your ankles behind you. Close both hands into fists and place on the ball, keeping your elbows straight but not locked. Keep your head up, back straight, and abs tight. Feather your breathing as you roll forward on the ball through a count of 10 seconds. Hold for 2 seconds at the MTP. Return to starting position through a count of 10 seconds. Without resting, repeat three times.

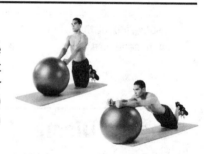

Russian Twist on Swiss Ball

Sit on the ball with your knees bent, feet about hip-width apart for balance. Keep your chin up and abs tight as you lean back slightly, engaging your abs. While holding a medicine ball, extend your arms away from your chest and turn to one side to begin exercise. Feather your breathing as you slowly rotate your torso as far as possible to the other side through a count of 10 seconds. Hold and squeeze for 2 seconds at the MTP. Rotate back to the other side through a count of 10 seconds. Without resting, repeat three times.

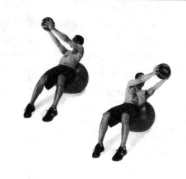

WEEK 7

As you gear up to start your week, use these tips based on your Life Priority to create extra inner drive and motivation. They are customized to your age category, but I recommend you read every one of them. You'll find valuable information in each tip, no matter what your age.

20 to 35 PRIME TIME

Cologne

You can have a ripped body, wear nice clothes, and say all the right things, but none of that will make someone want to get as close to you as the right cologne will. Ultimately it's your *pheromones*—odorless chemical substances your body releases—that create chemistry, but the right scent could help draw someone in. Studies have revealed that certain scents can be sexually arousing. Women respond to the scents of licorice and cucumber. Men are aroused by the scents of lavender, pumpkin pie, and cinnamon. You don't have to start carrying candy or spices in your pockets, but be sure to get cologne that doesn't scare anyone off! Since different scents can react differently with each person's skin, try some free samples first. Collect a few on the tabs handed out in stores and find some you like. Then ask for samples of your favorites. Try them out at home and even take them for a test run to a club. Of course, if you have a significant other, get that person's opinion first! Three popular fragrances for guys: Acqua Di Gio by Giorgio Armani®, John Varvatos Cologne, and Fierce by Abercrombie & Fitch®.

35 to 50 STAY YOUNG

Break Bad Habits Now

If you are a smoker, chances are you don't need me to tell you smoking is bad for you. So instead let me tell you it's *terrible* for you. But there's good news: Quitting today can benefit you in only a matter of hours. Twelve hours after you quit smoking, your carbon dioxide level adjusts to normal. And in just two weeks, your circulation improves along with your lung function. Getting your workouts in will help you stick to quitting. One study done in Austria determined that 80 percent of people who exercised while trying to stop smoking were able to stay committed to quitting. Even if you're not a smoker, I bet you've carried over some bad habits into your late thirties and forties. But let me tell you, the longer you hang on to bad habits, the harder they are to give up. Use your free day to have a few drinks if that's your guilty pleasure, but I suggest keeping your alcohol consumption to a minimum the rest of the week. Alcohol not only makes it tougher to get your six-pack abs but also can do some damage to vital organs, such as your liver, increase triglyceride levels, and cause hypoglycemia. If you're going to have a drink, aim for a glass of red wine, because of its antioxidant properties, but be sure to add cardio to your routine to balance out the extra calories.

50-Plus LONGEVITY

Give Wheatgrass a Shot

You've probably sworn off tequila shots at this point in your life, but there's one shot you should actually *start* taking: wheatgrass. Wheatgrass is full of good stuff, including vitamin A, vitamin B, and vitamins C and E. But the most important benefits come from what makes it green—chlorophyll. This pigment has a molecular structure similar to that of our own blood cells, which is why it's considered a blood builder. It's also known to be effective at detoxifying the blood and helping cleanse vital organs, such as your liver and intestines. Research has suggested that wheatgrass also could be beneficial in the prevention of cancer. With its antibiotic properties, it helps fight bacteria and toxins that pollute the body, and it helps promote the growth of new, healthy cells. One other surprising advantage: It can help neutralize odors. Toxins in our body are what cause odor, and drinking cleansing shots of wheatgrass can help eliminate the some of these smells, such as body odor. It's even worked on balancing out not-so-fresh breath from drinking coffee or alcohol or eating potent foods like garlic. You can buy 2- or 4-ounce "shots" of wheatgrass at Jamba Juice stores and grocery stores such as Whole Foods.

MONDAY

Push-Up on Swiss Ball (Easy)

Begin with the ball about 3 feet in front of you; then place your hands on the ball about a foot apart, fingers pointing forward. Balance on your knees and cross your ankles and extend your arms. Slowly lower yourself toward the ball through a count of 10 seconds. Hold and squeeze for 2 seconds at the MTP (about 2 inches from the ball). Return to starting position through a count of 10 seconds. Without resting, repeat three times. Rest for 30 seconds and then repeat the entire sequence.

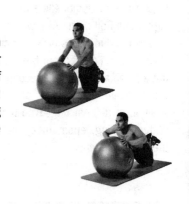

Flat Barbell Press

Hold the barbell and lie on the ball so that it comfortably supports your shoulder blades. Extend your arms in front of you, pressing the weight up. Feather your breathing as you lower the weight through a count of 10 seconds. Hold for 2 seconds at MTP (about 1 inch above your chest). Press the barbell back to starting position through a count of 10 seconds. Without resting, repeat three times. Rest for 30 seconds and then repeat the entire sequence.

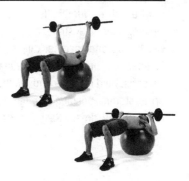

Incline Unilateral Dumbbell Press

Grasp a dumbbell in one hand and lie on the ball so that your head and neck are supported. Allow your hips to drop almost to the ground. Press the weight up with one hand, keeping your free hand on your hip. Feather your breathing as you slowly lower the weight toward your chest through a count of 10 seconds. Hold and squeeze for 2 seconds at the MTP (about 2 inches above your chest). Return to starting position through a count of 10 seconds. Without resting, repeat once more on this side and then switch sides and complete 2 more reps for a total of 4. Rest for 30 seconds and then repeat the entire sequence.

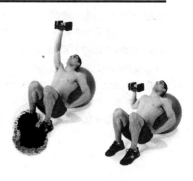

Incline Dumbbell Fly

Hold a pair of dumbbells and lie on the ball with your head and neck supported. Roll down the ball until your hips drop almost to the ground. Extend the dumbbells over your chest, palms facing each other, elbows slightly bent. Feather your breathing as you lower the weights down and out through a count of 10 seconds. Hold for 2 seconds at the MTP (when your arms are open in a "T" position). Raise the weights back to starting position in a "bear hug" type motion through a count of 10 seconds. Without resting, repeat three times. Rest for 30 seconds and then repeat the entire sequence.

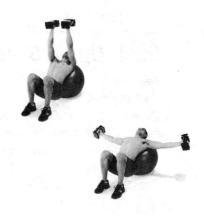

Standing Shoulder Press

Hold a pair of dumbbells and take a wide step forward with one foot, keeping your back straight, abs tight, and knees slightly bent. Extend the weights up and together directly over your head, palms facing forward. Feather your breathing as you lower the weights through a count of 10 seconds. Hold for 2 seconds at the MTP (chin level). Press the dumbbells up to starting position through a count of 10 seconds. Without resting, repeat three times. Rest for 30 seconds and then repeat the entire sequence.

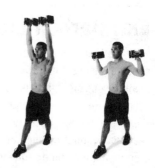

Chicken Wing

Hold a pair of dumbbells and stand with feet hip-width apart and knees slightly bent. Bend your elbows, holding the dumbbells in front of you at a 45-degree angle. Keep your forearms tight and feather your breathing as you raise your elbows up and out through a count of 10 seconds. Hold and squeeze for 2 seconds at the MTP. Return to starting position through a count of 10 seconds. Without resting, repeat three times. (Note: Be sure to relax yo   ck and avoid shrugging the shoulders.)

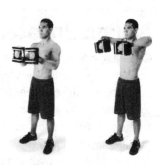

Front Delt Raise

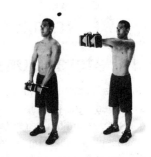

Hold a pair of dumbbells and stand up straight with your chest up and abs tight. Feather your breathing as you raise the dumbbells up with slightly bent elbows for a count of 10 seconds. Hold for 2 seconds at the MTP (about eye level). Lower the weights to starting position through a count of 10 seconds. Without resting, repeat three times. Rest for 30 seconds and then repeat the entire sequence.

Seated V-Up

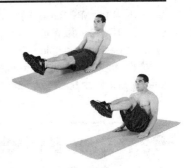

Sit on the ground with your arms slightly behind you, elbows bent, and fingertips pointed forward. Start with your knees together, legs extended, and heels off the ground about 2 inches. Support your upper body weight with your palms. Feather your breathing as you pull your knees into your chest for a count of 10 seconds. Hold and squeeze for 2 seconds at the MTP. Return to starting position through a count of 10 seconds, keeping your abs tight. Without resting, repeat three times.

Swiss Ball Crunch with Elevated Feet

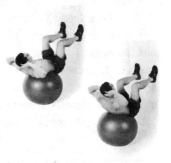

Sit on the ball about 2 feet away from a wall, arms crossed. Walk your feet out and place them against the wall. Feather your breathing as you crunch up through a count of 10 seconds, using only your abs. Hold and squeeze for 2 seconds at the MTP. Return to starting position through a count of 10 seconds. Without resting, repeat three times. (Note: The range of motion is significantly shorter on this exercise so be sure to adjust your pace.)

Bicycle Crunch

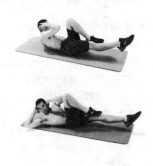

Lie flat on your back. Place your hands behind your head and raise your heels about 2 inches from the ground, keeping your chin up and abs tight throughout the exercise. Bring your right elbow to your left knee and feather your breathing as you rotate to the other side for a count of 10 seconds. Hold and squeeze for 2 seconds at the MTP (where your left elbow meets your right knee). Return to starting position through a count of 10 seconds. Without resting, repeat three times.

WEDNESDAY

Unilateral Dumbbell Pull-Over

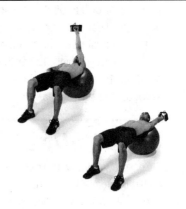

Grasp a dumbbell and lie on the ball with your head and neck supported. Keep your hips up and abs tight throughout the exercise. With one arm, extend the weight over your chest, keeping a slight bend in the elbows; place other arm on your hip. Feather your breathing as you lower the weight behind your head through a count of 10 seconds. Hold for 2 seconds at the MTP. Raise the weight back to starting position through a count of 10 seconds. Without resting, repeat once more on this side then switch sides and complete 2 more reps for a total of 4. Rest for 30 seconds and then repeat the entire sequence. (Note: How far you can stretch your arms back will determine your MTP.)

Bent-Over Barbell Row (Overhand Grip)

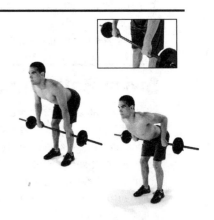

Hold the barbell with your arms extended, using the overhand grip. Stand with your feet hip-width apart. Bend at the waist as if you were about to tie your shoes; then lift only your chin and chest, creating a slight arch in your back. Keeping a bend in your knees, feather your breathing as you pull the weight up toward your hips in a fluid rowing motion through a count of 10 seconds. Hold and squeeze your shoulder blades together for 2 seconds at the MTP. Lower your arms to starting position through a count of 10 seconds. Without resting, repeat three times. Rest for 30 seconds and then repeat the entire sequence.

Bent-Over Dumbbell Row (Standard Grip)

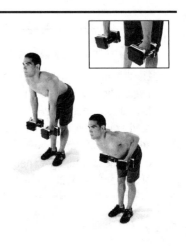

Hold a pair of dumbbells, arms extended, palms facing each other. Stand with your feet hip-width apart. Bend at the waist as if you were about to tie your shoes; then lift only your chin and chest, creating a slight arch in your back. Bend your knees slightly. Feather your breathing as you pull the dumbbells up in a fluid rowing motion through a count of 10 seconds, keeping your elbows close to your body. Hold and squeeze your shoulder blades together for 2 seconds at the MTP. Lower your arms to starting position through a count of 10 seconds. Without resting, repeat three times. Rest for 30 seconds and then repeat the entire sequence. (Note: Keep your elbows close to your body throughout the exercise.)

Barbell Dead Lift

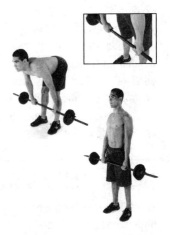

Grip the barbell with one palm facing forward, one palm facing back, and your feet about 6 to 8 inches apart. Bend over at the waist as if you were about to tie your shoes, knees slightly bent. Lift your chin and chest, creating a slight arch in your back. Feather your breathing as you lift your upper body through a count of 10 seconds, driving through your heels and using your lower back and hamstrings. Hold for 2 seconds at the MTP (at the top of the movement). Return to starting position through a count of 10 seconds. Without resting, repeat three times. Rest for 30 seconds and then repeat the entire sequence.

Standing Dumbbell Curl

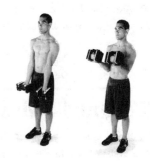

Hold a pair of dumbbells, palms facing out. Stand with your feet shoulder-width apart and your arms extended by your sides, knees slightly bent. Feather your breathing as you curl the dumbbells up through a count of 10 seconds. Hold and squeeze for 2 seconds at the MTP. Keep your elbows tight against your body as you lower the weights for 10 seconds to starting position. Without resting, repeat three times. Rest for 30 seconds and then repeat the entire sequence. (Note: Keep your elbows tight against your sides throughout the exercise.)

Barbell Preacher Curl

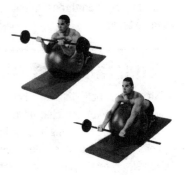

Hold the barbell and rest over the ball with your knees on the floor and a 6- to 8-inch gap between your arms. Lift your arms to starting position with your elbows bent at about a 90-degree angle. Feather your breathing as you lower the weight through a count of 10 seconds. Hold for 2 seconds at the MTP. Lift the barbell to starting position through a count of 10 seconds. Without resting, repeat three times. Rest for 30 seconds and then repeat the entire sequence.

Hammer Curl

Holding a pair of dumbbells, stand with your feet shoulder-width apart, your arms extended slightly in front of your thighs, palms facing each other, and knees slightly bent. Feather your breathing as you curl the weights up through a count of 10 seconds, keeping your palms facing each other. Hold and squeeze for 2 seconds at the MTP. Lower the weights to starting position through a count of 10 seconds. Without resting, repeat three times. Rest for 30 seconds and then repeat the entire sequence.

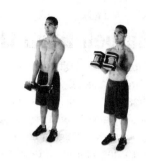

Swiss Ball Ab Roll

Kneel on a mat in front of a ball and cross your ankles behind you. Close both hands into fists and place on the ball, keeping your elbows straight but not locked. Keep your head up, back straight, and abs tight. Feather your breathing as you roll forward on the ball through a count of 10 seconds. Hold for 2 seconds at the MTP. Return to starting position through a count of 10 seconds. Without resting, repeat three times.

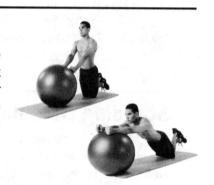

Weighted Swiss Ball Crunch

Sit on the ball with your feet on the floor and hold a medicine ball under your chin. Walk your feet out until your hips are slightly lower than your knees but your lower back is still firmly supported. Feather your breathing and, using only your abs, slowly crunch up through a count of 10 seconds. Hold and squeeze for 2 seconds at the MTP. Lower yourself to starting position through a count of 10 seconds. Without resting, repeat three times.

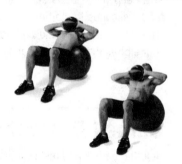

Russian Twist on Swiss Ball

Sit on the ball with your knees bent, feet about hip-width apart for balance. Keep your chin up and abs tight as you lean back, engaging your abs. While holding a medicine ball, extend your arms away from your chest and turn to one side to begin exercise. Feather your breathing as you slowly rotate your torso as far as possible to the other side through a count of 10 seconds. Hold and squeeze for 2 seconds at the MTP. Rotate back to the other side through a count of 10 seconds. Without resting, repeat three times.

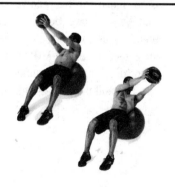

FRIDAY

Barbell Squat

Stand with your feet hip-width apart and hold a weighted barbell across your shoulders. Keep your back straight, abs tight, and head up. Feather your breathing as you squat through a count of 10 seconds. Hold for 2 seconds at the MTP. Push through your heels as you stand and return to starting position through a count of 10 seconds. Without resting, repeat three times. Rest for 30 seconds and then repeat the entire sequence.

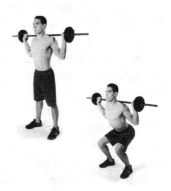

Swiss Ball Squat

Place the ball against a wall and position yourself with the ball supporting your middle to upper back. Hold a pair of dumbbells with your arms against your sides. Move your feet forward about 1 foot, keeping them about hip-width apart. Feather your breathing as you slowly squat down through a count of 10 seconds. Hold for 2 seconds at the MTP (when your knees are at a 90-degree angle). Return to starting position through a count of 10 seconds. Without resting, repeat three times. Rest for 30 seconds and then repeat the entire sequence.

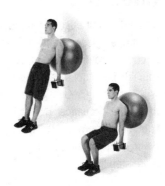

Barbell Sumo Squat

Rest the barbell across your back and stand with your feet about two times wider than shoulder-width apart, toes turned out to the sides, and knees aligned over the toes. Feather your breathing as you squat through a count of 10 seconds. Hold for 2 seconds at the MTP. Push through your heels to return to starting position through a count of 10 seconds. Without resting, repeat three times. Rest for 30 seconds and then repeat the entire sequence.

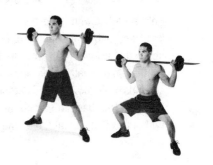

Split Squat with Swiss Ball

Grip an empty barbell, placing it across the back of your shoulders. Stand about 3 feet in front of a ball; then place the top of one foot on the ball for balance. With your back straight, chest up, and abs tight, feather your breathing as you bend your front knee, lowering yourself toward the ground through a count of 10 seconds. Keep your front knee from extending beyond your toe. Hold for 2 seconds at the MTP (when there is about a 90-degree bend in the front knee). Return to starting position through a count of 10 seconds. Repeat once more and then switch sides and complete 2 more reps for a total of 4. Rest for 30 seconds and then repeat the entire sequence. (Note: To avoid injury, make sure that your front knee stays aligned with your toes and doesn't bend farther than a 90-degree angle.)

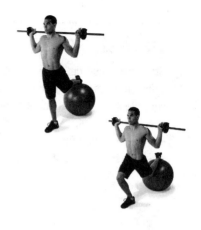

Chair Dip

Sit on the front edge of a sturdy chair, hands close to your sides, fingers forward, and legs extended. Feather your breathing as you lower yourself through a count of 10 seconds. Hold for 2 seconds at the MTP. Push yourself back up to starting position through a count of 10 seconds. Without resting, repeat three times. Rest for 30 seconds and then repeat the entire sequence. (Note: The MTP will depend on how flexible your shoulders are. Your MTP will be about 1 inch above your most flexible point. If this exercise is too difficult, move your feet closer to your body for more stability.)

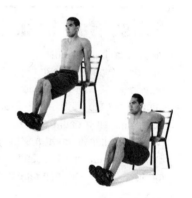

Close-Grip Barbell Press

Hold a barbell with a close grip, and lean back onto a ball so that your head and neck are supported. Elevate your hips slightly and keep your abs tight. Extend your arms in front of you, pressing the weight up. Feather your breathing as you lower the barbell through a count of 10 seconds. Hold for 2 seconds at the MTP (about 1 inch above your chest). Press the bar back to starting position through a count of 10 seconds. Without resting, repeat three times. Rest for 30 seconds and then repeat the entire sequence.

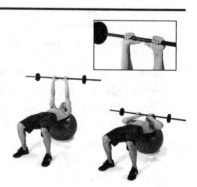

Barbell Skull Crusher

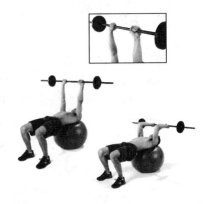

Hold a barbell and lie on the ball so that your head and neck are supported. Elevate your hips slightly and keep your abs tight. Extend the barbell straight up with your palms facing out. Drop your arms back toward your head slightly. Feather your breathing as you bend your elbows and lower the weight through a count of 10 seconds. Hold for 2 seconds at the MTP (a few inches above your forehead). Raise the barbell to starting position through a count of 10 seconds. Without resting, repeat three times. Rest for 30 seconds and then repeat the entire sequence.

Medicine Ball Pull-Over

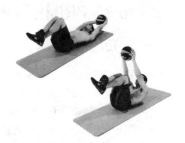

Lie on a mat and bring your knees up to a 90-degree angle. Grasp a medicine ball and extend it over your head, keeping a slight bend in your elbows. Keep your abs tight and feather your breathing as you raise the ball over your head and crunch up through a count of 10 seconds. Hold for 2 seconds at the MTP. Lower the ball to starting position through a count of 10 seconds. Without resting, repeat three times.

Jackknife

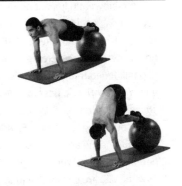

Stand about 3 feet in front of the ball and place your palms on the ground, hands shoulder-width apart. Put one foot on the ball about mid-shin level. Once you are stabilized, place the other foot on the ball, keeping your head forward, spine straight, and abs tight. Slowly pull your knees up to your chin through a count of 10 seconds as you concentrate on maintaining stability by squeezing your abs tight. Hold and squeeze for 2 seconds at the MTP. Return to starting position through a count of 10 seconds. Without resting, repeat three times.

Lying Oblique Twist

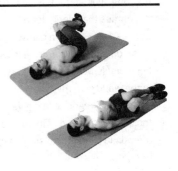

Lie on your back with your arms outstretched, palms facing down. Raise your knees up to a 90-degree angle and drop your knees down to one side. Feather your breathing as you rotate your knees to the other side through a count of 10 seconds. Hold and squeeze for 2 seconds at the MTP (when your knees are a few inches from the ground). Rotate to the other side through a count of 10 seconds. Without resting, repeat three times.

WEEK 8

As you gear up to start your week, use these tips based on your Life Priority to create extra inner drive and motivation. They are customized to your age category, but I recommend you read every one of them. You'll find valuable information in each tip, no matter what your age.

20 to 35 PRIME TIME

Pep Talk

Give yourself a pep talk. Coaches do this all the time to get teams fired up to face opponents or to make a comeback. Why shouldn't you do it to get pumped for a big meeting, a workout, or a date—or even just to face the day? The things you say to yourself greatly impact how you feel. If you keep saying to yourself, "I'm so nervous," you really will *be* nervous. Instead, think about how you want to feel, and create a power mantra or pep talk for yourself. Use words like *strong, powerful, confident, unstoppable, focused, successful, fired up, bold, fearless*—the list could go on, but you get the idea. Pick words that trigger your adrenaline and make you feel ready to handle anything. When you get up in the morning or when you are getting ready to go out or into a meeting, look at yourself in the mirror and repeat the phrase that works for you: "I'm unstoppable and fearless." "I am in control." "I am going to win." "I can do this." Customize a mantra for yourself. Positive "self-talk" really works. The best athletes in the world give themselves pep talks to get emotionally ready for a big game—and you can too. If you still need help finding motivation, I offer daily coaching to stay on track at BodyatHome.com.

35 to 50 STAY YOUNG

Stay Social

Hanging out with your buddies on a Friday night isn't just fun. It can add years to your life. Studies have shown that maintaining healthy friendships and relationships can lower your blood pressure, make you feel relaxed, and even let you live longer. Isolation can not only get a little boring but can lead to depression and anxiety as you get older. Whether you're single, married, or in a relationship, maintaining an active social life is important. A healthy relationship with another person allows time for you to miss someone. Heading to a ball game or to the beach with your friends but without your significant other can make you want to rush back home and make your significant other eager for your return. If you're single, get your friends to try activities with you that will help you meet more than just a casual fling. Don't be afraid to get creative. Try a cooking class. Even if barbecue is the only thing you're into, brush up on your grilling techniques while you strike up casual conversations. Or check out a different gym for a yoga class. You'll de-stress and perhaps bump into your next date.

50-Plus LONGEVITY

Add Antioxidants

You've probably heard plenty about antioxidants, but how much do you really know about them? Since they're so important to maintaining good health, a basic understanding of what they do is worth having. There's a process that occurs in our bodies called *oxidation*. It happens when we do just about everything—when we eat, breathe, go outside, exercise, and so on. It's a completely natural process. When oxidation occurs, chemical by-products called *free radicals* are released. Think of free radicals as incomplete particles that roam your body looking to beat up healthy cells so they can steal an electron from them and become complete. Free radicals can lead to deterioration of joints and bones, the breakdown of your organs, visible signs of aging, and even cancer. The key to combating these nasty bullies? Consuming enough antioxidants to slow or prevent oxidation. Try to eat vegetables and fruits in an array of colors to help ensure you get enough antioxidants. Get beta-carotene from orange foods such as mangoes, carrots, and cantaloupe; lutein from green, leafy vegetables such as kale and spinach; and lycopene from pink and red foods such as tomatoes, watermelon, apricots, and pink grapefruit.

Incline Barbell Press

Hold the barbell with your palms facing out and lie on the ball so that your head and neck are supported. Allow your hips to drop almost to the ground. Press the weight up over your nose, keeping a slight bend in the elbows so that the upper chest is targeted. Feather your breathing as you lower the weight through a count of 10 seconds. Hold for 2 seconds at the MTP (when the barbell is only a couple of inches from your chest). Press the bar up to starting position through a count of 10 seconds. Without resting, repeat three times. Rest for 30 seconds and then repeat the entire sequence.

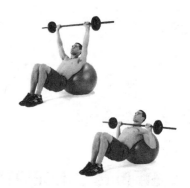

Unilateral Flat Dumbbell Press

Grasp a dumbbell in one hand and lie on the ball so that your head and neck are supported, keeping your hips and abs tight. Press the weight up with one hand, keeping your free hand on your hip. Feather your breathing as you slowly lower the weight toward your chest through a count of 10 seconds. Hold and squeeze for 2 seconds at the MTP (about 2 inches above your chest). Return to starting position through a count of 10 seconds. Without resting, repeat once more on this side and then switch hands and complete 2 more reps for a total of 4. Rest for 30 seconds and then repeat the entire sequence.

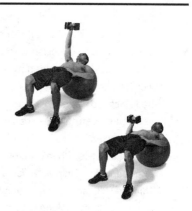

Flat Barbell Press

Hold the barbell and lie on the ball so that it comfortably supports your shoulder blades. Extend your arms in front of you, pressing the weight up. Feather your breathing as you lower the weight through a count of 10 seconds. Hold for 2 seconds at the MTP (about 1 inch above your chest). Press the barbell back to starting through a count of 10 seconds. Without resting, repeat three times. Rest for 30 seconds and then repeat the entire sequence.

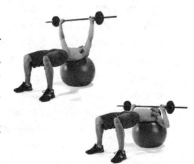

Push-Up on Swiss Ball (Difficult)

Begin with the ball in front of you about 3 feet, and place your hands on the ball about a foot apart, fingers pointing forward. Extend your arms and get your balance. Slowly lower yourself toward the ball through a count of 10 seconds. Hold and squeeze for 2 seconds at the MTP (about 2 inches from the ball). Return to starting position through a count of 10 seconds. Without resting, repeat three times. Rest for 30 seconds and then repeat the entire sequence.

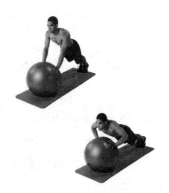

Standing Barbell Military Press

Hold the barbell and stand with your feet slightly apart, knees slightly bent, back straight, abs tight, and chin up. Extend the barbell up and directly over your head, palms facing forward. Feather your breathing as you lower the weight through a count of 10 seconds. Hold for two seconds at the MTP (chin level). Press the barbell up to starting position through a count of 10 seconds. Without resting, repeat three times. Rest for 30 seconds and then repeat the entire sequence.

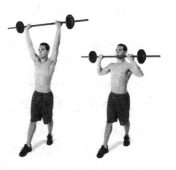

Standing Lateral Raise

Hold a pair of dumbbells and stand with your feet together, back straight, and abs tight. With your arms against your sides and elbows slightly bent, feather your breathing as you raise the weights up through a count of 10 seconds. Hold and squeeze for 2 seconds at the MTP ("T" position). Lower the weights to starting position through a count of 10 seconds. Without resting, repeat three times. Rest for 30 seconds and then repeat the entire sequence.

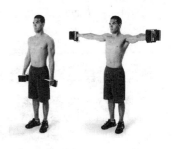

Bent-Over Rear Delt Raise

Hold a pair of dumbbells, palms facing each other. Bend at the waist as if you were about to tie your shoes; then lift only your chin and chest, creating a slight arch in your back. Feather your breathing as you raise the weights to your sides through a count of 10 seconds. Hold and squeeze for 2 seconds at the MTP. Lower the weights to starting position through a count of 10 seconds. Without resting, repeat three times. Rest for 30 seconds and then repeat the entire sequence.

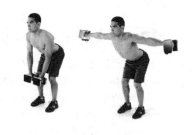

Double Crunch

Lie on a mat and place your hands behind your head, elbows up, chin up, and abs tight. Pull your heels toward your butt as far as you can. Using your upper abs, feather your breathing as you crunch up while simultaneously pulling your knees in through a count of 10 seconds. Hold and squeeze for 2 seconds at the MTP. Return to starting position through a count of 10 seconds, never letting your upper back touch the ground. Without resting, repeat three times. (Note: The range of motion on this exercise is very short so be sure to adjust your speed so that you hit the MTP on the count of 10.)

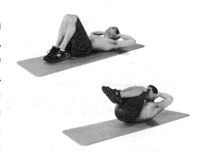

Reaching Crunch

Sit on the ball with your feet on the floor. Walk your feet out until your hips are slightly lower than your knees but your lower back is still firmly supported. Grasp a medicine ball and extend your arms toward the ceiling. Feather your breathing and, using your abs only, slowly crunch up through a count of 10 seconds, keeping the ball pointed toward the ceiling. Hold and squeeze for 2 seconds at the MTP. Lower yourself back to starting position through a count of 10 seconds. Without resting, repeat three times.

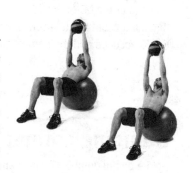

Bicycle Crunch

Lie flat on your back. Place your hands behind your head and raise your heels about 2 inches from the ground, keeping your chin up and abs tight throughout the exercise. Bring your right elbow to your left knee and feather your breathing as you rotate to the other side for a count of 10 seconds. Hold and squeeze for 2 seconds at the MTP (where your left elbow meets your right knee). Return to starting position through a count of 10 seconds. Without resting, repeat three times.

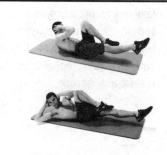

WEDNESDAY

Unilateral Dumbbell Pull-Over

Grasp a dumbbell and lie on the ball with your head and neck supported. Keep your hips up and abs tight throughout the exercise. With one arm, extend the weight over your chest, keeping a slight bend in the elbows; place other arm on your hip. Feather your breathing as you lower the weight behind your head through a count of 10 seconds. Hold for 2 seconds at the MTP. Raise the weight back to starting position through a count of 10 seconds. Without resting, repeat once more on this side and then switch arms and complete 2 more reps for a total of 4. Rest for 30 seconds and then repeat the entire sequence. (Note: How far you can stretch your arms back will determine your MTP.)

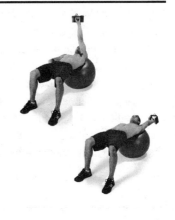

Swiss Ball Row

Hold a pair of dumbbells and lie on the ball so that it is at the middle of your waist. Extend your arms in front of you and raise your head and chest, creating a slight arch in the back. Feather your breathing as you pull the dumbbells up and back toward your hips in a rowing motion through a count of 10 seconds. Hold and squeeze the shoulder blades together at the MTP for 2 seconds. Return to starting position through a count of 10 seconds. Without resting, repeat three times. Rest for 30 seconds and then repeat the entire sequence.

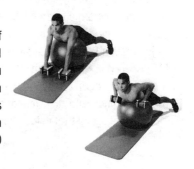

Bent-Over Dumbbell Row (Underhand Grip)

Hold a pair of dumbbells, using the underhand grip, arms extended. Stand with your feet hip-width apart. Bend at the waist as if tying your shoes. Raise your head and chest to create a slight arch in the back. Bend your knees slightly. Feather your breathing as you pull the dumbbells up in a fluid rowing motion through a count of 10 seconds, keeping your elbows close to your body. Hold and squeeze your shoulder blades together for 2 seconds at the MTP. Lower your arms to starting position through a count of 10 seconds. Without resting, repeat three times. Rest for 30 seconds and then repeat the entire sequence.

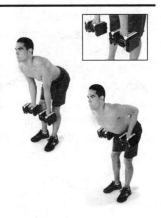

Barbell Dead Lift

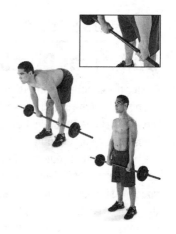

Grip the barbell with one palm facing forward, one palm facing back, and your feet about 6 to 8 inches apart. Bend over at the waist as if you were about to tie your shoes, knees slightly bent. Lift your chin and chest, creating a slight arch in your back. Feather your breathing as you lift your upper body through a count of 10 seconds, driving through your heels and using your lower back and hamstrings. Hold for 2 seconds at the MTP (at the top of the movement). Return to starting position through a count of 10 seconds. Without resting, repeat three times. Rest for 30 seconds and then repeat the entire sequence.

Standing Barbell Curl (Close Grip)

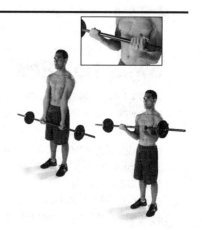

Hold the barbell using the close grip. Stand with your feet shoulder-width apart and your arms extended by your sides, knees slightly bent. Feather your breathing as you curl the barbell up through a count of 10 seconds to just past a 90-degree angle. Hold and squeeze for 2 seconds at the MTP. Keep your elbows tight against your body as you lower the weight through a count of 10 seconds. Without resting, repeat three times. Rest for 30 seconds and then repeat the entire sequence. (Note: Keep the elbows tight against your sides throughout the exercise.)

Standing Side Curl

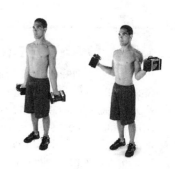

Hold a pair of dumbbells with your palms turned out, elbows to your side. Keep your chest up, feet hip-width apart, knees slightly bent, and abs tight throughout the exercise. Feather your breathing as you curl the weights up through a count of 10 seconds. Hold and squeeze for 2 seconds at the MTP. Lower the weights to starting position through a count of 10 seconds until your arms are completely straight (do not lock your elbows). Without resting, repeat three times. Rest for 30 seconds and then repeat the entire sequence.

Dumbbell Preacher Curl

Hold a pair of dumbbells and rest over the ball with your knees on the floor and a 6- to 8-inch gap between your arms. Lift your arms to starting position, with your elbows bent at about a 90-degree angle. Feather your breathing as you lower the weights through a count of 10 seconds. Hold for 2 seconds at the MTP. Lift the dumbbells to starting position through a count of 10 seconds. Without resting, repeat three times. Rest for 30 seconds and then repeat the entire sequence.

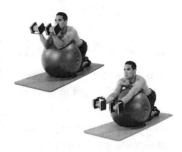

Jackknife

Stand about 3 feet in front of the ball and place your palms on the ground, hands shoulder-width apart. Put one foot on the ball about mid-shin level. Once you are stabilized, place the other foot on the ball, keeping your head forward, spine straight, and abs tight. Slowly pull your knees up to your chin through a count of 10 seconds as you concentrate on maintaining stability by squeezing your abs tight. Hold and squeeze for 2 seconds at the MTP. Return to starting position through a count of 10 seconds. Without resting, repeat three times.

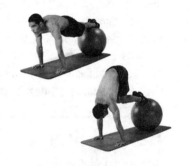

Medicine Ball Pull-Over

Lie on a mat and bring your knees up to a 90-degree angle. Grasp a medicine ball and extend it over your head, keeping a slight bend in your elbows. Keep your abs tight and feather your breathing as you raise the ball over your head and crunch up through a count of 10 seconds. Hold for 2 seconds at the MTP. Lower the ball to starting position through a count of 10 seconds. Without resting, repeat three times.

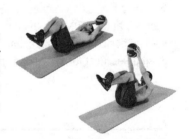

Russian Twist on Swiss Ball

Sit on the ball with your knees bent, feet about hip-width apart for balance. Keep your chin up and abs tight as you lean back, engaging your abs. While holding a medicine ball, extend your arms away from your chest and turn to one side to begin exercise. Feather your breathing as you slowly rotate your torso as far as possible to the other side through a count of 10 seconds. Hold and squeeze for 2 seconds at the MTP. Rotate back to the other side through a count of 10 seconds. Without resting, repeat three times.

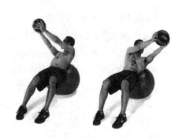

FRIDAY

Split Squat with Swiss Ball

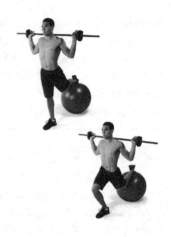

Grip an empty barbell, placing it across the back of your shoulders. Stand about 3 feet in front of a ball; then place the top of one foot on the ball for balance. With your back straight, chest up, and abs tight, feather your breathing as you bend your front knee, lowering yourself toward the ground through a count of 10 seconds. Keep your front knee from extending beyond your toe. Hold for 2 seconds at the MTP (when there is about a 90-degree bend in the front knee). Return to starting position through a count of 10 seconds. Repeat once more and then switch sides and perform 2 more reps for a total of 4. Rest for 30 seconds and then repeat the entire sequence. (Note: To avoid injury, make sure that your front knee stays aligned with your toes and doesn't bend farther than a 90-degree angle.)

Barbell Squat

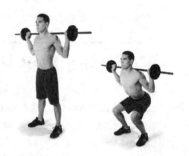

Stand with your feet hip-width apart and hold a weighted barbell across your shoulders. Keep your back straight, abs tight, and head up. Feather your breathing as you squat through a count of 10 seconds. Hold for 2 seconds at the MTP. Push through your heels as you stand and return to starting position through a count of 10 seconds. Without resting, repeat three times. Rest for 30 seconds and then repeat the entire sequence.

Barbell Lunge

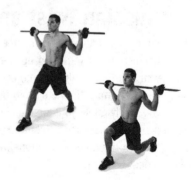

Hold a barbell across your back and stand in a lunge position. Keep your back straight, chest up, and abs tight. Feather your breathing as you drop your back knee toward the ground through a count of 10 seconds. Hold for 2 seconds at the MTP (about 1 inch above the ground). Return to starting position through a count of 10 seconds. Without resting, repeat one more time on this leg and then perform 2 more reps on the other side for a total of 4. Rest for 30 seconds and then repeat the entire sequence. (Note: To avoid injury, make sure that your front knee stays aligned with your toes and doesn't bend farther than a 90-degree angle.)

Swiss Ball Hamstring Curl

Lie on your back with your arms at your sides, palms flat on the floor. Place your heels on the ball, knees straight but not completely locked; then lift your butt and hips off the ground. With your abs tight, feather your breathing and bend your knees as you roll the ball toward your butt with your heels. Hold for 2 seconds at the MTP. Return to starting position through a count of 10 seconds. Without resting, repeat three times. Rest for 30 seconds and then repeat the entire sequence.

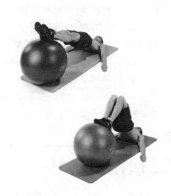

Barbell Skull Crusher

Hold a barbell and lie on the ball so that your head and neck are supported. Elevate your hips slightly and keep your abs tight. Extend the barbell straight up with your palms facing out. Drop your arms back toward your head slightly. Feather your breathing as you bend your elbows and lower the weight through a count of 10 seconds. Hold for 2 seconds at the MTP (a few inches above your forehead). Raise the barbell to starting position through a count of 10 seconds. Without resting, repeat three times. Rest for 30 seconds and then repeat the entire sequence.

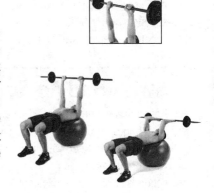

Overhead Barbell Triceps Extension

Grasp the barbell, palms facing out. Sit on a ball with your chest up, back straight, feet together. Extend your arms with your elbows slightly bent, keeping your biceps close to your head. Feather your breathing as you drop the bar back through a count of 10 seconds. Hold for 2 seconds at the MTP (when your elbows are at about a 90-degree angle). Press the bar up to starting position through a count of 10 seconds. Without resting, repeat three times. Rest for 30 seconds and then repeat the entire sequence.

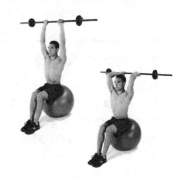

Diamond Push-Up

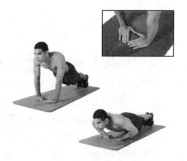

Lie on a mat with your hands in the "diamond" position. Press up to starting position, keeping your back straight, abs tight, and head up. Feather your breathing as you lower your body through a count of 10 seconds, allowing your elbows to move outward. Hold for 2 seconds at the MTP (about 2 inches above the ground). Push your body back to starting position through a count of 10 seconds. Without resting, repeat three times. Rest for 30 seconds and then repeat the entire sequence.

Seated V-Up

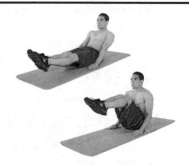

Sit on the ground with your arms slightly behind you, elbows bent, and fingertips pointed forward. Start with your knees together, legs extended, and heels off the ground about 2 inches. Support your upper body weight with your palms. Feather your breathing as you pull your knees into your chest for a count of 10 seconds. Hold and squeeze for 2 seconds at the MTP. Return to starting position through a count of 10 seconds, keeping your abs tight. Without resting, repeat three times.

Swiss Ball Ab Roll

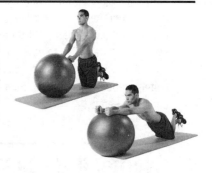

Kneel on a mat in front of a ball and cross your ankles behind you. Close both hands into fists and place on the ball, keeping your elbows straight but not locked. Keep your head up, back straight, and abs tight. Feather your breathing as you roll forward on the ball through a count of 10 seconds. Hold for 2 seconds at the MTP. Return to starting position through a count of 10 seconds. Without resting, repeat three times.

Barbell Twist

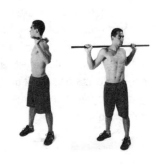

Grip an empty barbell, placing it across the back of your shoulders. Stand with your legs about 3 feet apart. Twist your upper body to one side. With your chin up and abs squeezed tight, feather your breathing as you slowly twist to the other side through a count of 10 seconds. At the MTP of your twist, hold and squeeze for 2 seconds. Return to starting position through a count of 10 seconds. Without resting, repeat three times. (Note: If you can do more than 4 reps, you're not squeezing your abs hard enough throughout the exercise.)

Gut-Free for Life

"This program has helped me put my life back on track! I highly recommend Body at Home™ to anyone looking to get back in shape and look their best long term."

—RIK BARAN, BODY AT HOME™ STAR, LOST 7 POUNDS

Congratulations on a phenomenal eight weeks! Go ahead and pat yourself on the back—in fact, maybe even flex your muscles in the mirror and say, "I did this." Making the commitment to your body and losing your gut is no small achievement. Be proud of yourself.

Now that you've created a body you can really be proud of, you want to know how to make those results last. The most important thing is for you to view this as your new life—there's no looking back. Body at Home™ is a *lifestyle* change, which means it's not something you should stop after eight weeks. Working out three times a week and making smart food choices should be just like some of your other good habits—such as brushing your teeth or changing the oil in your car. If you go right back to your old ways of ignoring your body and your health, your body is not going to magically maintain itself—and you're going to go right back to feeling tired and out of shape. The only way to prevent going backward is to stay committed to living a healthier, stronger, and better life—I know you can do it. Maintaining this new lifestyle is going to ensure that you continue to build new muscle mass, keep off the beer belly, and live a life of health and vitality.

The first thing to consider is where you are with your goal. Did you reach your goal weight or hit a biceps measurement you were striving for? Or do you have a bit to go still? Either way, you've come a long way from where you were eight weeks ago, and you need to reward yourself. Maybe go to a ball game or get a massage or buy that new "toy" you've been eyeing. The hard part is behind you. Take a day or two off to rest, recuperate, and motivate yourself to continue moving forward with your new lifestyle.

If you have achieved your goal, then the key for you is maintenance. Since you're not trying to lose weight, you may want to consider adding some calories to your diet. This doesn't mean beer and nachos. Add calories from quality food sources. Have some additional fruit with breakfast or maybe add in a bit more healthy fat. Now, with the workouts, it's up to you if you want to start a new 8-Week Challenge. You may start the program from the beginning, or you can mix it up to suit your own preferences. If you want to challenge yourself, take your workouts to the gym to put yourself in a motivating environment. The plan will continue to build muscle for you as long as you keep raising your intensity level. Customize the plan so that it will continue to work for you long-term. Here are some options for maximizing your results as you move forward:

Option 1—Repeat: If you liked the structure of the workouts and had great success with them, don't mess with a good thing; just flip back to week one and start over. I recommend reviewing your logs from week eight and working forward from there. That way you'll continue to challenge your muscles and create new mass and definition.

Option 2—Odds and Evens: To mix it up a bit, move the workouts around and create a new structure. Do the odd-numbered workouts for your first four weeks, and then do the even-numbered workouts in your last four weeks, or vice versa. Here's how the program would shape up:

WEEK	WORKOUTS
Week 1	Workouts 1, 2, 3
Week 2	Workouts 7, 8, 9
Week 3	Workouts 13, 14, 15
Week 4	Workouts 19, 20, 21
Week 5	Workouts 4, 5, 6
Week 6	Workouts 10, 11, 12
Week 7	Workouts 16, 17, 18
Week 8	Workouts 22, 23, 24

Option 3—Try My 12-Second Sequence™: If you want to try something entirely new, check out the eight-week program from my *12-Second Sequence™* book. It requires gym time in the final four weeks. The 12-Second Sequence™ is in a circuit-training format, which means no rest between sets. That's what gives it some great built-in cardio benefits. But if you prefer to stay out of the gym, stick with Option 1 or Option 2.

If you haven't reached your ultimate goal, don't feel frustrated. Depending on your personal goal, you may have just a little bit longer distance to travel to get there. I suggest you start another 8-Week Challenge as soon as possible. Remember to reward yourself with a short break, but don't let yourself go so long that you fall back into your old ways. It's important to start right back up with the workouts. They are now an essential part of your life, and they will continue to help you live a stronger, healthier, and happier life. Continue to focus on your goals, and even take your goals up a notch to keep yourself moving forward.

Here are some additional tips to help you stay motivated:

- *Make new goals.* As I mentioned, don't be afraid to take it up a notch! If you don't set new goals for yourself along the way, it's inevitable that you will lose motivation to continue this new lifestyle. Consider using a trip or an upcoming event that you really want to look and feel great for—maybe a high school reunion or an alumni game. Or perhaps you want to add 2 inches to your biceps. Try to create a specific goal. You can even use Body at Home™ as a springboard into other physical activities.

- *Get your buddies on board.* Try to get a friend to do the workouts with you. Having someone there to challenge you will force you to really push yourself. Or, if you prefer to work out alone, set up a friendly bet, such as first guy to reach his goal gets tickets to the big game. Bringing a little competition into anything always adds some good motivation.

- *Look for an online network.* There are tons of fitness forums that you can join to get answers to any questions or to stay connected with other people who are working as hard as you to get fit. At BodyatHome.com, there are some great member boards that you can join. Find out what other guys are doing to keep their workouts challenging.

- *Three is the magic number.* Eating every three hours is essential even if you're trying only to maintain your weight and not lose more. Your metabolism will stay revved, you'll avoid energy crashes throughout the day, and you'll keep your blood sugar in check. Plus, you won't be stuffing yourself at three main meals each day.

- *Tie your continued success to health.* If you're getting fit for health reasons, let numbers motivate you. For example, if you've had problems with cholesterol or high blood pressure or any other health indicators, keep getting checked. Create a goal to get those numbers down, and use upcoming screenings to motivate yourself. Some of my clients saw their cholesterol numbers go way down. Let your health become what continues to drive you forward.

Bottom line: You have done some amazing work on your body these past eight weeks. Congratulate yourself for your dedication and commitment to your body—I know sometimes you really have to push yourself to stick with it. Be proud of what you've accomplished: not only what you have to show for all your hard work on the outside (your V-Shape), but the giant steps you've taken toward living a long, healthy life filled with energy and strength. It's crucial that you maintain this new lifestyle. It will allow you to live your best life possible. Plus, looking and feeling good is contagious—you will inspire others around you to get fit and rock their best body.

 BODY AT HOME™ STAR Jonathan Austin

Height: 6'5" | Age: 29 | Gained: 6 pounds of lean muscle

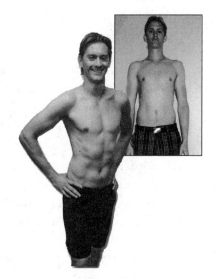

"Before this program, I did go to the gym and eat rather well; a hamburger here and there when I was dashing off to school was my only dietary downfall. Yet I never felt that I was really getting the body I wanted. I have always been skinny and I have always felt rather intimidated by the buff guys working out at the gym. I rarely ventured to the hard-core section of bench presses and free weights that no guy could lift.

"Now that I've built up muscle and feel stronger, I feel much more confident. I go to the gym now and feel comfortable getting on machines and lifting weights—I don't hold back!"

Do This

· Enjoy the new experience with a program that's really going to give you the results you want.

· Plan out your meals ahead of time; even spend some time on Sunday scheduling your meals for the week.

· Pick a time of day to schedule your workouts and stick to it throughout the program. This really helps you stay committed to them.

(10) BODY AT HOME™ STAR   Michael McKibben

Height: 5'9" | **Age:** 32 | **Lost:** 10 pounds (Plus restored 1 pound of lean muscle)

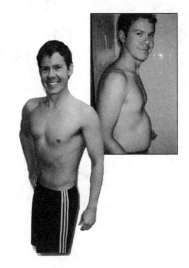

"While I have always been interested in fitness, I never quite had the tools to get the body I wanted; I was just thin, never ripped. I also lacked energy, couldn't sleep, and was always hungry. Body at Home™ is the owner's manual our bodies should have come with! It's so simple that everyone can follow it. It has really changed my life—I now have tons of energy at all hours of the day and I feel great. My health has been flawless since starting the program, my stomach is tight, my chest is defined, and seeing myself in the mirror still shocks me—but now in a good way! People notice the glow in my face and constantly compliment me. I'm finished my eight weeks, but I'm sticking with what I learned for life!"

Do This

· Write down your meals on the Eating Planner log. It's so much easier to keep track!

· Put your goals on the fridge and look at them every day.

· Wear an "A-frame" type of T-shirt so you can actually see your muscles. They will get bigger and leaner, and you will be encouraged by the results every time you work out!

8 Frequently Asked Questions

"I have so much more energy and stamina that my activity level after work has picked up and I require less sleep than I did previously. I haven't felt this good or been this fit since my 30s."

—RON COURTOIS, BODY AT HOME™ STAR, LOST 14 POUNDS

Will I really lose 10 pounds in two weeks?

Absolutely! Following the Body at Home™ program will not only help you lose 10 pounds from your gut, but help you build your chest, add inches to your arms, and develop a strong and powerful V-Shape. The key is consistency with the exercise program and the diet. Really take the first two weeks to push yourself and let your body become adjusted to the program. You will be amazed at the results you see. And remember, be sure to measure your waist as well track your results off the scale.

Do I really have to follow the eating plan, or can I just do the strength training to lose my gut?

Although the strength training is critical to building lean muscle on your entire body, without proper nutrition your body will not have the ingredients to build muscle. Think of the food you eat as the materials to build the house, and think of strength training as the work that adds shape and definition. Each is essential to the other, and doing one without the other will not create the best results. By combining strength training and proper eating, you are going to ensure your results and maximum success!

Do I have to do morning cardio?

Although the Body at Home™ plan is based solely on strength training three times a week, some of my most successful clients have used cardio in the morning to achieve even better results. The amount of morning cardio you do depends on your body type. Refer to Chapter 4 for information on body types, and follow what's recommended based on whether you are an endomorph, a mesomorph, or an ectomorph. Because of your body type, you might not need any cardio, or you may have to do cardio every day. I recommend morning cardio because research studies have revealed that morning cardio on an empty stomach burns more fat, especially belly fat, than cardio done after eating. Plus, you're more likely to take your walk in the morning before the stress of work piles on or other distractions start to pop up.

Will these exercises make me sore, and if so, how do I deal with it?

There are a number of reasons why you could become sore from resistance training, including your previous level of fitness and activity, your age, and the intensity of your workouts. If this is the first time you have exercised or it has been a while since you last hit the weights, there's a good chance that these exercises will cause your muscles to become sore. The soreness occurs because you are causing microscopic tears in your muscle fibers when you strength-train. The pain you feel on the days following intense exercise is from these minute tears and is called *delayed onset muscle soreness*. It is normal and can last between one and seven days following your workout. As these tears heal, your muscles will become stronger; and as your muscles adapt over time, the soreness will lessen after your workouts.

Here are some things you can do to help lessen soreness. Be sure you are allowing time to warm up, cool down, and stretch properly before and after your workouts. Be sure you are drinking enough water throughout the day, and stay active. Keeping your blood flowing by doing some light cardio, getting a massage, or doing any light physical activity on the days following your workout will help. Even doing some of those unwanted house chores can help relieve a little of the pain!

What if I don't feel my muscles burning?

If you're counting correctly throughout your 10-second motions and 2-second holds, you should feel a significant burn when you finish each set. If you aren't feeling that burn, your form or your intensity may not be at the ideal level. To make sure that you get the most out of your workouts, make sure that you maintain proper form. You should feel the intensity of each move on the muscle you're working. Don't let surrounding muscles support your movements. When you do a biceps curl, for example, you should feel the full weight of the dumbbell on your biceps, not in your back or shoulders. Bad form not only cheats you out of an effective workout but also puts you at risk for debilitating injuries.

Will the supplements and exercises make me more aggressive or be harmful to me?

No. None of the supplements is going to make you more aggressive or be harmful. In particular, creatine, L-glutamine, and nitric oxide do not alter your hormones and do not have any mood-altering side effects. Each of these supplements is naturally produced by the body in various quantities. You are pushing your body, and supplementing helps your body recover properly and more efficiently. Remember, check with your doctor if you want to be sure about what you can take.

I want rock-hard abs and big arms! Can I just do exercises for those specific muscles and skip the others in the workouts?

No. You cannot exercise only those muscles and achieve 100 percent results. In order build muscle mass and burn fat so those muscles pop, including your abs and arms, you have to work *your entire body*. Missing exercises or entire workouts will cause imbalances within your body and fail to create the results you desire. Lifting your entire body will release more testosterone and growth hormone, which help you to build muscle while your body rests and repairs itself. If you are lifting only your abs and arms, your body releases less of these hormones, and although you might build some muscle, the results will be less effective than they will be if you complete the full Body at Home™ program.

Can I strength-train more than three times a week?

No. Doing more than three workouts a week could impede your results and slow your progress. Your muscles grow while they are at rest, so too much resistance training can do more harm than good. If you feel the exercises are not hard enough, you might need to use heavier weights and increase your intensity. If you really want to do something more, cardio can be the option, depending on your body type. You can do more cardio in the afternoons to help speed up your results. Remember, you should do only 20 minutes of cardio in the morning before breakfast. Any other cardio should be done after you have nourished your body so you will have the proper energy to push yourself. Adding cardio later in the day will be good for your heart and burn more calories. Be sure to refer to Chapter 4 to find your body type and the proper amount of cardio for you.

Can I go to the gym and do these workouts there if I want to?

Yes. Although the program has been designed to be done entirely at home, you can go to the gym to do the exercises. You can even substitute exercises with different machines, benches, and weights, but make sure you are working the body part indicated in the plan. If you are supposed to be working your chest, be sure to do a chest exercise. If you are supposed to be working your legs, be sure you are doing a leg exercise to replace the move. The gym can be an extra motivator because you are changing your environment. Sometimes it is easy to sabotage yourself and not do the exercises at home, perhaps because you are tired or your favorite show is on. Leaving your house and going to the gym every once in a while could keep you on track and focused. Two gyms I recommend and trust are Bally Total Fitness and David Barton gyms. For more information and to find one of these gyms near you, go to ballyfitness.com or davidbartongym.com.

How can I avoid overeating at night?

Most of the time, especially if we're eating every three hours all day, eating late at night is less about hunger and more about some other stuff we might be going through. Sometimes we're stressed or just plain bored and entertain ourselves with a big bowl of popcorn or a few beers. I've learned that nighttime is when most of my clients are likely to sabotage all their hard work. You can log on to BodyatHome.com and chat with any buddies you've made. Maybe go for a walk with your spouse or hit that punching bag a few times until the cravings pass. Focus on your commitment and you will be successful.

Do I have to drink the whey shakes for my snacks?

As I mentioned, whey protein shakes are your ideal snacks on this plan. Whey protein shakes are the best way to feed your muscles what they need to build and repair themselves after your workouts. The next best option is low-fat (2 percent) cottage cheese. One-half cup has only 100 calories, has only 2 grams of fat, and provides over 15 grams of good protein. But remember, you are here to lose your gut in just two weeks . . . you need to keep it simple and effective and whey protein is truly the best.

Will this program promote a healthy digestive system?

If your digestive system is working properly, you probably are having two or three bowel movements a day; but dehydration, the types of foods you eat, and even when you eat all play a role in digestive health. The Body at Home™ program will help keep you "regular" for the following reasons: Eating portioned meals every three hours will prevent your digestive system from being overloaded. Your diet will be high in fiber from your whole grains and vegetables. Because you will be eating less toxic food, your digestive track will work less. Also, you will be more "regular" because you are drinking half your body weight in ounces of water a day. Plus, exercise and physical activity will ensure your digestive system is moving food properly along with better blood flow.

I've heard steroids can accelerate muscle growth and recovery. Would taking steroids accelerate my progress?

Steroids are not the answer! Too many people are looking for a fast and easy fix. Steroids could help you add muscle, but at a serious cost to your health. Steroids are extremely harmful to your body and the risks outweigh the benefits tenfold. Side effects of steroids include liver failure, cardiovascular disease, depression, increased body fat, aggression, gynecomastia (development of breast-like tissue), acne, oily skin, hypertension, reduction of testosterone, prostate hypertrophy, and thyroid disease. Short-term gains from the use of steroids are dwarfed by the possible health problems steroids bring about. Good old-fashioned hard work, dedication, and commitment are the only healthy and safe ways to increase muscle mass safely and effectively.

I'm naturally slim and don't need to lose fat. Will this program help me become stronger and more toned?

Absolutely! Since you don't need to lose weight, you'll see results much more quickly. This program will increase your muscle definition and make you stronger and more fit. It will give you ripped abs, a bigger chest, toned legs, and defined arms. Check with your doctor to be sure you're eating enough calories, though. Since you already have a high metabolism, you may need to consume more than this program recommends.

I've hit a plateau. How can I lose more weight or build more muscle?

Plain and simple, plateaus are frustrating. You work so hard and see no change on the scale or in your measurements. But don't get discouraged! All you need to do is change your program around a bit. Think about your eating plan. Are you writing down everything you eat? It is very likely that you are consuming more than you think you are. Make sure you are getting the right portions. Many times we have too many carbs at one sitting and not enough protein. Try increasing the intensity of your strength training or add more walking to your routine. To burn more calories, try walking up some hills if you've been walking on level ground. Mixing up your routine will help you break through a plateau in no time.

What if I fall off the eating plan and eat a bag of chips or have a few beers? Or what if I miss one of my workouts? Do I have to start over?

No. When you eat too much or miss a workout, accept it and get back on track tomorrow. If it's your friend's birthday and you have a few drinks, or if you're out for Mexican food and you eat too many tortilla chips, you're not going to undo all your hard work. Regroup and look forward, not back.

I'm over 50, and I've been inactive for most my life. Is it too late for me to do this program and get in shape?

No! It's never too late to improve muscle tone and eliminate body fat. In fact, resistance training is particularly important for men as they get older, because it improves strength and helps combat the wear and tear of age.

I advise you to talk to your doctor before starting the program, to make sure that you're in good health and able to complete the Body at Home™ exercises. Once you get the go-ahead, you're on your way!

15 BODY AT HOME™ STAR   Chris Matthews

Height: 5'10" | **Age:** 37 | **Lost:** 15 pounds

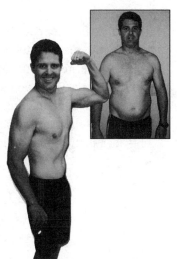

"I have been an active individual most of my life. While I'm in great aerobic shape, I've always trained under the work harder not smarter method, which produced roller-coaster results in my weight and fitness. I've tried several diets, but I was not able to sustain the results I wanted. Body at Home™ finally convinced me that I could make a lifestyle change.

"This plan provides the right balance between diet and exercise and fits right into my active lifestyle. I have seen a significant increase in my strength and aerobic fitness. This plan left me feeling more energized on a regular basis—I was even much sharper at work and at home. Body at Home™ has raised my overall quality of life and given me a fitness foundation."

Do This

· Take the workouts seriously.

· Spend some quality time in front of your mirror. Muscles you never thought existed will start popping up in a few short weeks and that is a great confidence booster!

· Make a weekly meal plan and shopping list; incorporate some new food choices to spice things up a little.

RESOURCES FOR HIM

TOOLS FOR STAYING ON TRACK

The Eating Planner and Workout Logs on the following pages will help keep you organized during the two weeks of the Quick-Start Phase and then will help keep you on track through the Power Phase. You will use the Eating Planner every day, so make at least 14 copies of it for the first two weeks. Plus, you will need at least two copies of each Workout Log (Days 1, 2, and 3) to get you through the Quick-Start Phase. Photocopy these charts, three-hole-punch them, and place them in a binder. You can also stay organized throughout your challenge with downloadable logs that you can find at BodyatHome.com.

EATING PLANNER

This plan will ensure leaner muscle and a higher metabolism.

Breakfast>time_____   Description

○	**PROTEIN** (5oz)	
○	**CARBS** (½ cup or 1 slice of bread)	
○	**FRUIT** (1 cup)	
○	**FAT** (1 teaspoon)	

Snack>time_____   Description

○	**WHEY PROTEIN SHAKE** (1 scoop)	

Jorge recommends Jorge's Packs™ for your protein drinks. **>** See list of other recommended snacks at the back of the book.

Lunch>time_____   Description

○	**PROTEIN** (5oz)	
○	**CARBS** (½ cup or 1 slice of bread)	
○	**VEGGIES*** (2 cups)	
○	**FAT** (1 teaspoon)	

Snack>time_____   Description

○	**WHEY PROTEIN SHAKE** (1 scoop)	

Dinner>time_____   Description

○	**PROTEIN** (5oz)	
○	**VEGGIES*** (2-4 cups)	
○	**FAT** (1 teaspoon)	

Snack>time_____   Description

○	**WHEY PROTEIN SHAKE** (1 scoop)	

*Veggies = nonstarchy vegetables.

Water (eight 8-oz cups)   ○ ○ ○ ○ ○ ○ ○ ○

Multivitamin   ○

DAY 1

DATE_____

Start Time_____ Finish Time_____

TOTAL TIME_____

Select weights so that by the end of the 4th rep of each exercise you feel an intensity level of 8.

	Muscle Group	Exercise	Weight Used	Intensity Level	set 1	set 2
LARGE	CHEST					
	CHEST					
	CHEST					
	CHEST					

At this point you should be about 6 minutes into your workout.

SMALL	SHOULDERS					
	SHOULDERS					
	SHOULDERS					

At this point you should be about 14 minutes into your workout, including 2 minutes of transition time.

ABS	ABS					
	ABS					
	ABS					

At this point in your workout you should be at 20 minutes. Congratulations! YOU DID IT!

BONUS CARDIO 20-MINUTE MORNING POWER WALK ◯

After my workout I feel _____

(e.g., confident, strong)

DAY 2

DATE_____

Start Time_____ Finish Time_____

TOTAL TIME_____

Select weights so that by the end of the 4th rep of each exercise you feel an intensity level of 8.

	Muscle Group	Exercise	Weight Used	Intensity Level	set 1	set 2
LARGE	BACK					
	BACK					
	BACK					
	BACK					

At this point you should be about 6 minutes into your workout.

	Muscle Group	Exercise	Weight Used	Intensity Level	set 1	set 2
SMALL	BICEPS					
	BICEPS					
	BICEPS					

At this point you should be about 14 minutes into your workout, including 2 minutes of transition time.

	Muscle Group	Exercise	Weight Used	Intensity Level	set 1	set 2
ABS	ABS					
	ABS					
	ABS					

At this point in your workout you should be at 20 minutes. Congratulations! YOU DID IT!

BONUS CARDIO 20-MINUTE MORNING POWER WALK ○

After my workout I feel _____

(e.g., confident, strong)

DAY 3

DATE_____

Start Time_____ Finish Time_____

TOTAL TIME_____

Select weights so that by the end of the 4th rep of each exercise you feel an intensity level of 8.

Muscle Group	Exercise	Weight Used	Intensity Level	set 1	set 2
LEGS					
LEGS					
LEGS					
LEGS					

At this point you should be about 6 minutes into your workout.

TRICEPS					
TRICEPS					
TRICEPS					

At this point you should be about 14 minutes into your workout, including 2 minutes of transition time.

ABS					
ABS					
ABS					

At this point in your workout you should be at 20 minutes. Congratulations! YOU DID IT!

LARGE **SMALL** **ABS**

BONUS CARDIO 20-MINUTE MORNING POWER WALK ◯

After my workout I feel _____

(e.g., confident, strong)

WEEKLY JOURNEY TO SUCCESS

	Monday	Tuesday	Wednesday	Thursday	Friday	Saturday	Sunday	
	DAY 1 WORKOUT 1	**DAY 2** DAY OFF	**DAY 3** WORKOUT 2	**DAY 4** DAY OFF	**DAY 5** WORKOUT 3	**DAY 6** DAY OFF	**DAY 7** DAY OFF	WEEK 1
	DAY 8 WORKOUT 1	**DAY 9** DAY OFF	**DAY 10** WORKOUT 2	**DAY 11** DAY OFF	**DAY 12** WORKOUT 3	**DAY 13** DAY OFF	**DAY 14** DAY OFF	WEEK 2
	DAY 15 WORKOUT 1	**DAY 16** DAY OFF	**DAY 17** WORKOUT 2	**DAY 18** DAY OFF	**DAY 19** WORKOUT 3	**DAY 20** DAY OFF	**DAY 21** DAY OFF	WEEK 3
	DAY 22 WORKOUT 1	**DAY 23** DAY OFF	**DAY 24** WORKOUT 2	**DAY 25** DAY OFF	**DAY 26** WORKOUT 3	**DAY 27** DAY OFF	**DAY 28** DAY OFF	WEEK 4
	DAY 29 WORKOUT 1	**DAY 30** DAY OFF	**DAY 31** WORKOUT 2	**DAY 32** DAY OFF	**DAY 33** WORKOUT 3	**DAY 34** DAY OFF	**DAY 35** DAY OFF	WEEK 5
	DAY 36 WORKOUT 1	**DAY 37** DAY OFF	**DAY 38** WORKOUT 2	**DAY 39** DAY OFF	**DAY 40** WORKOUT 3	**DAY 41** DAY OFF	**DAY 42** DAY OFF	WEEK 6
	DAY 43 WORKOUT 1	**DAY 44** DAY OFF	**DAY 45** WORKOUT 2	**DAY 46** DAY OFF	**DAY 47** WORKOUT 3	**DAY 48** DAY OFF	**DAY 49** DAY OFF	WEEK 7
	DAY 50 WORKOUT 1	**DAY 51** DAY OFF	**DAY 52** WORKOUT 2	**DAY 53** DAY OFF	**DAY 54** WORKOUT 3	**DAY 54** DAY OFF	**DAY 56** SUCCESS!	WEEK 8

*Please photocopy and place on your refrigerator. As you complete your workouts, cross off the days so you can see your success!

7-DAY MENU PLANNER

This is a sample planner.

Day 1

Breakfast:	**Protein Oatmeal**
Snack:	½ cup of low-fat cottage cheese
Lunch:	**Chinese Chicken Salad**
Snack:	Whey protein shake
Dinner:	**Turkey Meatloaf**
Snack:	Whey protein shake

Day 2

Breakfast:	**Blueberry Banana Smoothie**
Snack:	Whey protein shake
Lunch:	**French Bread Pizzas**
Snack:	½ cup Muscle Milk 'n Oats™
Dinner:	**Black Pepper Pork with Balsamic Glaze**
Snack:	Whey protein shake

Day 3

Breakfast:	**Cottage Cheese with Fruit and Toast**
Snack:	Whey protein shake

Lunch:	**Meatball Subs**
Snack:	Instone High Protein Pudding™
Dinner:	**Salmon with Grilled Vegetable Salad**
Snack:	Whey protein shake

Day 4

Breakfast:	**Spinach Feta Frittata**
Snack:	Chef Jay Trioplex Protein Cookies™
Lunch:	**Shrimp Caesar Salad with Body at Home™ Caesar Dressing**
Snack:	Whey protein shake
Dinner:	**Boneless Buffalo "Wings"**
Snack:	Whey protein shake

Day 5

Breakfast:	**Breakfast Burritos**
Snack:	Whey protein shake
Lunch:	**Steak Sandwiches with Body at Home™ Blue Cheese Dressing**
Snack:	Ostrim™ high-protein ostrich snacks
Dinner:	**Filet Mignon with Puréed Cauliflower and Sautéed Spinach**
Snack:	Whey protein shake

Day 6

Breakfast:	**Steak and Eggs**
Snack:	Muscle Milk® Bar
Lunch:	**Scallop and Prosciutto Pizza**
Snack:	Whey protein shake
Dinner:	**Body at Home™ Burger**
Snack:	Whey protein shake

Day 7

Breakfast:	**Sausage and Egg Sandwich**
Snack:	Schwartz Labs Protein Pancake Mix™
Lunch:	**BBQ Chicken Pita Sandwiches**
Snack:	Whey protein shake
Dinner:	**Turkey Chili**
Snack:	Whey protein shake

Note: Remember to refer to the Bonus Items section (page 341) for the Ideal Foods List and the Fast and Frozen Foods List for additional ideas and suggestions.

BODY AT HOME™ RECIPES

Breakfast

Blueberry Banana Smoothie

Breakfast Burritos

Cottage Cheese with Fruit and Toast

Protein Oatmeal

Sausage and Egg Sandwich

Spinach Feta Frittata

Steak and Eggs

Lunch

BBQ Chicken Pita Sandwiches

Chinese Chicken Salad

French Bread Pizzas

Meatball Subs

Scallop and Prosciutto Pizza

Shrimp Caesar Salad with Caesar Dressing

Steak Sandwiches with Blue Cheese Dressing

Dinner

Body at Home™ Burger

Black Pepper Pork with Balsamic Glaze

Boneless Buffalo "Wings"

Filet Mignon with Puréed Cauliflower and Sautéed Spinach

Salmon with Grilled Vegetable Salad

Turkey Chili

Turkey Meatloaf

Blueberry Banana Smoothie

Combine all ingredients in a blender and purée until smooth. If the mixture is too thick, thin it with a bit of water. Serve.

Serves 1
COOKING TIME: 5 minutes

½ very ripe banana
1 cup frozen blueberries
½ cup light vanilla soymilk
1½ scoops vanilla protein powder
1 teaspoon flaxseed oil

Breakfast Burritos

Heat a large nonstick skillet over medium heat and spray with cooking spray. Add the bell pepper to the skillet and season with salt and pepper. Sauté for 1 minute. Add the tomatoes and spinach and sauté for 30 seconds. Whisk together the eggs and egg whites in a medium bowl and pour over the vegetables in the skillet. Cook until soft curds form, stirring occasionally. Remove from the heat and season with salt and pepper.

Heat the tortillas in the microwave. Divide the egg mixture among the tortillas and roll into burrito shapes. Serve with the oranges.

Serves 4
COOKING TIME: 10 minutes

Cooking spray
1 bell pepper, any color, diced
Salt and freshly ground black pepper
2 Roma tomatoes, diced
2 cups baby spinach
9 eggs
7 egg whites
4 Mission® 96% Fat-Free Tortillas
4 oranges, peeled and sectioned

Cottage Cheese with Fruit and Toast

Serves 4
COOKING TIME: 5 minutes

2 cups diced fruit
   (strawberries, melon,
   apple, pear, etc.)
4 cups 2% cottage cheese
4 slices whole-wheat bread,
   toasted
4 teaspoons flaxseed oil

In a large bowl, stir together the fruit and cottage cheese. Divide among four bowls. Drizzle the toasted bread with flaxseed oil. Serve each person one bowl of cottage cheese and one slice of toast.

Protein Oatmeal

Serves 4
COOKING TIME: 15 minutes

1 teaspoon kosher salt
2 cups rolled oats
3 scoops unflavored protein
   powder
4 cups blueberries
4 teaspoons flaxseed oil

In a medium saucepan over medium heat, bring 3½ cups water to a boil and add salt. Stir in the oats and protein powder and bring back to a boil. Reduce heat to low and simmer, uncovered, stirring occasionally, until the oatmeal is tender, 10 to 15 minutes. Remove from heat and stir in the blueberries and flaxseed oil. Divide among four bowls and serve.

Sausage and Egg Sandwich

Heat a large nonstick skillet over medium heat and spray with cooking spray. Add the sausage patties and cook until browned and heated through, 4 minutes per side. Place one patty on each of four English muffin halves.

Spray the skillet again with cooking spray and carefully crack the eggs into the pan. Fry until the whites are set and the yolk is still runny, 1 to 2 minutes per side. Place one egg on each sausage patty and top with the other English muffin half.

Mix the cottage cheese with the blueberries and divide among four bowls.

Serve each person one sandwich and one bowl of cottage cheese.

Serves 4
COOKING TIME: 10 minutes

Cooking spray
4 soy-based sausage-style patties
4 whole-wheat English muffins, toasted
4 eggs
2 cups 2% cottage cheese
1 cup blueberries

Spinach Feta Frittata

Preheat broiler.

Heat a large, nonstick, oven-safe skillet over medium heat and spray with cooking spray. Add onion and garlic and sauté until tender, 2 minutes. Add the potato and spinach and season with salt and pepper. Carefully stir until combined. Pour the beaten eggs into the skillet and stir gently to evenly distribute the fillings. Cook until the bottom is set, 2 to 3 minutes. Sprinkle with the feta and place under the broiler until cooked through, 4 to 5 minutes.

Slice the frittata into four wedges and serve with the apples.

Serves 4
COOKING TIME: 10 minutes

Cooking spray
¼ medium onion, diced
1 garlic clove, minced
1½ cups diced cooked potato
1 box frozen chopped spinach, thawed and squeezed dry
Salt and freshly ground black pepper
12 eggs, lightly beaten
¼ cup crumbled feta cheese
4 apples

Steak and Eggs

Serves 4
COOKING TIME: 15 minutes

Cooking spray
Four 4-ounce beef tenderloin
    filets, trimmed of all visible
    fat
Salt and freshly ground black
    pepper
4 eggs
2 slices whole-wheat bread,
    toasted
2 cups cubed cantaloupe

Heat a nonstick skillet over medium-high heat and spray with cooking spray. Season the steaks with salt and pepper and add to the skillet. Sear the steaks to desired doneness, 4 to 5 minutes per side for medium rare. Place the steaks on a plate and tent with foil to keep warm.

Reduce heat to medium-low and spray again with cooking spray. Carefully break eggs into the pan and fry until the whites are set and the yolk is still runny, 1 to 2 minutes per side.

Serve each person one steak with one egg, half a slice of toast, and ½ cup of cantaloupe.

LUNCH

BBQ Chicken Pita Sandwiches

Serves 4
COOKING TIME: 10 minutes

1 cup prepared barbecue
    sauce
1 pound cooked chicken
    breast meat, shredded
2 tablespoons reduced-fat
    mayonnaise
1 teaspoon cider vinegar
1 teaspoon Dijon mustard
2 cups shredded cabbage
    slaw mix
Salt and freshly ground black
    pepper
2 whole-wheat pita breads,
    split into four halves
4 medium oranges, peeled
    and sectioned

Bring the barbecue sauce to a simmer in a large saucepan over medium heat. Add the shredded chicken and simmer until the chicken is heated through, 5 to 7 minutes.

In a medium bowl, mix together the mayonnaise, vinegar, and mustard. Add the slaw and toss to combine. Season to taste with salt and pepper.

Divide the chicken mixture among the pita pockets and top with the slaw. Serve with the oranges.

Chinese Chicken Salad

Combine all ingredients in a large bowl and toss to combine. Season to taste with salt and pepper. Serve.

Serves 4
COOKING TIME: 5 minutes

20 ounces cooked chicken breast meat
6 cups mixed salad greens
6 cups prepared cabbage slaw mix
½ cup shredded carrots
3 green onions, sliced
1 red bell pepper, thinly sliced
¼ cup cilantro leaves, roughly chopped
½ cucumber, thinly sliced
½ cup low-fat Asian-style salad dressing
2 cups cooked brown rice
Salt and freshly ground black pepper

French Bread Pizzas

Preheat oven to 425° F.

Heat a large nonstick skillet over medium heat and add the sausage. Sauté until browned and crumbled. Add the onion, pepper, and garlic and sauté until the vegetables are tender. Remove from the heat.

Stir together the tomato paste, 1 tablespoon of water, salt, pepper, oregano, and crushed red pepper in a small bowl.

Slice the rolls in half lengthwise and scoop out the insides to create a shell. Spread the shells with the tomato mixture and place on a sheet pan. Divide the sausage mixture among the four pizza shells.

Sprinkle each pizza with 1 tablespoon Parmesan. Bake the pizzas until the filling is heated through and the bread is toasted, 10 minutes.

Toss the greens with the dressing in a large bowl.

Serve each person one pizza and one salad.

Serves 4
COOKING TIME: 20 minutes

1 pound hot or sweet turkey Italian sausage
½ medium onion, sliced lengthwise into ¼-inch strips
1 green bell pepper, sliced lengthwise into ¼-inch strips
2 garlic cloves, minced
2 tablespoons tomato paste
Pinch each salt, pepper, sugar, dried oregano, and crushed red pepper flakes
Two 12-inch crusty French rolls
4 tablespoons grated Parmesan cheese
12 cups mixed salad greens
½ cup fat-free vinaigrette salad dressing

Serves 4

COOKING TIME: 20–30 minutes

Cooking spray

½ onion, finely diced

4 garlic cloves, minced

½ cup finely chopped
  mushrooms, about 4 large

1 teaspoon each kosher salt
  and freshly ground black
  pepper

1 egg

2 tablespoons nonfat milk

¼ cup chopped fresh parsley

1 teaspoon crushed red
  pepper flakes

1 tablespoon Worcestershire
  sauce

20 ounces ground turkey
  breast

2 cups prepared marinara
  sauce

2 tablespoons olive oil

12 cups mixed greens

¼ cup fat-free vinaigrette
  salad dressing

4 reduced calorie hot dog
  buns

4 tablespoons grated
  Parmesan cheese

Meatball Subs

Heat a large nonstick skillet over medium heat and spray with cooking spray. Add the onion, garlic, and mushrooms and season with ½ teaspoon salt and ½ teaspoon pepper. Sauté until the vegetables are tender and the mushrooms have given off most of their liquid. Remove from heat and set aside to cool.

In a large bowl, combine the egg, milk, parsley, remaining salt and pepper, crushed red pepper, Worcestershire sauce, and onion mixture and stir to blend. Add the ground turkey breast and gently fold to combine. Shape the mixture into spheres the size of Ping-Pong balls. You should have about sixteen meatballs.

Heat the marinara sauce in a large saucepan over medium heat.

Add the olive oil to the skillet that the onion mixture cooked in and heat over medium-high heat. Fry the meatballs in batches, taking care not to crowd the pan. Brown the meatballs on all sides and add to the marinara sauce. Simmer the meatballs in the sauce until cooked through, 15 minutes.

Toss the greens with the dressing and divide among four salad plates.

Spoon four meatballs into each hot dog bun and spoon sauce over the top. Sprinkle each sandwich with 1 tablespoon grated Parmesan and serve with the salads.

Scallop and Prosciutto Pizza

Preheat oven to 450°F.

Spread the pizza sauce on the shell, leaving a 1-inch border around the edges. Sprinkle with the mozzarella. Scatter the scallops, prosciutto, onion, and tomatoes on the shell. Season with salt and pepper. Top with Parmesan. Bake until the scallops cook through and the cheese is browned and bubbly. Sprinkle with the basil and slice into four pieces.

In a large bowl, toss the greens with the dressing and divide among four plates.

Serve each person one slice of pizza and one salad.

Serves 4
COOKING TIME: 10 minutes

¼ cup prepared pizza sauce

1 Boboli® Thin Crust pizza shell

2 ounces part-skim mozzarella cheese, shredded

12 ounces bay scallops, patted dry

4 ounces thinly sliced prosciutto, sliced into thin ribbons

¼ red onion, thinly sliced

2 Roma tomatoes, diced

Salt and freshly ground black pepper

1 ounce Parmesan cheese, grated

¼ cup chopped fresh basil

12 cups mixed salad greens

¼ cup fat-free vinaigrette dressing

Serves 4

COOKING TIME: 10 minutes

Cooking spray

20 ounces medium shrimp, peeled and deveined

Salt and freshly ground black pepper

12 cups chopped romaine lettuce

2 cups seasoned croutons

½ cup Caesar Dressing (recipe follows)

4 tablespoons grated Parmesan cheese

4 lemon wedges

Shrimp Caesar Salad

Heat a grill or grill pan over medium-high heat and spray with cooking spray. Season the shrimp with salt and pepper and place on the grill. Cook the shrimp until browned on the exterior and opaque throughout.

While the shrimp grill, toss the lettuce and croutons with the dressing. Top the salad with the grilled shrimp and sprinkle with Parmesan. Serve with lemon wedges.

Makes 1 cup

6 ounces light silken tofu

1 teaspoon anchovy paste or Worcestershire sauce

Juice of ½ lemon

2 tablespoons grated Parmesan

1 garlic clove

2 tablespoons extra virgin olive oil

Salt and pepper

Caesar Dressing

Combine the tofu, anchovy paste, lemon juice, Parmesan, and garlic in a blender. Purée until smooth, and stream in olive oil. Thin the dressing with water to desired consistency. Season to taste with salt and pepper.

Steak Sandwiches with Blue Cheese

Serves 4
COOKING TIME: 10–15 minutes

Preheat oven to 500°F.

Heat a large oven-safe skillet over high heat and spray with cooking spray. Season the beef liberally with salt and pepper. Add the beef to the skillet and sear on all sides to form a golden brown crust. Place the skillet in the oven and roast until the meat reaches an internal temperature of 125°F for medium rare, 10 to 15 minutes. Place the roast on a plate and tent with foil to keep warm. Rest the beef for 10 minutes.

Toast the bread and spread with mustard. Thinly slice the beef and divide among the slices of toast. Drizzle each sandwich with 1 tablespoon of the blue cheese dressing. Top with the onion and the arugula.

Toss the greens with the vinaigrette in a large bowl. Divide among four salad plates.

Serve each person one open-faced sandwich with one salad.

Cooking spray
20 ounces beef tenderloin, trimmed of all visible fat
Coarse salt and freshly ground black pepper
4 slices whole-wheat bread
4 teaspoons Dijon mustard
¼ cup Blue Cheese Dressing (recipe follows)
4 thin slices red onion
1 cup baby arugula
12 cups mixed greens
¼ cup fat-free vinaigrette salad dressing

Blue Cheese Dressing

Makes ¾ cup

Combine the mayonnaise, yogurt, buttermilk, half the cheese, Worcestershire, lemon juice, and garlic in a blender or food processor, and purée until smooth. Stir in remaining cheese. Season to taste with salt and pepper.

¼ cup fat-free mayonnaise
¼ cup fat-free plain yogurt
2 tablespoons low-fat buttermilk
2 ounces crumbled blue cheese
Dash Worcestershire sauce
1 teaspoon freshly squeezed lemon juice
1 garlic clove
Salt and pepper

Body at Home™ Burger

Serves 4
COOKING TIME: 15 minutes

Cooking spray
1½ pounds 95% lean ground beef
1 egg white
2 tablespoons Worcestershire sauce
2 teaspoons garlic powder
2 teaspoons kosher salt
1 teaspoon freshly ground black pepper
12 cups mixed salad greens
¼ cup fat-free vinaigrette dressing
4 teaspoons mustard
4 slices tomato
4 slices red onion
12 large leaves red leaf lettuce

Heat a grill or grill pan over medium heat and spray with cooking spray.

Combine the ground beef with the egg white, Worcestershire, garlic powder, salt, and pepper. Mix gently until all the seasonings are incorporated. Divide into four equal patties.

Grill the hamburger patties until they're cooked through, 5 to 6 minutes on each side. Remove burgers from heat and let rest for 5 minutes.

While the burgers rest, toss the salad greens with the dressing in a large bowl. Divide among four salad plates.

Spread each burger with mustard and top with slices of tomato and onion. Wrap each burger in three lettuce leaves.

Serve one burger with one salad.

Black Pepper Pork with Balsamic Glaze

Bring 2 inches of water to a boil in a large stockpot and add a steamer basket. Add the broccoli and cover. Steam until the broccoli is tender, 6 to 8 minutes.

Slice the pork tenderloin into 2-inch medallions and pound to ½-inch thickness. Season with salt and pepper.

Heat a large skillet over medium-high heat and spray with cooking spray. Add the pork to the skillet and sear until well browned and still pink in the middle, 1 to 2 minutes per side. Remove from the heat and tent with foil to keep warm. Add the vinegar and chicken broth to the pan and bring to a boil. Scrape the bottom of the pan with a wooden spoon to loosen any brown bits. Reduce the sauce by half and swirl in the butter. Return the pork to the skillet and turn to coat with the sauce.

Serve each person one-quarter of the pork with sauce and 2 cups of steamed broccoli.

Serves 4
COOKING TIME: 10 minutes

8 cups broccoli florets
1½ pounds pork tenderloin, well trimmed
1 teaspoon kosher salt
2 tablespoons coarsely crushed black pepper
Cooking spray
½ cup balsamic vinegar
½ cup low-sodium chicken broth
1 tablespoon butter

Boneless Buffalo "Wings"

Combine the chicken with the hot sauce in a large ziptop bag. Marinate for at least an hour and up to 8 hours.

Heat a grill or grill pan over medium-high heat and spray with cooking spray. Add the chicken pieces to the grill and cook, turning once, until cooked through, about 3 to 4 minutes per side.

Toss the greens with the carrots, celery, and dressing. Divide among four plates.

Serve each person one-quarter of the chicken with extra sauce for dipping and one salad.

Serves 4
COOKING TIME: 10 minutes

1½ pounds chicken breast tenders
1 cup Frank's® RedHot® Original Cayenne Pepper Sauce
Cooking spray
12 cups mixed greens
½ cup diced carrot
½ cup diced celery
¼ cup blue cheese salad dressing (see page 331)
Extra hot sauce for dipping

Serves 4
COOKING TIME: 10–15 minutes

2 heads cauliflower, cut into
  florets
2 tablespoons butter
2 tablespoons skim milk
Salt and pepper
Four 6-ounce beef tenderloin
  filets, well trimmed
Cooking spray
4 garlic cloves, thinly sliced
12 cups baby spinach

Filet Mignon with Puréed Cauliflower and Sautéed Spinach

Bring a large pot of salted water to a boil and add the cauliflower. Reduce heat to medium and simmer until tender. Add the cauliflower to a blender or food processor and purée until smooth. Add the butter and milk and pulse until well combined. Season to taste with salt and pepper. Keep warm.

Season the steaks with salt and pepper. Heat a grill or grill pan over high heat and spray with cooking spray. Add the steaks to the grill and cook to desired doneness, 3 to 4 minutes per side for medium rare. Remove from the heat and tent with foil to keep warm.

While the steaks rest, heat a large nonstick skillet over medium heat and spray with cooking spray. Add the garlic and sauté until golden. Add the spinach, in batches if necessary, and sauté until wilted. Season to taste with salt and pepper.

Divide the steaks, cauliflower, and spinach among four plates and serve.

Salmon with Grilled Vegetable Salad

Heat a grill or grill pan over medium heat and spray with cooking spray. Scrape the brown gills from the inside of the mushroom caps. Season the vegetables with salt and pepper and add to the grill. Cook until browned and softened, but don't overcook! Remove from the grill while they still retain some texture. Set aside until cool enough to handle.

Chop the veggies into bite-size pieces and place in a large bowl. Whisk together the vinegar, mustard, and oil and toss with the veggies.

Turn the grill up to high and spray again with cooking spray. Season the salmon with salt and pepper and place on the grill. Cook to desired doneness, 3 to 4 minutes per side for medium, turning once.

Serve each person one salmon fillet and one-quarter of the veggie salad.

Serves 4
COOKING TIME: 15 minutes

Cooking spray

2 Portobello mushroom caps

2 zucchini, sliced lengthwise into ½-inch planks

2 yellow squash, sliced lengthwise into ½-inch planks

1 red onion, sliced into ½-inch slices, rings kept intact

1 medium eggplant, sliced lengthwise into ½-inch planks

2 red or yellow bell peppers, halved and seeded

Salt and freshly ground black pepper

2 tablespoons red wine vinegar

1 tablespoon Dijon mustard

2 tablespoons extra virgin olive oil

Four 6-ounce salmon fillets (preferably wild Alaskan salmon)

Turkey Chili

Serves 4

COOKING TIME: 15 minutes

2 tablespoons olive oil

1½ pounds ground turkey breast

1 teaspoon kosher salt

1 teaspoon freshly ground black pepper

1 onion, diced

8 garlic cloves, minced

1 jalapeño pepper, seeded and minced

2 tablespoons chili powder

½ teaspoon cayenne pepper (or more to taste)

2 teaspoons cumin

2 teaspoons dried oregano

1 cup (or more) low-sodium chicken broth

1 cup canned black beans, drained and rinsed thoroughly

12 cups mixed salad greens

¼ cup fat-free vinaigrette salad dressing

2 ounces reduced-fat cheddar cheese, shredded

½ cup chopped fresh cilantro

Heat the olive oil in a large stockpot over medium heat. Add the turkey breast and season with salt and pepper. Brown the turkey, stirring occasionally, until it is about half cooked. Add the onion, garlic, jalapeño, chili powder, cayenne, cumin, and oregano and stir to combine. Cook until no pink remains in the turkey and add 1 cup chicken broth. Add more if necessary to reach desired consistency. Bring mixture to a boil and reduce heat to low. Simmer over low heat for 10 minutes. Stir in the black beans and simmer until heated through. Taste for seasoning and adjust if necessary.

In a large bowl, toss the greens with the dressing. Divide among four salad plates.

Divide the chili among four bowls and top with the cheese and cilantro. Serve with the salad.

Turkey Meatloaf

*Preheat the oven to 400° F.

Heat a large nonstick skillet over medium heat and spray with cooking spray. Add the onion, garlic, and bell pepper and season with a ½ teaspoon each of salt and pepper. Sauté until tender and add spinach. Sauté until wilted and remove the pan from the heat to let cool.

In a large bowl, mix together the cooled onion mixture, ground turkey, remaining salt and pepper, egg, vinegar, tomato paste, Worcestershire, parsley, basil, and crushed red pepper until well combined. Do not overmix or the meatloaf will be tough.

Line a baking sheet with parchment paper or aluminum foil (if using foil, spray with cooking spray). Mound the turkey mixture into the center of the pan and pat into an oval shape. Spread with the mustard. Bake until the meatloaf is brown and crusty and the interior reaches 160° F, 25 to 30 minutes. Let rest for 10 minutes.

Toss the greens with the lemon juice and flax oil and divide among four plates.

Slice the meatloaf into four pieces and serve with the salad.

Serves 4
COOKING TIME: 25–30 minutes

Cooking spray
½ large onion, minced
5 garlic cloves, minced
1 red bell pepper, diced
1 teaspoon kosher salt
1 teaspoon freshly ground black pepper
2 cups baby spinach, packed
1½ pounds ground turkey
1 egg
1 tablespoon balsamic vinegar
1 tablespoon tomato paste
2 tablespoons Worcestershire sauce
2 tablespoons chopped fresh parsley
2 tablespoons chopped fresh basil
1 teaspoon crushed red pepper
2 tablespoons whole-grain mustard
12 cups mixed salad greens
Juice of half a lemon
4 teaspoons flaxseed oil

This routine is designed to cut out all excuses. You can do it anywhere at any time with just a Swiss ball (these deflate and pack easily). So it's perfect if you're traveling or stuck in your office and can't get home to work out. It takes only 33.5 minutes and will provide you with an intense and effective workout. Complete one set of 4 reps, rest 30 seconds, and then complete the second set. You will do only one set of the abs exercises, but you still should incorporate a 30-second rest between moves. Use this workout to get started today!

Quadriceps Flex

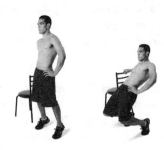

Stand with feet shoulder-width apart. Grasp a sturdy chair for support at about hip level. Feather your breathing as you bend your knees and allow your body to fall backward, letting your heels come off the floor, through a count of 10 seconds. Hold and squeeze your quads for 2 seconds at the MTP (when your knees are near the floor). Return to starting position through a count of 10 seconds. Without resting, repeat three times. Rest for 30 seconds and then repeat the entire sequence.

Swiss Ball Hamstring Curl

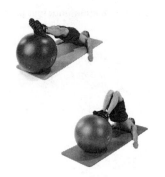

Lie on your back with your arms at your sides, palms flat on the floor. Place your calves and heels on the ball, knees straight but not locked. Tighten your abs and lift your butt and hips off the ground. Feather your breathing and bend your knees as you roll the ball toward your butt with your heels. Hold for 2 seconds at the MTP. Return to starting position through a count of 10 seconds. Without resting, repeat three times. Rest for 30 seconds and then repeat the entire sequence.

Push-Up

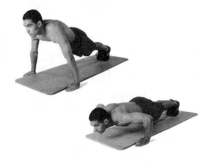

Lie on a mat with your hands slightly wider than shoulder-width apart and your fingers pointing forward. Press up to starting position, keeping your back straight, abs tight, and head up. Feather your breathing as you lower your chest toward the floor through a count of 10 seconds. Hold for 2 seconds at the MTP. Push your body back to starting position through a count of 10 seconds, keeping your elbows slightly bent. Without resting, repeat three times. Rest for 30 seconds and then repeat the entire sequence.

Hyperextension

Lie facedown on the ball with your hips supported and your hands behind your head. Bend at the waist. Feather your breathing as you lift your upper body through a count of 10 seconds, using your lower back. Hold for 2 seconds at the MTP. Return to starting position through a count of 10 seconds. Without resting, repeat three times. Rest for 30 seconds and then repeat the entire sequence.

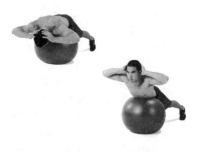

V Push-Up

Stand with your feet shoulder-width apart, bend forward, and walk your hands out to create an upside-down "V" with your body. Keep your abs tight and feather your breathing as you lower your head and upper body toward the mat through a count of 10 seconds. Hold for 2 seconds at the MTP. Press back up through a count of 10 seconds. Without resting, repeat three times. Rest for 30 seconds and then repeat the entire sequence.

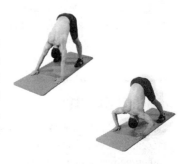

Diamond Push-Up

Lie on a mat with your hands in the "diamond" position. Press up to starting position, keeping your back straight, abs tight, and head up. Feather your breathing as you lower your body through a count of 10 seconds, allowing your elbows to move outward. Hold for 2 seconds at the MTP (about 2 inches above the ground). Push your body back to starting position through a count of 10 seconds. Without resting, repeat three times. Rest for 30 seconds and then repeat the entire sequence.

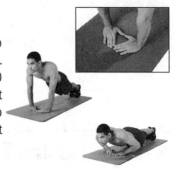

Chair Dip

Sit on the edge of a sturdy chair with your hands behind you and fingers forward grasping the front edge of the chair. Flex your feet so that your weight is on your heels and slide yourself away from the chair. Feather your breathing as you lower yourself through a count of 10 seconds. Hold for 2 seconds at the MTP. Push yourself back up to starting position through a count of 10 seconds. Without resting, repeat three times. Rest for 30 seconds and then repeat the entire sequence. (Note: The MTP will depend on how flexible your shoulders are—about 1 inch above your most flexible point.)

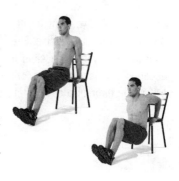

Double Crunch

Lie on a mat or towel. Place your hands behind your head, elbows up, chin up, and abs tight. Pull your heels toward your butt as far as you can. Using your upper abs, feather your breathing as you crunch up while simultaneously pulling your knees in through a count of 10 seconds. Hold and squeeze for 2 seconds at the MTP. Return to starting position through a count of 10 seconds, never letting your upper back touch the ground. Without resting, repeat three times. (Note: The range of motion on this exercise is very short so be sure to adjust your speed so that you hit the MTP on the count of 10.)

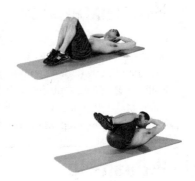

Toe Reach

Lie on your back. Cross your legs, flex your feet, and extend your legs into the air. With your arms extended and chin up, feather your breathing as you crunch up, reaching toward your toes through a count of 10 seconds. Hold and squeeze for 2 seconds at the MTP. Lower yourself to starting position, keeping your shoulder blades from touching the ground through a count of 10 seconds. Without resting, repeat three times.

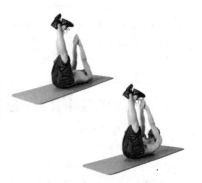

Seated Russian Twist

Sit on the floor with your knees bent, feet together. Keep your chin up and abs tight as you lean back slightly, engaging your abs. Extend your arms away from your chest with your palms pressed together and turn to one side to begin exercise. Feather your breathing as you slowly rotate your torso as far as possible to the other side through a count of 10 seconds. Hold and squeeze for 2 seconds at the MTP. Rotate back to the other side through a count of 10 seconds. Without resting, repeat three times.

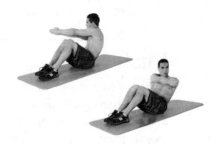

BODY AT HOME™ BONUS ITEMS

IDEAL FOODS LIST

Here's a list of the best foods to choose when you're creating your own meals. Be sure to stick to the recommended serving size (which is alongside each food group listing) for each meal to ensure your success. Serving sizes listed are per meal.

Protein

- 95% lean beef
- Beef tenderloin
- Chicken/turkey breast (skinless)
- Eggs (whole)
- Fish
- Lamb
- London broil
- Low-fat cottage cheese
- Ostrich
- Pork tenderloin
- Round steak
- Shellfish

Carbohydrate (½ cup or 1 slice of bread)

- Brown rice
- Buckwheat
- Sweet potatoes
- Wheat germ
- Whole-grain flour
- Whole-grain cereal
- Whole-wheat bread
- Whole-wheat pasta
- Whole-wheat tortilla
- Wild rice

Vegetables (Nonstarchy) (2 to 4 cups)

- Alfalfa sprouts
- Asparagus
- Bell peppers
- Broccoli
- Brussels sprouts
- Cabbage
- Cauliflower
- Celery
- Chiles
- Cucumber
- Eggplant
- Garlic
- Green beans
- Green onions
- Lettuce
- Mushrooms
- Radishes
- Spinach
- Squash
- Tomatoes
- Watercress
- Zucchini

Fat (1 teaspoon)

- Almonds (6)
- Almond butter
- Avocado ($\frac{1}{8}$)
- Cashews (6)
- Flaxseed oil
- Olive oil
- Peanut butter
- Peanuts (10)

Fruit (1 item or 1 cup diced)

- Apples
- Blackberries
- Blueberries
- Grapefruit
- Grapes
- Lemon
- Lime
- Melon
- Peaches
- Pears
- Strawberries

Snacks (3 per day)

- Jorge's Packs™ Whey Protein Shake
- Low-fat cottage cheese ($\frac{1}{2}$ cup)
- 1 ounce beef jerky
- $\frac{1}{2}$ cup chopped cooked chicken breast meat
- 3 ounces tuna or salmon (canned or pouch)
- $1\frac{1}{2}$ cups edamame
- 6 ounces plain nonfat yogurt
- $\frac{1}{2}$ cup Muscle Milk 'n Oats™
- Schwartz Labs Protein Pancake Mix™ (2 pancakes)
- Instone High Protein Pudding™ (1 container)
- Chef Jay Trioplex Protein Cookie™ (1 cookie)
- Ostrim™ high-protein ostrich snacks (1 pack)
- Muscle Milk® Bar (1 bar)

Freebies

- Water
- Club soda
- Mineral water
- Coffee (minimize; no more than 1 cup a day)
- Diet soda (minimize; no more than one 12-ounce drink a day)

Sugar Substitutes

- Stevia
- Xylitol

Sweets (No more than one serving size as indicated on product nutrition label)

- Sugar-free candies
- Sugar-free gum
- Sugar-free gelatin desserts

Flavor Enhancers (Add to taste)

- Low-sodium broth
- Garlic
- Herbs (fresh or dried)
- Lemon or lime juice
- Mustard
- Pickles
- Salsa
- Spices
- Low-sodium soy sauce
- Vinegar
- Worcestershire sauce

FAST AND FROZEN FOODS LIST

I'm very busy, so I understand that sometimes you need to pick up something to eat on the go. Here are some of the best choices at some popular restaurants that you'll most likely find where you live.

BREAKFAST

Fast Food

- Subway® Western Egg with Cheese Breakfast Sandwich (1)
  Add a piece of fruit.
- McDonald's® Egg McMuffin® (1)
  Add a piece of fruit.
- Denny's® Veggie Cheese Omelet with Egg Beaters® (1)
  Add a piece of fruit.

Frozen Food

- Weight Watchers® Smart Ones® English Muffin Sandwich (1)
  Add a whey protein shake and a piece of fruit.
- Lean Pockets® Bacon, Egg, and Cheese (1)
  Add a whey protein shake and a piece of fruit.
- Lean Pockets® Sausage, Egg, and Cheese (1)
  Add a whey protein shake and a piece of fruit.

LUNCH

Fast Food

· Arby's® Santa Fe Salad with Grilled Chicken (1)
  Add 1 serving of Light Buttermilk Ranch Dressing.
· Baja Fresh® Shrimp Tacos (2)
  Add a side salad (2 cups) and a squeeze of lemon for dressing.
· Blimpie® Turkey Sub, 6-inch on wheat (1)
· Burger King® TenderGrill® Chicken Filet Salad (1)
  Add one serving of Ken's® Fat Free Ranch Dressing.
· Chick-fil-A® Chicken Cool Wrap® (1)
  Add a side salad (2 cups) and a squeeze of lemon for dressing.
· Chick-fil-A® Southwest Chargrilled Chicken Salad (1)
  Add a squeeze of lemon for dressing, half a packet of Garlic and Butter Croutons, and a small order of
  Hearty Breast of Chicken Soup.
· Chipotle Bol with Barbacoa (1)
  Ask for double lettuce, fajita vegetables, red tomatillo salsa, and black beans. No rice.
· Dairy Queen® Grilled Chicken Sandwich (1)
  Add a Side Salad with 1 serving of Fat Free Italian Dressing.
· KFC® Tender Roast® Sandwich Without Sauce (1)
  Ask for 2 additional servings of grilled chicken and add a House Side Salad with Hidden Valley® Golden Italian Light Dressing.
· McDonald's® Asian Salad with Grilled Chicken
  Ask for an additional serving of chicken and a side of Butter Garlic Croutons. Add a squeeze of lemon for
  dressing.
· Rubio's Fresh Mexican Grill® Mahi Mahi Taco (1)
  Ask for 2 additional servings of mahi mahi and add side salad (2 cups) with 2 tablespoons salsa for dressing.
· Rubio's Fresh Mexican Grill® Carne Asada Street Tacos (2)
  Ask for an additional serving of carne asada and add a half side order of pinto beans and a side salad (2
  cups) with 2 tablespoons salsa as dressing.
· Rubio's Fresh Mexican Grill® HealthMex® Chicken Taco (2)
  Ask for an additional serving of chicken and add a side salad (2 cups) with 2 tablespoons salsa as dressing.
· Subway® Club Sandwich, 6-inch, on whole wheat (1)
  Add a Veggie Delite salad with Fat Free Italian Dressing.

Frozen Food

- Lean Cuisine® Café Classics Chicken à L'Orange (1)
  Add a mixed green salad (2 cups) with a squeeze of lemon and 1 teaspoon flaxseed oil for dressing.
- Lean Cuisine® Casual Eating Classics™ Roasted Garlic Chicken Pizza (1)
  Add a mixed green salad (2 cups) with a squeeze of lemon and 1 teaspoon flaxseed oil for dressing.
- Lean Cuisine® One Dish Favorites™ Classic Five Cheese Lasagna (1)
  Add a mixed green salad (2 cups) with a squeeze of lemon and 1 teaspoon flaxseed oil for dressing.
- Healthy Choice® Flavor Adventures Chicken Tuscany (1)
  Add a mixed green salad (2 cups) with a squeeze of lemon and 1 teaspoon flaxseed oil for dressing.
- Healthy Choice® Flavor Adventures Grilled Whiskey Steak (1)
  Add a mixed green salad (2 cups) with a squeeze of lemon and 1 teaspoon flaxseed oil for dressing.

DINNER

Fast Food

- Chipotle Bol with Chicken (1)
  Ask for double lettuce, fajita vegetables, green tomatillo salsa, and tomato salsa. No rice or beans.
- Daphne's® Greek Chicken Salad (1)
  Ask for no pita and extra salad. Add a squeeze of lemon for dressing.
- KFC® Roasted Caesar Salad (1)
  Ask for an additional serving of roasted chicken and Hidden Valley® Light Golden Ranch Dressing.
- McDonald's® Bacon Ranch Salad with Grilled Chicken (1)
  Ask for an additional serving of grilled chicken and Newman's Own® Low-Fat Balsamic Vinaigrette.
- Subway® Grilled Chicken Breast and Spinach Salad (1)
  Ask for an additional serving of grilled chicken and Fat Free Italian Dressing.

Frozen Food

- Gorton's® Cajun Blackened Grilled Fillets (3)
  Add mixed green salad (3 cups) with lemon juice and 1 teaspoon flaxseed oil for dressing.
- Gorton's® Shrimp Temptations Scampi (2 servings)
  Add mixed green salad (3 cups) with lemon juice and 1 teaspoon flaxseed oil for dressing.
- Tyson® Mesquite Breast Fillets (Bagged) (2)
  Add mixed green salad (3 cups) with lemon juice and 1 teaspoon flaxseed oil for dressing.

Note: Visit BodyatHome.com for more fast and frozen food ideas.

I have tested a lot of products, and the following are my favorites. For more information on these products, visit BodyatHome.com.

BARLEAN'S® FLAXSEED OIL

All Barlean's® products are completely fresh and organic. Freshness is key, because flaxseed oil can turn rancid quickly—and when it's rancid it tastes awful! But Barlean's® Flaxseed Oils are guaranteed fresh.

- Flaxseed Oil
- Lignan Flaxseed Oil
- Omega Swirl—with a fruit smoothie look and taste
- Forti-Flax
- Greens

GOFIT™

I love GoFit™ products because they're convenient, safe, and comfortable. The Sportblock® combines eight pairs of dumbbells into one space-saving, easy-to-hold design. The GoFit™ exercise ball is burst-resistant up to 500 pounds, which means that you'll never have to worry about your safety while exercising with it. The GoFit™ Pilates mat is the softest, most comfortable mat out there. These three products are the ones that are featured in the exercises in this book.

- Sportblock® Adjustable Dumbbell Set and Sportblock Add-on Weight set
- Pilates mat
- Exercise balls (55 cm, 65 cm, and 75 cm)
- Portable Gym Kit

JORGE'S PACKS™ VITAMINS

One of my favorite things about these vitamins is that they come in single-serving, personalized packets—they even have your name printed on each little pack. They're portable and great for travel and everyday use. Plus, they contain everything that's right for you based on your custom online profile. I take mine with me everywhere I go! Visit jorgespacks.com to find out more.

JORGE'S PACKS™ WHEY PROTEIN POWDER

Jorge's Packs™ protein shakes are my favorite because they taste great and are rich in nutrients. They are delicious and the only ones that I drink each day for my three snacks. I love all the flavors, but my favorite is chocolate. It tastes just like chocolate milk. Available exclusively at jorgespacks.com.

- Chocolate
- Strawberry
- Vanilla

ABOUT THE AUTHOR

JORGE CRUISE used to be 40 pounds overweight. He constantly felt tired, old, and insecure about his weight. Today he is the author of three *New York Times* best-selling book series. More than 5 million copies of his books are in print, including *8 Minutes in the Morning, The 3-Hour Diet,* and his most recent, *The 12-Second Sequence.* He is recognized as America's leading health expert for busy people. Each Sunday his *USA WEEKEND Magazine* column is read by more than 50 million people in 600 newspapers nationwide. He has appeared on *The Oprah Winfrey Show,* CNN, *Good Morning America, The Today Show, Dateline NBC, The View, The Tyra Banks Show,* and VH1.

Jorge received his bachelor's degree from the University of California, San Diego (UCSD). He has fitness credentials from the Cooper Institute for Aerobics Research, the American College of Sports Medicine (ACSM), and the American Council on Exercise (ACE).

Jorge lives in San Diego with his wife and two sons.

You can contact Jorge at JorgeCruise.com.

INDEX

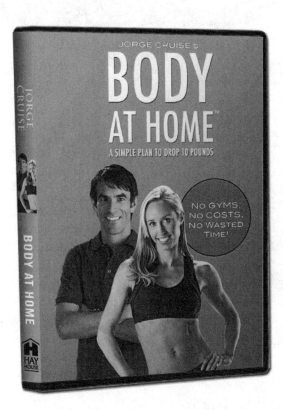
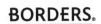 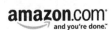 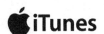
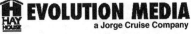

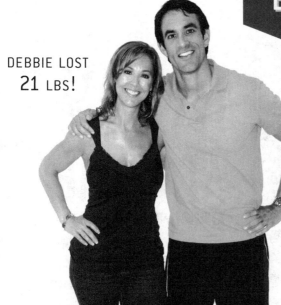